Radiology Fundamentals

Harjit Singh • Janet A. Neutze
Jonathan R. Enterline
Editors

Joseph S. Fotos • Brian Bentley
Associate Editors

Radiology Fundamentals

Introduction to Imaging & Technology

Fifth Edition

Springer

Editors
Harjit Singh, MD
Penn State Heart and Vascular Institute
Department of Radiology
Penn State Hershey Medical Center
Hershey, PA, USA

Janet A. Neutze, MD
Department of Radiology
Penn State Hershey Medical Center
Hershey, PA, USA

Jonathan R. Enterline, MD
Department of Radiology
Penn State Hershey Medical Center
Hershey, PA, USA

Associate Editors
Joseph S. Fotos, MD
Department of Radiology
Penn State Hershey Medical Center
Hershey, PA, USA

Brian Bentley, DO
Department of Radiology
Penn State Hershey Medical Center
Hershey, PA, USA

ISBN 978-3-319-10361-7 ISBN 978-3-319-10362-4 (eBook)
DOI 10.1007/978-3-319-10362-4
Springer Cham New York Heidelberg Dordrecht London

Library of Congress Control Number: 2014948464

Printed on acid-free paper

Springer is part of Springer Science+Business Media (www.springer.com)

To all those that ever wrote a book, I can now
empathize. To my family and wonderful wife,
Lindsey, for their endless love,
encouragement, and prayers.
– Jonathan R. Enterline

Are we there yet?! Thanks to the team
and to my family for staying the course
in this incredible journey.
– Janet A. Neutze

Thank you to the 5th edition team.
I couldn't have done it without you.
To my family, thank you for the support
and encouragement.
To Dad, thanks for watching over me.
– Harjit Singh

To my lovely wife, Melissa, thank you for
your love, encouragement and boundless
support. To all of those who have worked so
hard on this project over the years, thank
you. Your contributions will be appreciated
for years to come.
– Joseph S. Fotos

To all contributors, both past and present,
whose hard work made this book what it is,
thank you. To my family and incredible wife,
Elia, thank you for your patience,
understanding, and love.
– Brian Bentley

Preface to the Fifth Edition

The fifth edition of the *Radiology Fundamentals: Introduction to Imaging & Technology* is directed towards medical students, non-radiology housestaff, physician assistants, nurse practitioners, radiologist assistants and other allied health professionals as a curriculum guide to supplement their radiology education. This book serves only as an introduction to the dynamic field of radiology. The goal of this text is to provide the reader with examples and brief discussions of basic radiographic principles that should serve as the foundation for further learning. We hope that it will foster and further stimulate the process at the heart of medical education: self-directed learning.

Each edition continues to expand upon the first edition of the photocopied pages and films, written and organized by the original authors, Dr. William Hendrick and Dr. Carlton "Tad" Phelps. As mentors, Dr. Hendrick and Dr. Phelps of Albany Medical Center wanted a curriculum guide to reinforce the teaching concepts of their radiology elective. Dr. Harjit Singh, editor and author of much of the text of the first print edition, formalized the material in 1988. Our third edition, updated by faculty and students at Penn State Hershey, was a first effort at organizing and digitizing the information for publication. The fourth edition was an effort to expand and reinforce the original authors' work. Dr. Joseph Fotos and Dr. Jonathan Doud were new additions to the writing, illustrating, and editing side.

The fifth edition expands on the positive aspects of the fourth edition. The chapter lineup has changed and there is a new Pediatrics section.

Radiology continues to expand in breadth and depth. As consultants to our clinician colleagues, and from both cost and safety standpoints, radiologists need to know what they are doing. We hope this book, used in conjunction with lectures, electives, and discussions, is a start.

Hershey, Pennsylvania
July 2014

Harjit Singh, MD
Janet A. Neutze, MD
Jonathan R. Enterline, MD

Contents

Part VI Interventional Radiology Section

Part VII Musculoskeletal Section

Part VIII Neuroradiology Section

Part IX Pediatrics Section

Contributors

Original Authors

William J. Hendrick Jr., MD
Albany Medical Center
Albany, NY, USA

Carlton (Tad) Phelps, MD
Albany Medical Center
Albany, NY, USA

Harjit Singh, MD, FSIR
Penn State Hershey Medical Center
Hershey, PA, USA

Contributors to the Fifth Edition

Amit K. Agarwal, MD
Penn State Hershey Medical Center
Hershey, PA, USA

Brian S. Bentley, DO
Department of Radiology
Penn State Hershey Medical Center
Hershey, PA, USA

Karen L. Brown, MS
Penn State College of Medicine
Hershey, PA, USA

Allene S. Burdette, MD
Penn State Heart and Vascular Institute
Penn State Hershey Medical Center
Hershey, PA, USA

Rekha A. Cherian, DMRD, DNB, FRCR
Penn State Hershey Medical Center
Hershey, PA, USA

Jonathan R. Enterline, MD
Penn State Hershey Medical Center
Hershey, PA, USA

Joseph S. Fotos, MD
Department of Radiology
Penn State Hershey Medical Center
Hershey, PA, USA

Hassan M. Hal, MD, PhD
Penn State Hershey Medical Center
Hershey, PA, USA

Michael A. Hulse, DO, MS
Penn State Hershey Children's Hospital
Penn State Hershey Medical Center
Hershey, PA, USA

Carlos Jamis-Dow, MD
Penn State Hershey Medical Center
Hershey, PA, USA

Claudia J. Kasales, MD
Penn State Hershey Medical Center
Hershey, PA, USA

Steven H. King, MA
Penn State Hershey Medical Center
Hershey, PA, USA

Franklyn E. Luke, MB, CHB, FRCR
Penn State Hershey Medical Center
Hershey, PA, USA

Frank C. Lynch, MD, FSIR
Penn State Heart and Vascular Institute
Penn State Hershey Medical Center
Hershey, PA, USA

Julie A. Mack, MD
Penn State Hershey Medical Center
Hershey, PA, USA

Sosamma Methratta, MD
Penn State Hershey Children's Hospital
Penn State Hershey Medical Center
Hershey, PA, USA

Michael M. Moore, MD
Penn State Hershey Children's Hospital
Penn State Hershey Medical Center
Hershey, PA, USA

Janet A. Neutze, MD
Penn State Hershey Medical Center
Hershey, PA, USA

Tao Ouyang, MD
Penn State Hershey Medical Center
Hershey, PA, USA

Christine M. Peterson, MD
Penn State Hershey Medical Center
Hershey, PA, USA

Susann E. Schetter, DO
Penn State Hershey Medical Center
Hershey, PA, USA

Leslie B. Scorza, MD, FSIR
Penn State Heart and Vascular Institute
Penn State Hershey Medical Center
Hershey, PA, USA

Harjit Singh, MD, FSIR
Penn State Heart and Vascular Institute
Penn State Hershey Medical Center
Hershey, PA, USA

Mark Tulchinsky, MD
Penn State Hershey Medical Center
Hershey, PA, USA

Peter N. Waybill, MD, FSIR
Penn State Heart and Vascular Institute
Penn State College of Medicine
Penn State Hershey Medical Center
Hershey, PA, USA

Part I
Introductory Section

1 Patient Radiation Safety and Risk

Objectives:
1. Understand the difference between nonionizing and ionizing radiation
2. Understand the difference between stochastic and non-stochastic effects
3. Be able to discuss the concept of ALARA

Everyone is concerned about patient radiation dose. From 1993 through 2008, radiation dose attributed to medical radiation rose from 0.54 mSv to 3 mSv per capita. The largest component of the medical patient radiation dose was CT scanning (49 %). This is despite the fact that CT scanning makes up only 17 % of the total medical procedures that contributes to a patient's radiation dose.

Radiation dose for all diagnostic exams should be minimized to the lowest amount of radiation needed to produce a diagnostic quality exam.

What Is Radiation?

Radiation is emitted from unstable atoms. Unstable atoms are said to be "radioactive" because they release energy (radiation). The radiation emitted may be electromagnetic energy (x-rays and gamma rays) or particles such as alpha or beta particles. Radiation can also be produced by high-voltage devices, such as x-ray machines. X-rays are a form of electromagnetic energy with a wavelength that places it into an ionizing radiation category. In a diagnostic exam, these photons can penetrate the body and are recorded on digital or film medium to produce an image of various densities that show details inside the body.

H. Singh et al. (eds.), *Radiology Fundamentals: Introduction to Imaging & Technology*, DOI 10.1007/978-3-319-10362-4_1

Light, radio, and microwaves are nonionizing types of electromagnetic radiation. Radio waves are used to generate MR images. X-rays and gamma rays are *ionizing* forms of electromagnetic radiation and can produce charged particles (ions) in matter. When ionizations occur in tissue, they can lead to cellular damage. Most damage is repaired by natural processes. In some cases, the damage cannot be repaired or is not repaired correctly which can lead to biological effects.

There are two categories of biological effects related to radiation exposure:

Non-stochastic (also called deterministic)
Stochastic (also called probabilistic)

- *Non-stochastic* effects can occur when the amount of radiation energy imparted to tissue (dose) exceeds a threshold value. Below the threshold, no effect is observed. Above the threshold, the effect is certain.

  Examples:

  - Skin injury
  - Cataracts

- Stochastic effects can manifest at any dose, meaning there is no threshold below which the effect cannot occur. In reality, the probability of a stochastic effect increases as radiation dose imparted to the tissue increases.

  Examples:

  - Cancer
  - Leukemia

Where Do We Use Radiation in a Hospital?

Radiography:

- Fluoroscopy
- Mammography
- Cardiac catheterization
- Computed tomography
- Radiation therapy (linear accelerator)

Radioactive material:

- Nuclear medicine
- Radiation therapy

Listed below are three tables they provide an estimate of effective radiation dose from common diagnostic exams and interventional procedures (Tables 1.1, 1.2, and 1.3). As a reference standard, the average annual background radiation we all receive from the sun and soil is 3 mSv.

Table 1-1 Typical effective radiation dose from diagnostic x-ray-single exposure (Adapted with permission from Mettler et al. 2008)

Exam (Mettler et al. 2008)	Effective dose mSv (mrem)
Chest	0.1 (10)
Cervical spine	0.2 (20)
Thoracic spine	1.0 (100)
Lumbar spine	1.5 (150)
Pelvis	0.7 (70)
Abdomen or hip	0.6 (60)
Mammogram (2 view)	0.36 (36)
Dental bitewing	0.005 (0.5)
Dental (panoramic)	0.01 (1)
DEXA (whole body)	0.001 (0.1)
Skull	0.1 (10)
Hand or foot	0.005 (0.5)

Table 1-2 The dose a patient could receive if undergoing an entire procedure that may be diagnostic or interventional. For example, a lumbar spine series usually consists of five x-ray exams (Adapted with permission from Mettler et al. 2008)

Examinations and procedures	Effective dose mSv (mrem)
Intravenous pyelogram	3.0 (300)
Upper GI	6.0 (600)
Barium enema	7.0 (700)
Abdomen, kidney, ureter, bladder (KUB)	0.7 (70)
CT head	2.0 (200)
CT chest	7.0 (700)
CT abdomen/pelvis	10.0 (1,000)
Whole-body CT screening	10.0 (1,000)
CT biopsy	1.0 (100)
Calcium scoring	2.0 (200)
Coronary angiography	20.0 (2,000)
Cardiac diagnostic and intervention	30.0 (3,000)
Pacemaker placement	1.0 (100)
Peripheral vascular angioplasties	5.0 (500)
Noncardiac embolization	55.0 (5,500)
Vertebroplasty	16.0 (1,600)

Table 1-3 Typical effective radiation dose from nuclear medicine examinations (Adapted with permission from Mettler et al. 2008)

Nuclear medicine scan radiopharmaceutical (common trade name)	Effective dose mSv (mrem)
Brain (PET) 18F FDG	14.1 (1,410)
Brain (perfusion) 99mTc HMPAO	6.9 (690)
Hepatobiliary (liver flow) 99mTc sulfur colloid	2.1 (210)
Bone 99mTc MDP	6.3 (630)
Lung perfusion/ventilation 99mTc MAA & 133Xe	2.5 (250)
Kidney (filtration rate) 99mTc DTPA	1.8 (180)
Kidney (tubular function) 99mTc MAG3	2.2 (220)
Tumor/infection 67Ga	2.5 (250)
Heart (stress-rest) 99mTc sestamibi (Cardiolite)	9.4 (940)
Heart (stress-rest) 201Tl chloride	41.0 (4,100)
Heart (stress-rest) 99mTc tetrofosmin (Myoview)	11.0 (1,100)
Various PET Studies 18F FDG	14.0 (1,400)

What Are the Risks?

There is no threshold for stochastic effects so any imaging procedure or therapy that involves the use of radiation involves some risk. When performed properly, the risk is usually very small and is far outweighed by the medical benefit of having the procedure. Regardless, the concept of ALARA (keeping the radiation dose **as** **l**ow **as** **r**easonably **a**chievable) should always be employed to minimize the risk.

A small percentage of imaging and therapy studies performed in the hospital can potentially exceed threshold values for non-stochastic effects.

Radiation therapy and interventional fluoroscopy procedures may result in radiation doses that exceed the threshold dose for skin injuries, and less frequently for cataract induction. The procedures performed in these areas are often lifesaving, and every effort to minimize the magnitude of these effects is taken.

Resources

As you continue your career in medicine, you will specialize. Part of medicine, in virtually all areas of specialization, involves ordering x-rays or nuclear procedures for your patients.

In the news media, great attention has been paid to the increase in medical radiation dose to members of the public. Currently, there are discussions and debates

over the appropriateness of ordering certain exams without need. This will become a health system financial restraint as well as a public health question.
Some Resources to Look into:

ACR Appropriateness Criteria
http://www.acr.org/secondarymainmenucategories/quality_safety/app_criteria.aspx

Image Wisely Campaign (adult)
http://www.rsna.org/Media/rsna/upload/Wisely_525.pdf

Image Gently Campaign (pediatrics)
http://www.pedrad.org/associations/5364/ig/

Health Physics Society
http://hps.org/physicians/blog/
http://hps.org/publicinformation/asktheexperts.cfm

References

Mettler Jr FA, Huda W, Yoshizumi TT, Mahesh M. Effective doses in radiology and diagnostic nuclear medicine: a catalog. Radiology. 2008;248(1):254–63. Available from http://radiology.rsna.org/content/248/1/254.long. Accessed 8 May 2011.

National Council on Radiation Protection and Measurements. Ionizing radiation exposure of the population of the United States. Washington, DC: National Council on Radiation Protection and Measurements; NCRP Report No. 160; 2009. Summary of the report available at: http://www.ncrponline.org/Press_Rel/Rept_160_Press_Release.pdf. Accessed 8 May 2011.

2 Introduction to Radiology Concepts

Objectives:

1. Identify the four (4) naturally occurring densities visible on a conventional radiograph in order from the highest to lowest density
2. Define and give two examples of the silhouette sign on a frontal chest radiograph

Radiographic Densities

Let us disregard the anatomy seen on the radiograph for now and concentrate on basic radiographic principles. In Fig. 2.1, you can see examples of the four basic densities, bone, soft tissue, fat, and air, which are visible on a conventional radiograph.

Main Radiographic Densities

1. *Bone* – this is the most dense of the four basic densities and appears white or "radiodense" as radiologists prefer to say.
2. *Soft Tissue* – all fluids and soft tissues have the same density on a conventional radiograph. This density is slightly less than the bone but slightly greater than fat. One advantage of CT scanning is that various soft tissues and fluids can be discriminated as different radiographic densities to a much greater degree than conventional radiographs.
3. *Fat* – this density may seem the least obvious to you. Fat can be seen interposed between various soft tissue and fluid densities. Abdominal fat allows us to see

H. Singh et al. (eds.), *Radiology Fundamentals: Introduction to Imaging & Technology*, DOI 10.1007/978-3-319-10362-4_2

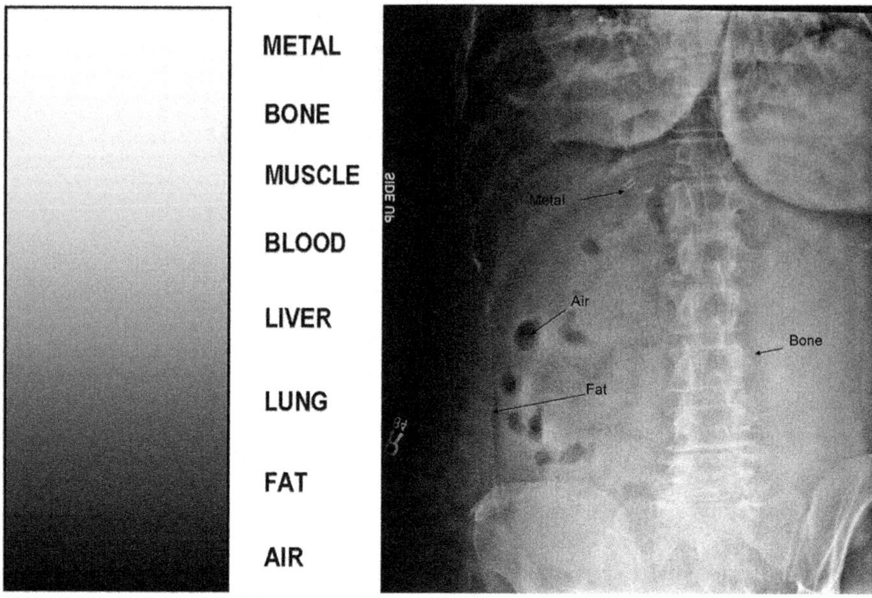

FIGURE 2.1 - RADIOGRAPHIC DENSITIES
Note how the four basic densities are visible on a chest radiograph

the edges of various soft tissue structures since the fat is slightly less dense than the organs themselves.

4. *Air* – the lungs, 'bowel gas' and the air surrounding the patient are examples of air densities. Air densities are generally quite dark, almost black, on the radiograph. Thus, the lungs are not radiodense but are instead said to be "radiolucent." Why does the air in the lungs appear less black (more radiodense) than the air around the patient? This is because the air density in the lungs is added to the densities of the superimposed chest wall structures.

There is an additional density on some radiographs which may be more dense than bone: metal density. This is not included in the above classification because it is not a naturally occurring density. Examples of metallic density on the radiograph include orthopedic hardware, the wire sutures in the sternum in the patients who have undergone cardiac surgery, and the wire leads seen in a pacemaker.

Radiographic densities are normally additive in an arithmetic way. This means that a soft tissue density which is twice as thick as an adjacent soft tissue structure will be twice as white. Conversely, a structure which is half as dense as an adjacent structure but twice as thick will demonstrate an identical radiographic density.

The Silhouette Sign

What is the effect of juxtaposition of structures of varying density upon each other? When two structures of *different densities* are adjacent (i.e., abutting each other), the interface between them will be clearly delineated on the radiograph. For example, the soft tissue density of the heart is clearly delineated from the air density of the lung along the cardiac border. However, when two structures of the *same density* are adjacent or overlapping, their margins cannot be distinguished. For example, when pneumonia fills the alveoli of the right lung with fluid, the lung becomes fluid density, the normal interface between the right heart border (soft tissue density) and the lung (air) may become invisible; the right heart border can no longer be seen (Fig. 2.2).

This is called the silhouette sign and is one of the most useful principles in radiology.

Other examples of the silhouette sign include the following:

1. The heart cannot be distinguished separately from the blood within the cardiac chambers because both have soft tissue/fluid density.
2. The dome of the liver and the inferior aspect of the right hemidiaphragm cannot be distinguished radiographically since both have soft tissue density. You would

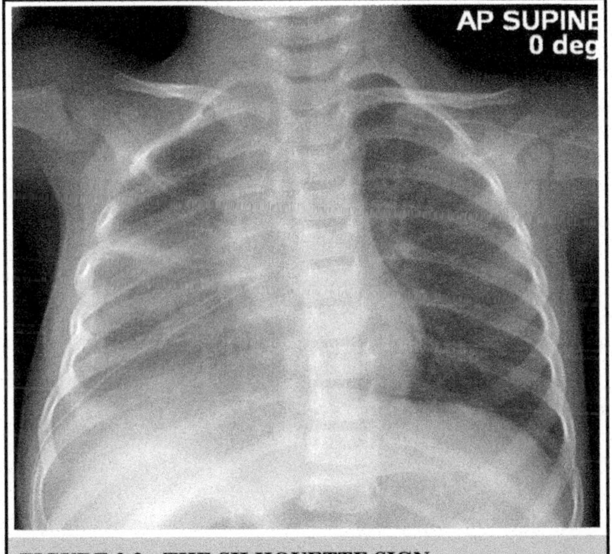

FIGURE 2.2 - THE SILHOUETTE SIGN
A right middle lobe pneumonia illustrates silhouetting of the right heart border by the area of consolidation. Compare to the crisp left heart border

only see the dome of the liver and the right hemidiaphragm separately when free intraperitoneal air is present. This is because the air density is interposed between the two soft tissue densities.

The silhouette sign will be used repeatedly in all sections of this course and in interpreting radiographs clinically. It is very important that you have a clear understanding of this principle.

3 CONVENTIONAL RADIOLOGY

Objectives:
1. State the convention for describing standard radiographic projections.
2. Explain why cardiac size differs on AP versus PA radiographs.
3. Define the "lordotic projection" view and two indications for its use.
4. Discuss how the following variables and techniques may alter the appearance of a conventional chest radiograph: underexposure, rotation, inspiration, and expiration.

The main purpose of this chapter is to demonstrate the effect of various technical factors on the appearance of conventional radiographs.

The Radiograph Projection

The radiographic projection is named according to the direction in which the x-ray beam passes through the body of the patient when the radiograph is taken (Fig. 3.1).

In other words, if the x-ray detector was placed behind the patient and the x-ray tube was placed in front of the patient, the x-rays would pass from the front of the patient through the back of the patient onto the x-ray detector in an anteroposterior (AP) radiograph. In a posterior-anterior (PA) radiograph, the detector is located along the anterior aspect of the patient's body with the x-ray tube posterior to the patient. In this situation, the x-ray beam passes through the patient from posterior to anterior.

H. Singh et al. (eds.), *Radiology Fundamentals: Introduction to Imaging & Technology*, DOI 10.1007/978-3-319-10362-4_3

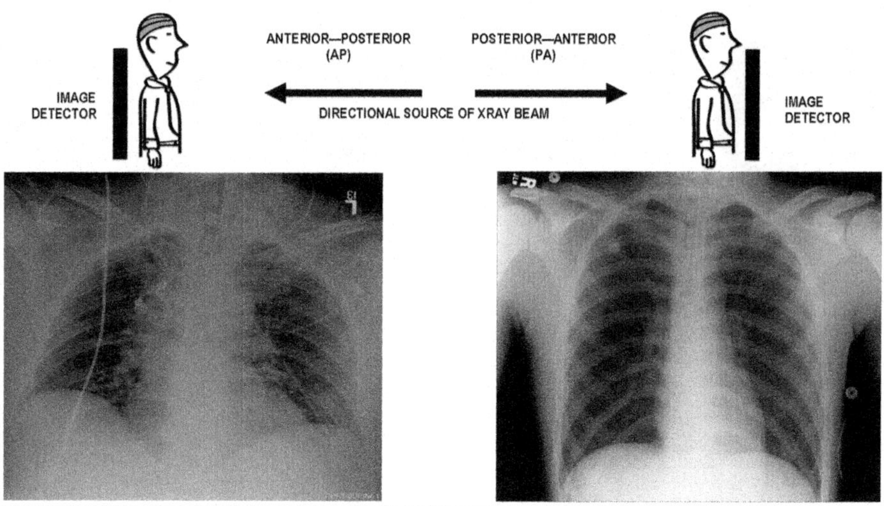

FIGURE 3.1 - THE AP AND PA VIEWS
How does this affect the appearance of various anatomical structures in the chest?

Note the difference in the size of the heart shadow between the AP and PA radiograph in Fig. 3.1. Because x-rays diverge from a point source, objects that are situated farther from the detector will cast a larger shadow. Since the heart is an anterior structure, it is magnified more on the AP radiograph because the anterior structures are farther from the radiographic detector. Demonstrate this principle for yourself by shining a flashlight on your hand so that it casts a shadow on the wall. The farther your hand is from the wall (which in this case acts like the x-ray detector), the more magnified and fuzzy the shadow becomes.

Next, look at Fig. 3.2. This is the "lordotic projection." With this projection, the x-ray source is angled toward the head and the clavicles project superior to the lung apex on the radiograph. This view is used to detect possible apical abnormalities such as tuberculosis or a lung tumor in the apex, called a Pancoast tumor. CT scans are now more commonly used because of increased sensitivity and specificity relative to the apical lordotic chest x-ray.

Look at Fig. 3.3. The heads of the clavicles and the spinous processes have been marked on the diagram. Since the clavicular heads are anterior structures and the spinous processes are quite posterior, they will move in opposite directions on the radiographs relative to a central axis of rotation. Using this principle of rotations, acquiring two radiographs, one in straight PA and one in slight rotation may help to determine the position of an abnormality in the lung.

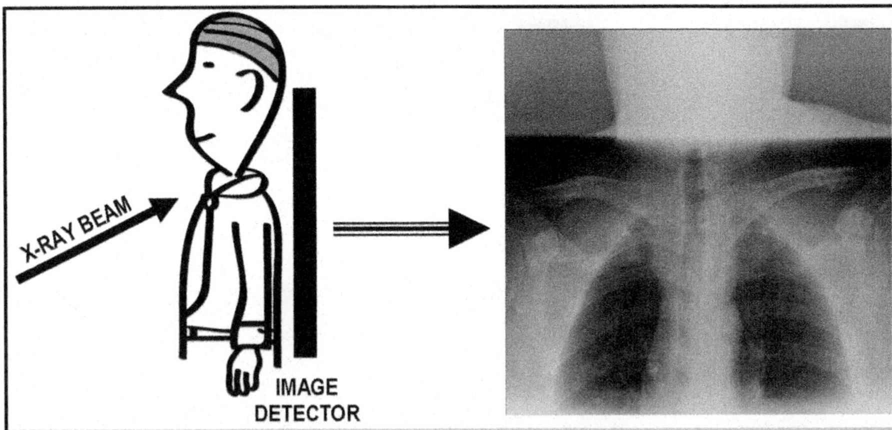

FIGURE 3.2 - THE LORDOTIC PROJECTION
The lordotic view is especially useful for visualizing the lung apices. The clavicles are projected cephalad, allowing a clear view of the lung apices

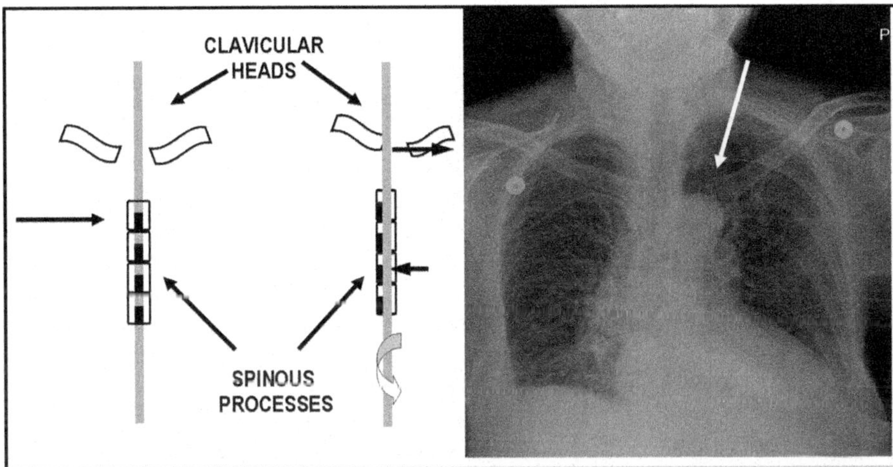

FIGURE 3.3 - ROTATION OF THE CHEST
In this illustration, note how the clavicle heads and spinous processes of the vertebral bodies appear in the AP position and with rotation of the chest to the left. On the chest x-ray, the *arrow points* to the left clavicular head, indicating that the patient is rotated to the left

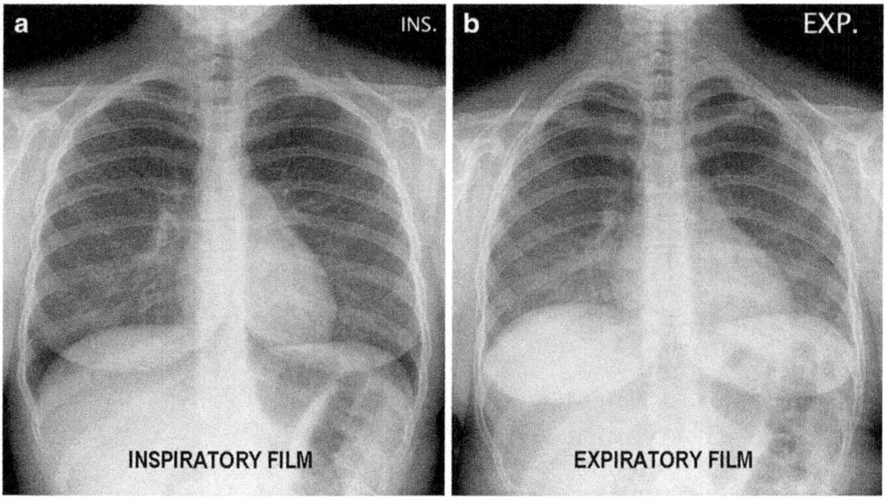

FIGURE 3.4 - INSPIRATORY AND EXPIRATORY FILMS
The radiographs here are those of inspiration (**a**) and expiration (**b**). Note the difference in the size of the lungs and their apparent difference in densities

Finally, note Fig. 3.4. The two radiographs were obtained within minutes of each other. Although this is an extreme example, it is important to realize that radiographs exposed at less than full inspiration produce artifactual crowding of the pulmonary vasculature which can simulate pulmonary edema.

In some situations, expiratory radiographs are intentionally obtained. The most common situation is when looking for a small pneumothorax. In this situation, the pneumothorax will become slightly larger relative to the lung as air is expired.

Next examine Fig. 3.5. Can you find examples of the four basic densities? Can you find examples of summation of radiographic densities due to superimposition of structures? Superimposed kidneys and stool-filled colon will be more dense than each structure by itself. Examples of the silhouette sign? Kidneys adjacent to liver or spleen will silhouette and obscure each other' margins.

And last, but certainly not the least, Fig. 3.6 is an image from a normal air contrast barium enema. This demonstrates how certain substances such as barium can be used to make certain anatomic structures more visible on the radiograph (in this case, barium and air in the large bowel).

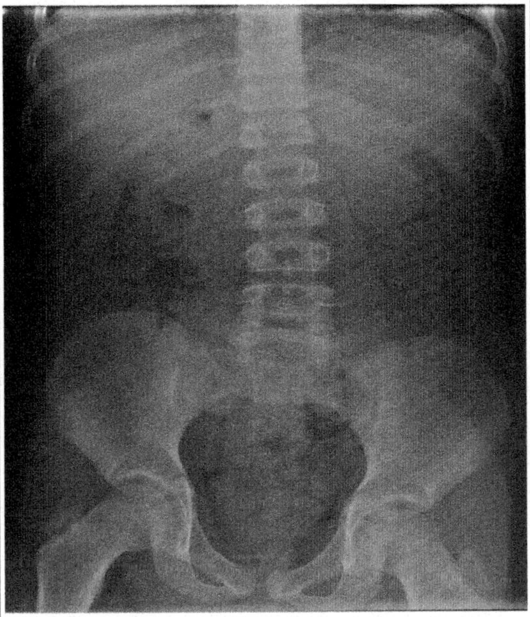

FIGURE 3.5 - NORMAL KUB

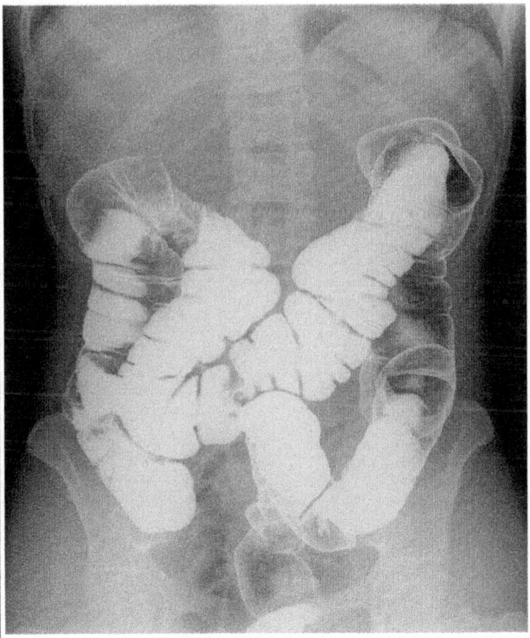

FIGURE 3.6 - NORMAL BARIUM ENEMA

4 ULTRASOUND

Objectives:
1. State the function of the transducer used in ultrasonography.
2. Define the term "sonolucent."
3. Give examples of structures that transmit sound well and that transmit sound poorly.

Ultrasound

Ultrasound uses no ionizing radiation, and it can image directly in any body plane. In practice, an ultrasonographer (either an ultrasound technologist called a sonographer or a physician) places gel on the patient's skin and moves a transducer across the surface of the patient's body. The gel forms an acoustic seal between the transducer and the skin for better transmission of sound, which results in better images.

The transducer can both send out and receive high-frequency sound waves, which transmit through, or reflect off, structures in the body. The returning sound waves are categorized by their intensity (referred to as echogenicity) and duration of time that it takes for them to return. It is the time that it takes for the echo to return from its encounter with an acoustic interface (a structure within the body which reflects sound) that allows its location within the image to be assigned (Fig. 4.1).

The intensity of the returning echo (echogenicity) of tissues varies greatly. Some tissues, like abdominal fat, are higher in echogenicity than other soft tissues. On the ultrasound image, such structures will appear whiter and are described as being increased in echotexture or "hyperechoic." Tissues/interfaces that return echoes of lower intensity are displayed as darker on ultrasound images and are described as

H. Singh et al. (eds.), *Radiology Fundamentals: Introduction to Imaging & Technology*, DOI 10.1007/978-3-319-10362-4_4

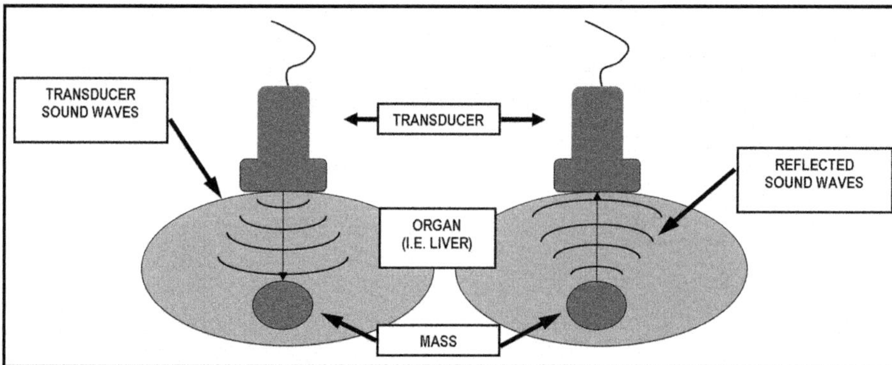

FIGURE 4.1 - ULTRASOUND
The ultrasound transducer acts similar to the sonar on a submarine. The transducer sends a short burst of high-frequency sound into the tissue. Some part of the sound is reflected back by the tissues, and the reflected signal is "read" by the transducer and an image is created

decreased in echotexture or "hypoechoic." By evaluating the echotexture of tissues, we can distinguish one organ from another and look for pathologic processes.

Fluid-filled structures (such as the gallbladder or urinary bladder) have few or no internal acoustic interfaces and hence appear clear black or sonolucent on ultrasound. Look at the simple cyst found when scanning the breast of a patient in Fig. 4.2. Note that the cyst depicted in this image is "anechoic," having no internal echoes. Sound waves traveling through the fluid-filled cyst lose less energy (since they encounter fewer acoustic interfaces). For this reason, they can pass through with more intensity when they reach the far wall of the cyst. This phenomenon is referred to as "acoustic enhancement" (arrows).

Some structures that are very dense, such as calcified structures or bone, will prevent sound waves from passing beyond them. As a result, there is no imaging information that can be obtained deep to those structures. A dark band-like "shadow" is produced beyond the echodense structure. This dark shadow can be quite prominent, helping identify even very small calcifications, such as kidney stones.

Orientation of the plane of section on an ultrasound image is indicated by the sonographer, who annotates the plane of section on images, either with text or with an indicator image.

Scans are normally viewed in "real time." This means that structures can be seen to move in the image (e.g., cardiac valves) and structures can pass into and out of the field of view. The images that the ultrasonographer records are only selected "frozen" images from an extensive examination. In some situations, it may be advantageous to record the examination in real time, known as a video or cine clip.

Ultrasound weakens or attenuates rapidly by the inverse square law with distance from the transducer; therefore, structures closer to the transducer are better visualized. Many transducers have been adapted to get them close to the imaged structures.

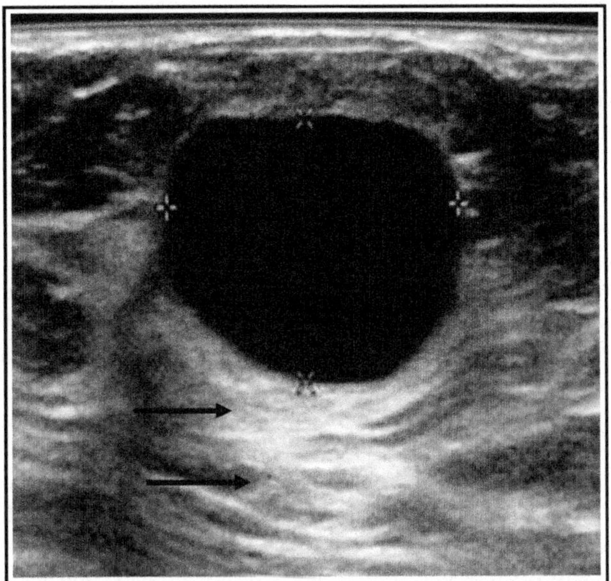

FIGURE 4.2 - SIMPLE BREAST CYST
"Anechoic" cyst having no internal echoes. Note the increased echodensity behind the cyst

$$X \propto \left(\frac{1}{D}\right)^2$$

FIGURE 4.3 - INVERSE SQUARE LAW
This is the inverse square law, as it applies to radiography, where X is the exposure at a given distance, D, from a radiation source. If, for example, the distance is doubled, the exposure would be one fourth of its original strength. The same law applies to the strength of the ultrasound beam

Transducers are included on endoscopes, allowing assessment of the duodenum, common bile duct, and pancreas. An endovaginal transducer provides very detailed imaging of the uterus and ovaries. Endorectal transducers allow high-resolution imaging of the prostate and rectum. By placing the transducer closer to the imaged object you can also use higher wavelengths of ultrasound, improving detail (Fig. 4.3).

Color and Power Doppler Imaging in Ultrasound

When an ultrasound beam encounters a moving structure a change in the pitch or frequency of the returning echo, compared to the echo sent out by the transducer, occurs. This is called the Doppler shift and it is encountered in real life when you hear a siren from a police car as it drives past you; the pitch or frequency of the sound you hear changes as the vehicle passes.

By using information generated by this Doppler shift, images can be generated, giving information about the speed and direction of the moving structure. This is most commonly used in evaluating blood vessels and blood flow. In conventional color Doppler, the displayed color identifies the direction of flow as well as the speed of flow. Power Doppler, which measures the concentration of moving structures, is more sensitive to low-flow states, but does not allow an evaluation of direction or speed.

Calculating the velocity of moving red blood cells numerically can allow an estimation of the diameter of the vessel in which the cells are flowing. This is the basis of arterial spectral (duplex) assessment of vessels such as the carotids. A spectral Doppler study will display grayscale images, color images, and waveform images of the vessel being evaluated. As the vessel lumen narrows, generally the velocity of red cells moving through it increases. By using multiple calculations along the path of the vessel, multiple velocity measurements and ratios of velocities can be calculated, allowing one to diagnose, quantify, and monitor focal areas of vascular narrowing.

Color/power Doppler and spectral imaging are used to assess for possible clot in veins, to evaluate areas of arterial narrowing/stenosis, and to determine if masses and organs have increased blood flow. You might see increased blood flow in a malignant tumor or reduced blood flow in a torsed testicle or ovary. Doppler imaging is also used to diagnose vascular malformations and assess for the presence of varicose veins.

Indications for Ultrasound Use

Ultrasound is most efficient in thinner individuals or when evaluating structures closer to the transducer. It does not require the use of ionizing radiation, but still should be used cautiously. Studies have shown that prolonged exposure to ultrasound can increase the temperature of tissue and that cavitation can occur when sound waves pass through a structure containing a gas bubble or air pocket (such as bowel and lung). Like any other imaging modality, ultrasound should be used judiciously, only when necessary, and by someone appropriately trained in the field.

Ultrasound is most commonly used to image specific organs such as the liver, gallbladder, kidneys, spleen, uterus/adnexa, and scrotum. Despite knowing the limitations of ultrasound when evaluating air- and fecal-filled bowel loops (and structures around them), ultrasound is being used increasingly to evaluate diseased bowel (which tends to be thicker and often fluid filled). With appropriate training, point-of-care ultrasound can aid in the detection of pneumothorax, pleural effusions or peritoneal fluid and in guiding the placement of central lines.

5 Computed Tomography

Objectives:

1. State how the densities on a CT scan are assigned.
2. Define the terms "pixel" and "voxel."
3. Compare and contrast the spatial and density resolution achieved with a CT scan with that of conventional radiographs.
4. State how to determine if contrast material is used when viewing a CT.

CT Imaging Orientation

Computed tomography (CT) uses ionizing radiation to create an image. This allows visualization of a greater variety of tissue structures beyond the four basic densities (air, bone, soft tissue, and fat) that are seen on a conventional radiograph. Unlike conventional x-rays, which utilize one projection to form an image, CT uses multiple small projections across the body and combines the information to form the image. It is this combining of the images that allows greater soft tissue detail to be displayed (Fig. 5.1).

Each individual picture of a computed tomography (CT) study is referred to as a section or an axial "slice." This is because the picture must be interpreted as if the patient has been completely sectioned in an axial plane, like a loaf of bread, with the viewer looking at the section from the feet towards the head.

H. Singh et al. (eds.), *Radiology Fundamentals: Introduction to Imaging & Technology*, DOI 10.1007/978-3-319-10362-4_5

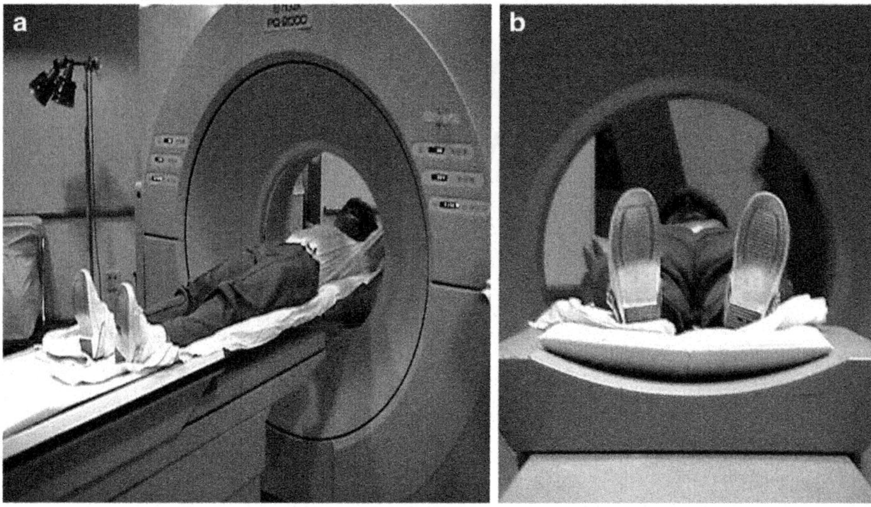

FIGURE 5.1 - COMPUTED TOMOGRAPHY (CT)
(**a**) The patient is placed in the CT gantry, and images are obtained in axial sections called "slices." (**b**) When reviewing the images, the radiologist interprets each image as if he/she were at the patient's feet, looking toward the patient's head

Pixels and Voxels

If you look closely at the CT scan, you will realize that the picture is actually made up of thousands of little squares called "pixels" (picture elements) (Fig. 5.2). Each pixel represents tissue that is about 1 mm or less on each of two sides and is assigned a grayscale value from 0 (black) to 255 (white). The grayscale value reflects how much of the x-ray beam that small piece of tissue (represented by the pixel) attenuated or blocked as it was passing through the patient. Darker shades (closer to black) represent structures that attenuate very little of the beam (like gas), while whiter shades represent structures that strongly attenuate the beam (like bone or calcification).

The thickness of the slice of a CT study is typically 1 mm or less, creating a three-dimensional volume element or "voxel" which is shaped like a cube. The word voxel is short for "volume pixel," the smallest distinguishable box-shaped part of a three-dimensional image. Pixel intensity represents an average from tissue within the "voxel." Although the spatial resolution of the CT scan is less than that of a conventional radiograph, the density resolution is much greater. Earlier models of CT scanners used the "step and shoot" method to acquire images. While lying on a motorized table, the patient was slowly moved into the scanning gantry, and a single slice was obtained while the patient was asked to hold his or her breath. These scanners,

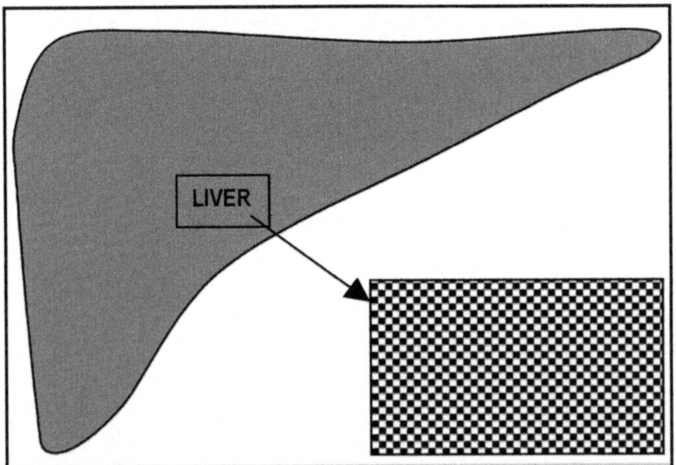

FIGURE 5.2 - CT PIXELS CONCEPT
As you look at the CT slice, it is important to keep in mind that each image is really made up of thousands of pixels (picture elements), each representing tissue about 1 mm^2

though remarkable for their generation, sometimes caused small pathology to be missed as patients would not hold their breath in the same fashion each time. These studies had long acquisition times.

Current generation scanners move the patient continuously through the scanning gantry during a single breath-hold. The patient is advanced while the x-ray tube continuously rotates, acquiring a data set that is much like a spiral in configuration (thus the name "spiral CT"). Current scans are performed much more rapidly than with the old "step and shoot" method. The data can then be reformatted into coronal, sagittal, and oblique planes. Current scanners have the capability of obtaining voxels of data so small that the reformatted images in other planes offer nearly identical resolution.

CT Values or Hounsfield Units (HU)

The amount of the x-ray beam that a particular voxel of tissue attenuates can be represented by a number called the Hounsfield unit, named after Sir Godfrey N. Hounsfield, an electrical engineer who won the Nobel Prize in 1979 for his pioneering work in the development of CT. By looking at the Hounsfield unit value of a structure you can get an idea of what types of tissue may be present (bone, calcification, water, blood, etc.). Also, by looking at changes in the Hounsfield unit value of tissue on images obtained before intravenous contrast compared to after intravenous contrast, you can determine how vascular a structure is. Listed below is a basic guide to HU values prior to contrast (Table 5.1).

Table 5.1 Typical HU for different tissues

Substance	Hounsfield units (HU)
Air	−1,000
Fat	−100
Water	0
Muscle/soft tissue	+40
Contrast	+130
Bone	+1,000

Contrast Studies

Intravenous contrast as well as oral and sometimes rectal contrast agents may be used in CT scans. The small "+C" label in the alphanumeric image of each section indicates that intravenous contrast was used. Also, if the aorta, kidneys, or ureter is radiopaque or white, it is a good indication that IV contrast was used. If the stomach or small or large bowel is radiopaque, oral contrast has been given.

Optimizing the Visualization of Specific Structures

Since CT scans are created from digital data, the grayscale display can be manipulated in such a way as to display the same information in various formats. These different formats are called window settings and amount to changing the total number of gray scales displayed and the value at which the gray scale is centered. Such changes determine which type of tissue is best displayed. Commonly used window settings include the soft tissue (mediastinal and abdomen), bone, and lung (pulmonary). In Fig. 5.3, you see the same image displayed using different windows. In the mediastinal window, soft tissue structures are discernable from each other. In the pulmonary window, the lung parenchyma is well seen, but the soft tissue structures all look the same. Additional electronic manipulation with filters and subtraction will provide more information and perhaps answer the clinical question that the raw images can only infer.

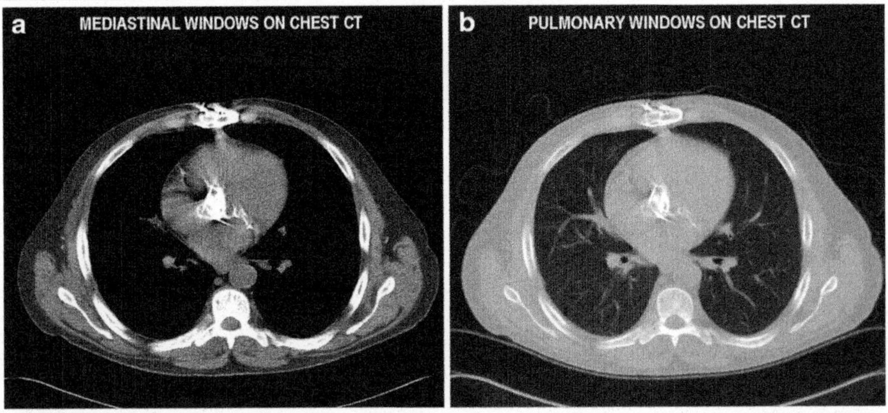

FIGURE 5.3 - CT SCAN OF THE CHEST
Note how the mediastinal windows (**a**) allow for optimal visualization of the mediastinal structures and the pulmonary windows (**b**) for lung parenchyma

6 MRI

Objectives:

1. Identify and characterize the tissue appearance of normal and common abnormal findings on CT and MRI.
2. State one advantage and three disadvantages that MRI has over CT.

Magnetic resonance imaging (MRI) has its greatest application in the fields of neuroradiology and musculoskeletal radiology.

To form a magnetic resonance image, the patient is placed in a strong uniform magnetic field. The magnetic field aligns hydrogen nuclei within the patient in the direction of the field. The nuclei are "disturbed" from this orientation by application of an external radiofrequency (RF) pulse. After the RF pulse is stopped, the hydrogen nuclei return to their alignment within the externally imposed magnetic field, giving off RF signals as they lose energy (Fig. 6.1).

The frequency of the RF signal emitted from the hydrogen nucleus as it returns to its orientation within the field is determined by the strength of that field. Therefore, the location of the RF signal given off by each hydrogen nucleus can be calculated. Each RF signal is analyzed by the computer for its intensity and other criteria. The signals are then assigned grayscale values (white to black) on the detector by the computer. Since this process of creating an image based on tissue characteristics is completely different from the absorption of x-rays by different tissues, MR images can show different types of pathologies and hence its utility. For example, MRI can discriminate soft tissue differences better than CT scans and is often used to define soft tissue abnormalities like herniated discs, ligament tears, and soft tissue tumors in the spine.

There are two basic sequences in MRI that are important to understand and recognize. These sequences are known as the T1-weighted and T2-weighted sequences.

H. Singh et al. (eds.), *Radiology Fundamentals: Introduction to Imaging & Technology*, DOI 10.1007/978-3-319-10362-4_6

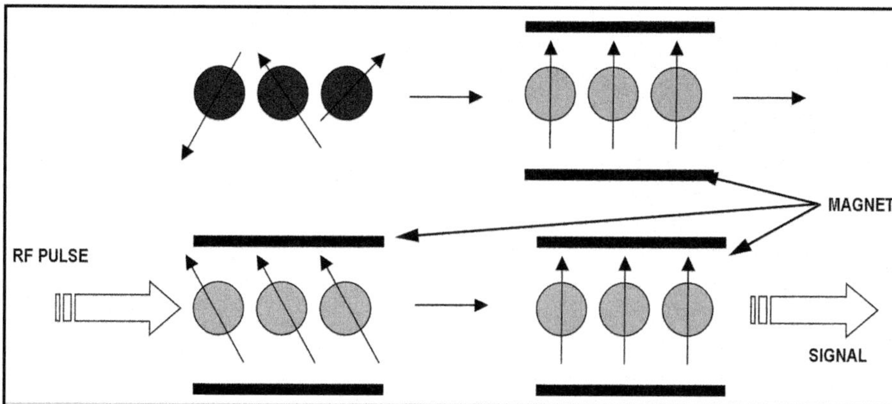

FIGURE 6.1 - MAGNETIC RESONANCE IMAGING: HYDROGEN NUCLEI
In their natural state, hydrogen atoms are spinning with their axes of rotation randomly oriented. When placed in a magnetic field, they align in a uniform direction. An RF pulse is applied, knocking the H-atoms out of their magnetic field orientation. Once the RF pulse is stopped, the atoms return to their previous alignment, giving off a signal which is then used to form the image

The "weighting" represents the exploitation of specific properties of hydrogen atoms that are exposed to a magnetic field. T1-weighted images classically demonstrate water as hypointense (dark) and fat as hyperintense (bright), with different soft tissues expressed as a gradient in between. In T2-weighted images, water is represented as hyperintense and fat as hypointense (again with soft tissues in the middle). Many of the more complicated sequences (gradient echo, FLAIR, etc.) are based on these basic sequences.

Advantages and Disadvantages of MRI

With the advent of multi-slice CT scanners, CT scans can be acquired or reformatted in many planes. Therefore, a prior advantage that MRI had, exclusive multiplane capacity, is nearly gone. However, MRI's clear advantage is that it uses no ionizing radiation. Disadvantages of MRI are that it is generally more costly than CT, is less available, and takes longer to perform. Another disadvantage is the inability to scan patients who have ferromagnetic material such as some shrapnel in them. These metallic fragments can actually move with the magnetic field and cause the patient significant discomfort or damage. Although MRI-compatible pacemakers are in development, generally speaking pacemakers are contraindicated because of their ferromagnetic properties; the MRI can heat the leads and inappropriately trigger the pacemaker. But some metal, based on location, type, or duration in place, may not be a contraindication to an MRI. Check with a radiologist if you are not sure if a device is MR compatible. Additionally, there are web resources that can ascertain the MR safety of different medical devices.

7 Introduction to Nuclear Medicine

Objectives:
1. Define the nuclear medicine (NM) specialty.
2. Be able to define key terms – isotope, radiopharmaceutical, gamma rays, gamma probe, gamma camera, planar imaging, etc.
3. Define how the component parts of a radiopharmaceutical and the route of its administration contribute to a diagnostic and therapeutic nuclear medicine.
4. Define unique characteristics of different imaging methods in nuclear medicine.

Introduction

The terms specific to nuclear medicine (NM) section will be displayed in *italics* when first mentioned, and the same abbreviations will be used from its first appearance to subsequent NM chapters. Only essential information is described in this book, but references to more detailed articles will be provided from publicly retrievable sources, including the Internet (e.g., Wikipedia) and medical journals.

Basic Definitions

Nuclear medicine (NM) is a medical specialty where practitioners are skilled in using radioactive isotopes for the diagnosis and therapy of disease. Isotopes are variants of stable elements that have an identical number of *protons* (p), which determines the atomic number and element's chemical characteristics, but differ in the

H. Singh et al. (eds.), *Radiology Fundamentals: Introduction to Imaging & Technology*, DOI 10.1007/978-3-319-10362-4_7

number of *neutrons* (n) (Wikipedia contributors 2013g). The sum of p and n equals the atomic mass. Some isotopes are radioactive, which means that they emit energy from the nucleus in the process of transformation to a more stable form – a process called *radioactive decay* (Wikipedia contributors 2013j). Every radioactive isotope decays exponentially with a specific rate that can be expressed as its *half-life* ($T_{1/2}$), which is the time required for an isotope to decay to half of its starting activity.

An example of iodine (I) may be helpful to illustrate the isotope concept (Wikipedia contributors 2013f). The stable element is ^{127}I, which contains 53 p and 74 n in its nucleus, thus having an atomic mass of 127. The common radioactive isotopes of iodine used in nuclear medicine are ^{123}I (p53, n70) and ^{131}I (p53, n78). These isotopes can be administered to patients in the simplest of chemical form, such as *sodium iodide salt* (also called *radioactive iodine*, *radioiodide*, or *radioiodine*). *Radiopharmaceutical* (RF) is another term for a chemical combination containing an isotope, where it is combined with (or *labeled* to) more complex molecules (pharmaceuticals), such as antibodies, hormones, or peptides, just to name a few. The pharmaceutical component of the RF would determine its biological distribution in the body, as well as its utility for diagnostic and/or therapeutic applications.

Radioisotopes and Radiopharmaceuticals

The most commonly used isotope in nuclear medicine is *metastable technetium-99* (^{99m}Tc). Its popularity is chiefly based on physical qualities, including the gamma ray emitted in the decay process that carries energy of 140 *kiloelectron volts* (KeV), which is ideally suited for efficient detection by NM imaging equipment. Another useful quality is its $T_{1/2}$ of 6 h, which is ideal for the majority of diagnostic applications. It also has advantageous chemical qualities which allow for convenient labeling to different pharmaceuticals, resulting in a wide array of RFs. Some of them are listed in Table 7.1. The biodistribution of RFs varies according to the route of administration. One of the oldest RFs is ^{99m}Tc-labeled sulfur colloid, which demonstrates how different routes of administration influence biodistribution and diagnostic utilization (Table 7.1). In general, the routes of RF administration include oral, intravenous, subcutaneous, intradermal, inhaled, and instilled into a body cavity or an organ through a catheter or a needle.

The use of different isotopes is also based on the type of rays (*photons*) they emit. These include *gamma* (Wikipedia contributors 2013e), *beta* (Wikipedia contributors 2013b), and *alpha* (Wikipedia contributors 2013a) photons. Gamma photons have the physical quality of a longer emission range (meters), and thus they are well suited for imaging. In contrast, alpha and beta photons travel very short distances (millimeters) before their energy is absorbed into tissues, which makes them ideal for *unsealed (internal) radiotherapy or radioisotope therapy* applications.

Table 7-1 Commonly used ^{99m}Tc-labeled radiopharmaceuticals in nuclear medicine

Radiopharmaceutical	Administration via	Test name	Main organ(s)/ system(s) tested	Physiologic function(s) tested
Tc-99m-diethylenetriaminepenta-acetic acid (DTPA)	Intravenous	Renal scan (scintigraphy)	Kidneys	Glomerular function, drainage
Tc-99m-diethylenetriaminepenta-acetic acid (DTPA)	Inhaled	Lung ventilation scan	Lung	Ventilation, ciliary clearance
Tc-99m-hydroxymethylene diphosphonate (HDP)	Intravenous	Bone scan (scintigraphy)	Bone	Osteoblast activity
Tc-99m-macroaggregated albumin (MAA)	Intravenous	Lung perfusion scan	Lung	Perfusion
Tc-99m-mebrofenin	Intravenous	Hepatobiliary ("HIDA") scan	Liver, biliary ducts, gallbladder	Bile production, gallbladder
Tc-99m-mercaptoacetyltriglycine (MAG3)	Intravenous	Renal scan (scintigraphy)	Kidneys	Tubular function, drainage
Tc-99m-methylene diphosphonate (MDP)	Intravenous	Bone scan (scintigraphy)	Bone	Osteoblast activity
Tc-99m-pertechnetate	Intravenous	Thyroid scan (scintigraphy)	Thyroid	Sodium iodine symporter
Tc-99m-pertechnetate	Intravenous	Salivary scan (scintigraphy)	Salivary glands	Saliva production, drainage
Tc-99m-pertechnetate	Intravenous	Meckel's scan	Stomach and bowel	Gastric mucosa
Tc-99m-red blood cells	Intravenous	Radionuclide ventriculography	Heart chambers	Wall motion, ejection fraction
Tc-99m-red blood cells	Intravenous	Gastrointestinal bleeding scan	Intestinal extravasation	Hemostasis
Tc-99m-sulfur colloid	Intravenous	Liver-spleen scan	Liver, spleen, bone marrow	Mononuclear phagocyte system
Tc-99m-sulfur colloid	Intradermal	Lymphangiography	Lymph vasculature and nodes	Lymphatic drainage
Tc-99m-sulfur colloid	Bladder catheter	Voiding cystourethogram (VCUG)	Bladder, ureters, kidney	Vesicoureteral valve
Tc-99m-sulfur colloid (cooked with eggs)	Orally	Gastric emptying test	Stomach	Gastric motility (emptying)

Detection, Imaging, and Quantification

The principle of gamma photon detection is based on its interaction with certain materials that produce a spark of light (or *scintillation* – Latin origin), which is converted into an electric pulse. This pulse is recorded as one *count*. The simplest method for clinical detection and quantification of gamma ray emissions is a *gamma probe* (Fig. 7.1a) (Wikipedia contributors 2013d). A smaller version of this instrument is available for the detection of radioactivity intraoperatively by a surgeon (Fig. 7.1b).

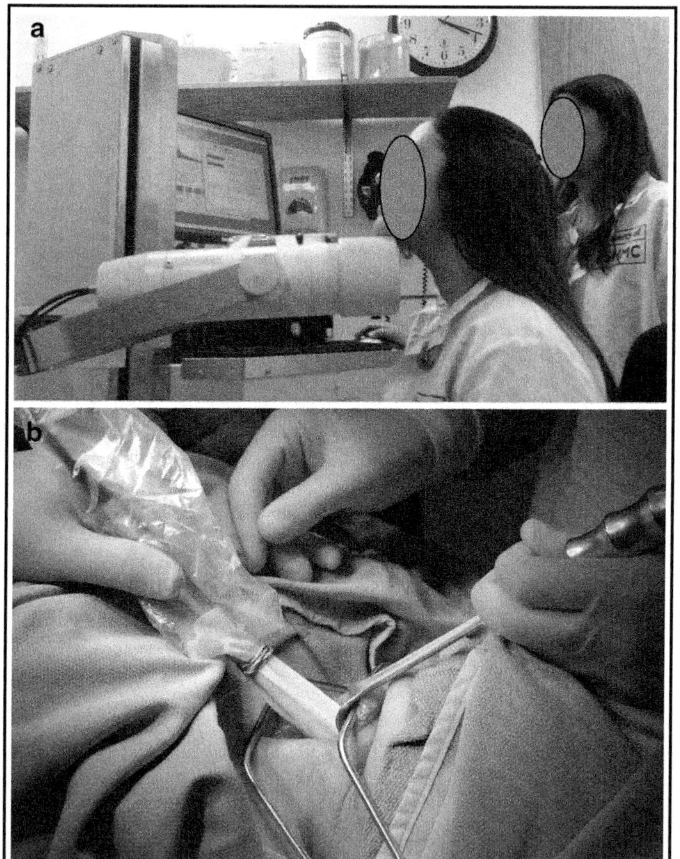

FIGURE 7.1 - GAMMA PROBES
The stationary thyroid gamma probe is shown measuring thyroid activity (**a**). This equipment is often used to calculate iodine-131 uptake. The handheld miniaturized gamma probe is used in the operating room to find radioactive thyroid tissue that was labeled before surgery (**b**).

This is useful in a number of circumstances when a focus targeted by a RF needs to be surgically excised, but cannot be readily distinguished from surrounding anatomy on visual inspection. These detectors provide no image, but simply count how many rays were detected per certain time, such as *counts per sec*, per min, per 5 min, etc. This relative unit (e.g., count/min) is directly proportional to the radioactivity in the emitting source.

Gamma camera (Wikipedia contributors 2013c) is essentially an array of probes that line a flat detector and is capable of capturing the distribution of the gamma-emitting RF within the body in a 2-dimensional (2-D) image, called a planar image (*scintigraphy*). Those images can be acquired in a *static* mode (single image, or a *spot* image, obtained for either a set time or number of counts) or *dynamic* mode (sequential frames – same as spot images, but set for a same amount of time each and acquired in uninterrupted succession), as exemplified in gastrointestinal NM chapter (Fig. 37.1, 37.2, and 37.3). The static mode can be adapted for the *whole-body imaging* obtained by slowly moving the camera head along the long axis of the body and capturing the image along its path (Fig. 7.2).

Specific to NM is the concept of emission imaging whereby imaged gamma rays (photons originating from the nucleus) are emitted from within the body. Some of those rays will be absorbed (attenuated) in the surrounding tissues. The less tissue that stands between the organ of interest and the camera detector, the fewer photons are lost and more of them make it to the detector, creating an informative image. For example, to image the sacrum during bone scanning, the detector would be optimally positioned closest to the patient's back – called *posterior view* (Fig. 7.2). If the image of anterior ribs, is desired, the front of the patient would be facing the detector – called *anterior view*. The posterior view would be less useful in depicting the anterior portion of the ribs, as most of the photons would be attenuated. In conventional radiology (refer to conventional radiology chapter in the introduction section), x-rays (photons originating from de-excitation of electrons) are emitted from the tube that is outside the patient and transmitted through the imaged part of the body. Unlike NM imaging, there is a small difference if the tube is facing the patient's front with the detector at the back or vice versa.

The same camera can obtain multiple 2-D static images from evenly spaced angles around the body. A computer algorithm can then reconstruct a 3-dimensional (3-D) depiction of the RF biodistribution. This is called *single-photon emission computed tomography* (SPECT) (Wikipedia contributors 2013k). Newer cameras combine SPECT with a CT on one gantry (called SPECT/CT), which takes both SPECT and CT images. This enables the fusion of the two modalities into one blended image called a *fusion image*. The positron-emitting isotopes are imaged using another 3-D imaging technique, called *positron emission tomography* (PET) (Wikipedia contributors 2013i), which is routinely combined with a CT on the same gantry – called PET/CT camera and imaging. The newest advance is to combine PET with MRI, but only a few PET/MR cameras are in practice today. These 3-D modalities provide tomographic slices in the standard three planes for physiological/molecular tests (SPECT or PET), corresponding anatomical (usually CT or MRI) and fused slices. This type of molecular and

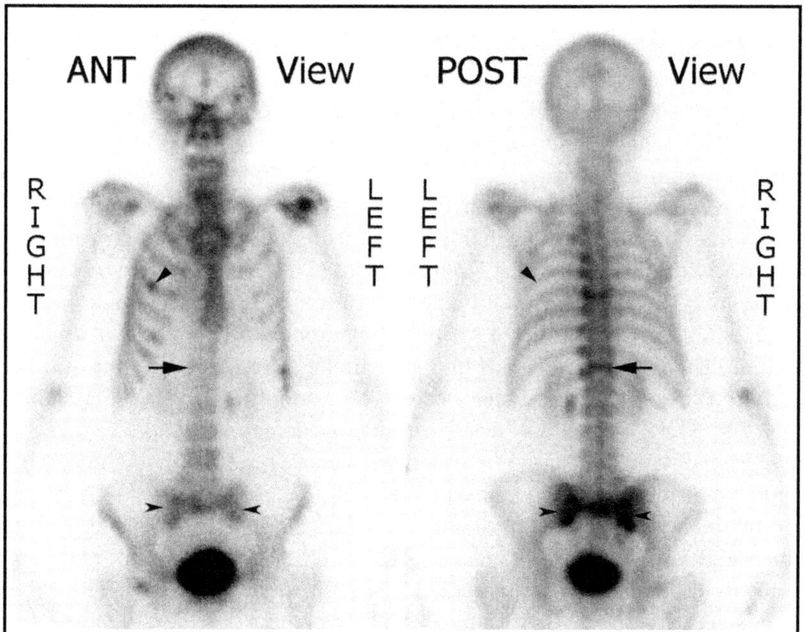

FIGURE 7.2 - BONE SCAN
Planar bone scan obtained in whole-body mode (lower extremities excluded here) in anterior (*ANT*) and posterior (*POST*) views. The most striking finding is the letter "H" shaped, intensely increased tracer uptake on the POST view over the upper sacral bone, which is best seen on the POST view (*concave-base arrowheads*). This configuration, called Honda sign, is typical for sacral insufficiency fracture. The same finding is much less intense on the ANT view due to the attenuation of a significant percent of photons (absorbed in soft tissues lying between the origin and the detector. A linear, mildly increased tracer uptake well seen on POST view (*arrow*) corresponds to the compressed superior end plate of the twelfth thoracic vertebra. This signal is totally attenuated on the ANT view. Similarly, the focal area of mildly increased uptake in the right anterior third rib (*straight-base arrowhead*) seen on ANT view cannot be seen on the POST view as a result of attenuation.

physiological information displayed on the background of exquisite anatomy has been more recently termed the *molecular imaging*. A simplified display of the physiological/molecular 3-D images (SPECT and PET) of the whole body can be achieved by projecting the most intense activity along parallel tracks piercing through the entire 3-D stack of slices onto a perpendicular 2-D plane. This is similar to the parallel rays of light going through the film of an old movie projector and displaying that image on a screen. Owning to this conceptual similarity, this imaging is called maximum intensity projection (MIP) (Wikipedia contributors 2013h). This projection can be done from any angle. Creating MIP images from evenly spaced angles all around the body (360°) produces a rotating object as if one is looking at the spinning whole body. This technique was invented by one nuclear medicine physician for display of SPECT information and now is used in most 3-D imaging techniques (MRI, CT, ultrasound), particularly PET (Wikipedia contributors 2013h).

Description of the imaging (scintigraphic) findings is based on relative intensity as compared to expected normal activity. It can be either increased (often called "hot spot") or decreased (termed "photopenic"). It is customary to describe severity of the scintigraphic findings as showing intensely or severely, moderately, mildly, and slightly increased or decreased radiotracer uptake. Pattern of the finding(s), such as fusiform or linear, focal or diffuse, is important in the consideration of a likely cause. Location is described using standard anatomical terms.

The organs of interest can be evaluated for dynamic handling of the RF by drawing regions of interest and creating curves of radioactivity over time (called *time-activity curves*). Those curves can be qualitatively described or mathematically analyzed (the most common metric is halftime of exponential activity disappearance). The activity of RF deposited in the paired organs (such as kidneys or lungs) according to their functions can be quantified as the percent each side contributes to the total function, which is called differential function. Such analyses are standard in renal scanning and quantitative lung function scintigraphy (see Chap. 39, "Pulmonary Nuclear Medicine").

References

Wikipedia contributors. Alpha particle. 30 Oct 2013 18:21 UTC; http://en.wikipedia.org/w/index.php?title=Alpha_particle&oldid=579504476. Accessed 10 Dec 2013 01:21 UTC, 2013a.

Wikipedia contributors. Beta particle. 9 Dec 2013 22:39 UTC; http://en.wikipedia.org/w/index.php?title=Beta_particle&oldid=585348060. Accessed 10 Dec 2013 01:20 UTC, 2013b.

Wikipedia contributors. Gamma camera. 4 Nov 2013 19:32 UTC; http://en.wikipedia.org/w/index.php?title=Gamma_camera&oldid=580198300. Accessed 10 Dec 2013 01:10 UTC, 2013c.

Wikipedia contributors. Gamma probe. 24 Sep 2013 10:52 UTC; http://en.wikipedia.org/w/index.php?title=Gamma_probe&oldid=574304543. Accessed 10 Dec 2013 01:18 UTC, 2013d.

Wikipedia contributors. Gamma ray. 4 Dec 2013 19:02 UTC; http://en.wikipedia.org/w/index.php?title=Gamma_ray&oldid=584563520. Accessed 10 Dec 2013 01:19 UTC, 2013e.

Wikipedia contributors. Iodine. 30 Nov 2013 18:00 UTC; http://en.wikipedia.org/w/index.php?title=Iodine&oldid=583934652. Accessed 3 Dec 2013 21:47 UTC, 2013f.

Wikipedia contributors. Isotope. 17 Nov 2013 23:25 UTC; http://en.wikipedia.org/w/index.php?title=Isotope&oldid=582119841. Accessed 21 Nov 2013 01:24 UTC, 2013g.

Wikipedia contributors. Maximum intensity projection. 28 Feb 2013 19:19 UTC; http://en.wikipedia.org/w/index.php?title=Maximum_intensity_projection&oldid=541316929. Accessed 08 Nov 2013, 2013h.

Wikipedia contributors. Positron emission tomography. 9 Dec 2013 22:50 UTC; http://en.wikipedia.org/w/index.php?title=Positron_emission_tomography&oldid=585349684. Accessed 10 Dec 2013 01:12 UTC, 2013i.

Wikipedia contributors. Radioactive decay. 20 Nov 2013 03:12 UTC; http://en.wikipedia.org/w/index.php?title=Radioactive_decay&oldid=582470982. Accessed 21 Nov 2013 01:20 UTC, 2013j.

Wikipedia contributors. Single-photon emission computed tomography. 4 Dec 2013 02:09 UTC; http://en.wikipedia.org/w/index.php?title=Single-photon_emission_computed_tomography&oldid=584460769. Accessed 10 Dec 2013 01:16 UTC, 2013k.

8 Cardiovascular and Interventional Radiology

Objectives:
1. Understand the concept behind digital subtraction angiography (DSA).
2. Be able to list the types of procedures performed in Cardiovascular and Interventional Radiology (CVIR).

In Cardiovascular and Interventional Radiology (CVIR), a combination of needles, wires, catheters, balloons, and stents is used to accomplish many things through small access points in the skin.

Digital Subtraction Angiography (DSA)

Arteriograms are used to diagnose the changes in the vasculature associated with disease (most commonly atherosclerosis and vasculitis) or injury (either iatrogenic or traumatic). The femoral artery is a commonly used entry point and is accessed at the level of the femoral head. At this location, its position is relatively superficial, and hemostasis can therefore be achieved with ease because the artery can be compressed against the femoral head once the procedure is completed. Different catheters are used to access the branch arteries requiring imaging. Once the catheter is in the appropriate vessel, iodinated contrast (often called "X-ray dye") is injected at a controlled rate and volume either via a power injector or by hand injection.

Imaging can be acquired on film radiographs (which are processed similarly to routine radiographs) or much more commonly with digital subtraction angiography (DSA). In DSA, images are processed with the help of a computer. The initial image has no contrast and is called the "mask." The X-ray images are then obtained in

H. Singh et al. (eds.), *Radiology Fundamentals: Introduction to Imaging & Technology*, DOI 10.1007/978-3-319-10362-4_8

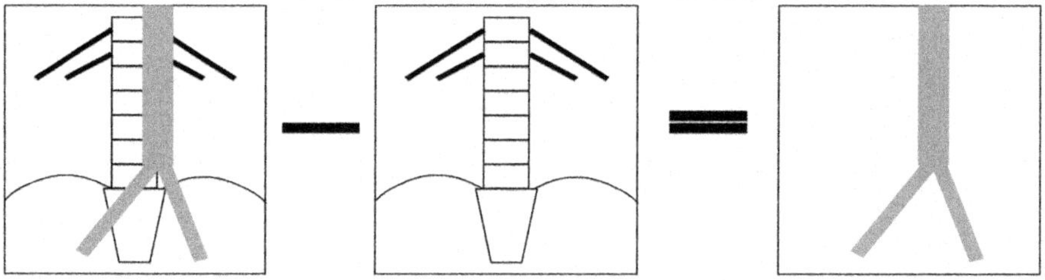

FIGURE 8.1 - DIGITAL SUBTRACTION ACQUISITION (DSA)
Contrast is injected in the patient's aorta, and images are acquired. Just before the contrast is injected, the computer acquired a mask, as seen in the *center*. As the contrast images are acquired, the computer subtracts the mask from the images leaving the only portion which has changed between the two, the intra-arterial contrast

rapid sequence while contrast is injected. The computer then digitally "subtracts" the mask from the subsequent images leaving only the contrast, thereby yielding finely detailed imaging of the vasculature (Fig. 8.1).

If an area of stenosis or narrowing is identified, it can be treated using percutaneous transluminal angioplasty (PTA), with or without the use of a metallic stent. If blood flow cessation is required in an area of bleeding (e.g., after trauma) or as preoperative embolization to reduce operative blood loss at subsequent surgery, a catheter can be advanced to the vessel requiring embolization. Various materials can be delivered into the artery to stop flow. Embolization materials include metallic coils, Gelfoam®, polyvinyl alcohol particles (PVA, which is fixed-size particulate material), alcohol, chemotherapeutic material, autologous clot, biocompatible glue, and other agents.

Central Venous Access

Central venous access can be accomplished in many different ways. There are catheters used for short-term to intermediate-term access such as the peripherally inserted central catheter (PICC) and the nontunneled central line. Long-term access catheters include tunneled infusion catheters and subcutaneous chest or arm ports. Dialysis access catheters, such as tunneled hemodialysis catheters, are also inserted in Interventional Radiology. Access can be obtained with either vascular ultrasound, contrast venography, carbon dioxide venography, or by using anatomic landmarks. With the use of real-time imaging (fluoroscopy), placement of the line can be quick, accurate, and safe. Difficult access pathways can be potentially treated with angioplasty (balloon dilation) if necessary as well.

More Interventional Radiology Procedures

Gastroenteric access can also be performed entirely percutaneously. The placement of gastrostomy tubes (G-tubes) or gastrojejunostomy tubes (G-J tubes) is accomplished with fluoroscopic guidance in a multi-planar fashion (many X-ray angles). The use of fluoroscopy allows the quick, accurate, and safe placement of gastroenteric tubes.

Placement of inferior cava filters can be performed through several access points, most often either the common femoral vein or the internal jugular vein. Careful evaluation of the inferior vena cava prior to filter placement should be performed to evaluate for variant anatomy and ensure proper positioning.

Genitourinary procedures are commonly performed in Interventional Radiology. The types of procedures include percutaneous nephrostomy placement (PCN), nephrostomy tube exchange, access for percutaneous nephrolithotomy (PCNL), placement and exchange of nephroureteral stents (NUS), and ureteral balloon dilation (ureteroplasty).

Women's health interventions represent a subset of procedures focusing on gynecologic issues. These procedures include uterine fibroid embolization, ovarian vein embolization for pelvic congestion syndrome, and fallopian tube recanalization.

Biliary procedures are commonly performed on patients who are clinically ill as a result of biliary obstruction. Percutaneous drainage with placement of an internal/external drainage catheter can be a precursor to surgical resection of a biliary or pancreatic mass. The biliary system frequently needs to be decompressed on a long-term basis, so biliary tube maintenance is also conducted by interventional radiology. If the patient is not an operative candidate, the interventional radiologist can place metallic stents (similar to those used in the arterial system) into the biliary system. This palliates symptoms and improves quality of life without the need for external drains.

These are many types of imaging studies and additional procedures that are performed by interventional radiologists:

1. Abscess drainage (using CT, ultrasound, and/or fluoroscopy)
2. Intraoperative cases (e.g., thoracic and abdominal aortic stent grafts)
3. Noninvasive cardiac and vascular imaging (e.g., cardiac MRI, coronary CT angiography, and duplex ultrasound)
4. Percutaneous oncologic interventions (e.g., transarterial chemoembolization, transarterial ^{90}Y radioembolization, radiofrequency ablation, and cryoablation)
5. Percutaneous biopsies (using CT, ultrasound, and/or fluoroscopy)
6. Minimally invasive venous procedures (e.g., endovenous laser or radiofrequency ablation, sclerotherapy, and phlebectomy)

The scope of Interventional Radiology is quite extensive and diverse. The various interventional procedures expand the diagnostic and therapeutic armamentarium for the clinical care team.

Part II
Chest Section

9 Heart and Mediastinum

Objectives:
1. Identify the structures that form the left and right mediastinal borders on a PA chest radiograph.
2. Know how cardiac size is assessed on a PA chest radiograph as well as technical factors that may affect this assessment.
3. Identify the radiographic divisions of the mediastinum and the differential diagnosis of abnormalities arising from each division.

Cardiac Contours

When evaluating the cardiopericardial outline and mediastinal contours, it is easiest to follow the right and left borders that these structures make with the aerated lung. Although the mediastinum is optimally visualized by various cross-sectional imaging techniques, the initial evaluation is often made on plain radiographs.

Review Fig. 9.1. The first convex segment along the left mediastinal border is formed by the aortic arch. The segment inferior to the aortic arch represents the main pulmonary artery. The large convex border inferiorly is formed by the left ventricle, with a small contribution from the left atrium. On the right, the superior vena cava is visualized superiorly. The right lateral border of the right atrium forms the convexity seen inferiorly. These contours can vary with age and certainly can change dramatically in abnormal situations. Any review of the cardiomediastinal silhouette should begin with an evaluation of these contours.

H. Singh et al. (eds.), *Radiology Fundamentals: Introduction to Imaging & Technology*, DOI 10.1007/978-3-319-10362-4_9

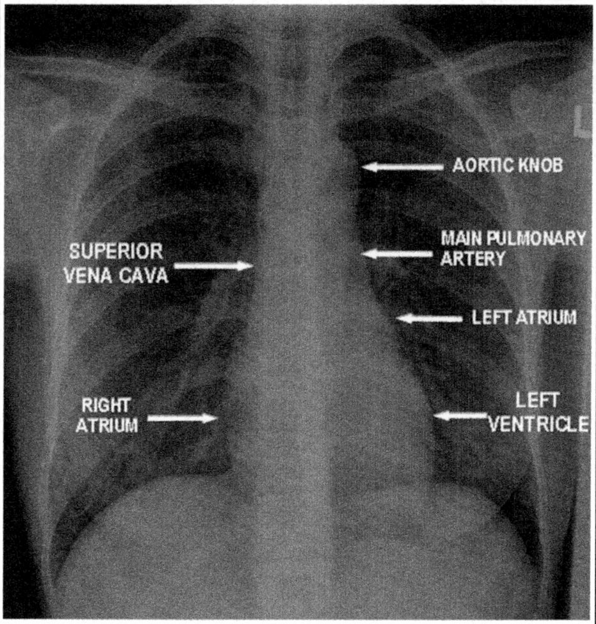

FIGURE 9.1 - MEDIASTINAL CONTOURS

Heart Size

The largest structure occupying the mediastinum is, of course, the heart. Recall from an earlier chapter that the cardiac size may vary depending on the projection of the radiograph (PA vs. AP). On an upright PA radiograph, the heart is said to be normal if its transverse diameter is no greater than 50–55 % of the transverse diameter of the internal bony thorax. This will not hold true on AP radiographs, since the heart will be artificially magnified. It may also not hold true in cases where the radiograph has been taken with a less than adequate inspiratory effort. Figure 9.2 demonstrates both a normal and an enlarged heart and shows examples of the points of measurement for both the heart and thoracic dimensions.

Mediastinal Structures and Compartments

In addition to the heart, great vessels, esophagus, and central airways, lymph nodes are present in the mediastinum. Lymph node enlargement can change the appearance of the mediastinum on a chest radiograph. Figure 9.3a shows where

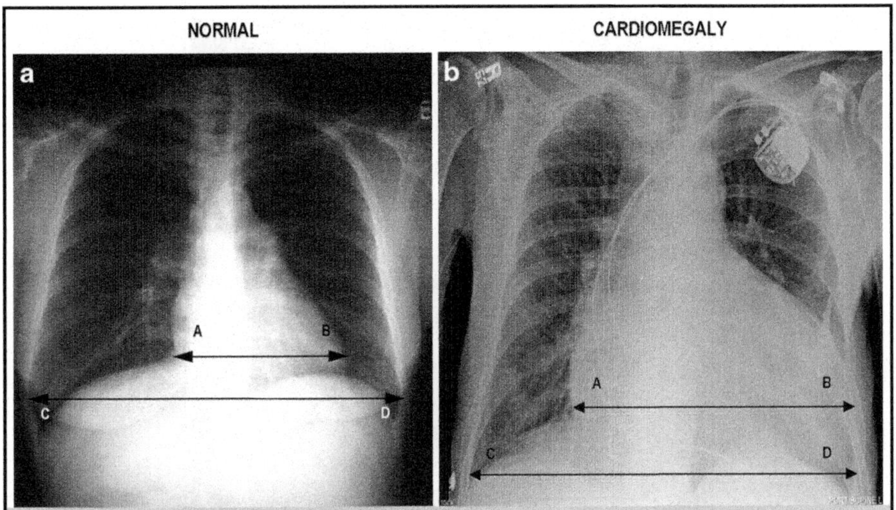

FIGURE 9.2 - MEASURING THE HEART
(**a**) When evaluating the size of the heart, *AB* (maximum heart size) should be 50–55 % of the measurement of *CD* (the maximum internal transverse thoracic diameter). (**b**) The image on the *right* shows marked enlargement of the cardiac silhouette with mild pulmonary vascular congestion. Note how the ratio of *AB* to *CD* is greater than 50 %

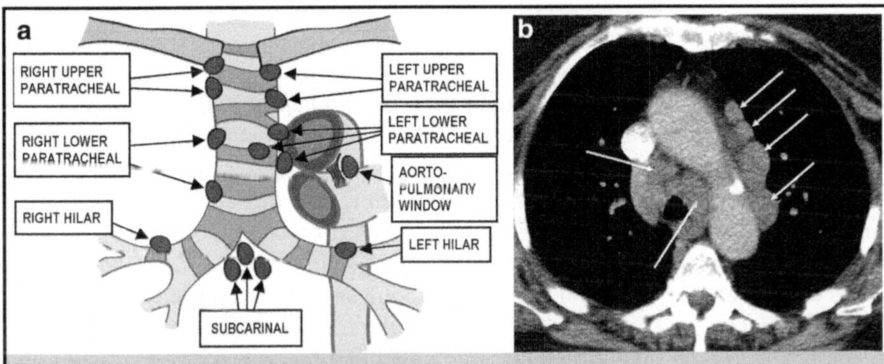

FIGURE 9.3 - LYMPH NODES OF THE MEDIASTINUM
In (**a**), the location of the lymph nodes in the chest are shown. Enlargement of these nodes can change the appearance of the mediastinum on a chest radiograph. In (**b**), mediastinal lymphadenopathy on an axial CT slice is demonstrated

mediastinal lymph nodes are located. Figure 9.3b is an axial CT image demonstrating enlarged lymph nodes around the aorta and superior vena cava.

Figure 9.4 shows a lateral view of the chest demonstrating the division of the mediastinum into three compartments: anterior, middle, and posterior. This is one of two commonly used methods to divide the mediastinum. The other method

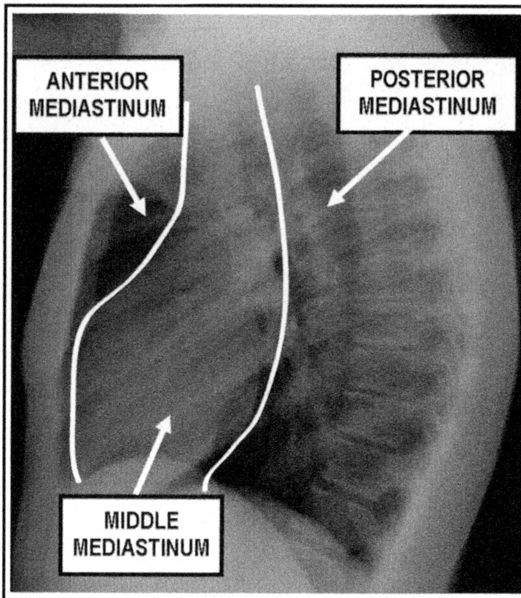

FIGURE 9.4 - MEDIASTINAL COMPARTMENTS
The subdivisions are the anterior, middle, and posterior mediastinum. These are important to the differential diagnosis of mediastinal pathology

(described by Felson) is not included in this chapter. These are not true compartments, but are useful in locating a mediastinal abnormality on the radiograph for a differential diagnosis.

The anterior compartment of the mediastinum is bounded anteriorly by the sternum and posteriorly by a line drawn along the anterior margin of the heart, ascending aorta, and brachiocephalic vessels. Normally, fat, thymic tissue and lymph nodes are present in this region. The middle compartment lies posterior to this. It is defined posteriorly by the posterior border of the trachea and the posterior surface of the heart. Middle mediastinal structures include the central airways, heart and great vessels, and lymph nodes. The posterior mediastinum lies posterior to this and contains the esophagus, descending aorta, and paravertebral tissues. Refer to Table 9.1 for mediastinal abnormalities by compartment.

The differential diagnosis for mediastinal masses is not as important as having a systematic method for reviewing conventional radiographs to decide whether what you are seeing is normal or abnormal. CT is almost universally employed as the next imaging step when a questionable mediastinal mass is appreciated on the plain radiograph. In some cases, MRI is being used for evaluation of mediastinal abnormalities as well.

Table 9-1 Mediastinal masses. A differential diagnosis of mediastinal masses may be made by the primary site of origin of the mass

Mediastinal division	Differential diagnosis
Anterior mediastinum	The four T's:
	Thyroid goiter
	Thymoma
	Teratoma
	"Terrible" lymphoma
Middle mediastinum	Lymphadenopathy
	Aortic aneurysms
	Thyroid goiter
	Bronchogenic and pericardial cysts
Posterior mediastinum	Neurogenic tumors
	Esophageal pathology
	Soft tissue tumors
	Descending aortic aneurysms
	Spinal infections and neoplasms

10 Cardiac CTA

Objectives:

1. Understand a typical indication for coronary CTA.
2. Be able to describe the steps in a coronary CTA exam.

CT scanners are now able to acquire images rapidly enough to "freeze" the heart in time and clearly delineate the coronary arteries. Their utility has been focused on the differentiation of patients with cardiac and noncardiac chest pain with an emphasis on those patients who have low to intermediate risk for coronary artery disease without EKG changes or enzyme elevation.

The patients are optimized for the coronary CT scan including the placement of a large-bore IV in the right arm (why the right arm?) and given oral or IV beta-blockers. Beta-blockers are contraindicated in the patients with:

- Known or suspected sick sinus syndrome
- Unexplained presyncope or collapse
- Current use of other antiarrhythmics
- Depressed left or right ventricular function
- History of bronchospastic disease, severe COPD
- Allergy to β-blockers

Finally, 800 mcg of sublingual nitroglycerin (SL NTG) is given just prior to contrast injection. Contraindications to the NTG include the following:

- Pronounced hypovolemia
- Inferior wall MI with RV involvement
- Elevated intracranial pressure
- Cardiac tamponade

H. Singh et al. (eds.), *Radiology Fundamentals: Introduction to Imaging & Technology*, DOI 10.1007/978-3-319-10362-4_10

- Constrictive pericarditis
- Severe aortic stenosis
- Hypertrophic obstructive cardiomyopathy
- Severe systolic hypotension

Contrast is usually injected at 6–8 cc/s for a total of 65–75 cc/s of nonionic contrast after bolus tracking technique (Fig. 10.1). Images are acquired during *diastole*, when the heart is filling passively but also has the least amount of motion (Fig. 10.2). If there is any ectopy, using certain imaging acquisition protocols, there can be significant artifact (Fig. 10.3) on the images. The images acquired are then viewed in both standard planes and on a 3D workstation (Fig. 10.4). Description of any plaque should include whether the plaque is noncalcified versus calcified versus mixed. Sensitivity and specificity for the 128 slice CT scanners are ~92 % and 95 %, respectively. It has a very good negative predictive value, and in that sense, it is very useful for the patient in the ED with convincing chest pain and no evidence of cardiac ischemia.

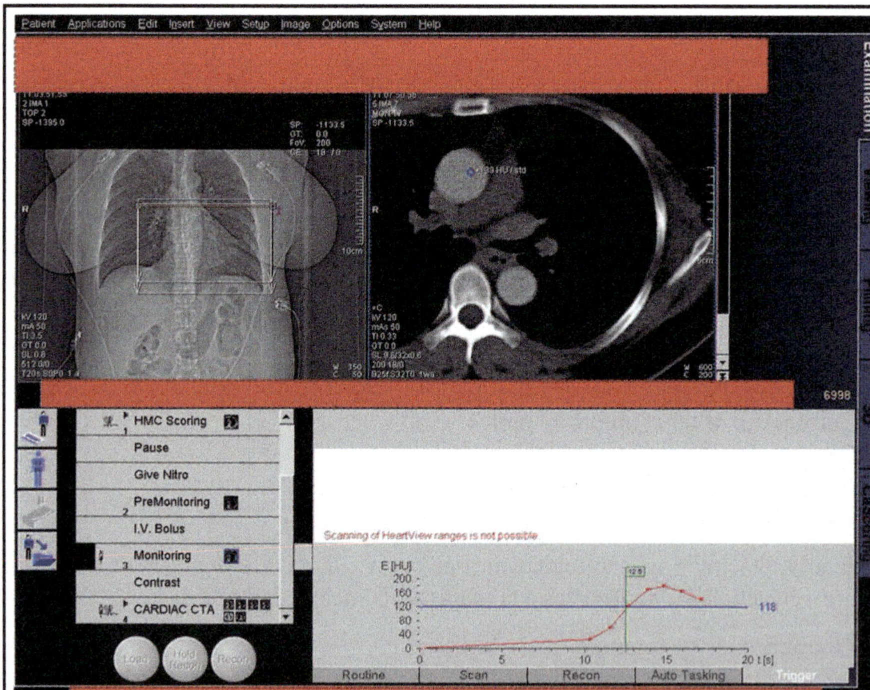

FIGURE 10.1 - Image from the planning screen of a cardiac CTA demonstrating the field of view (*upper left image*), the bolus tracking area in the ascending aorta (*upper right image*), the actual steps in the protocol (*lower left*), and the contrast-density curve (*lower right image*)

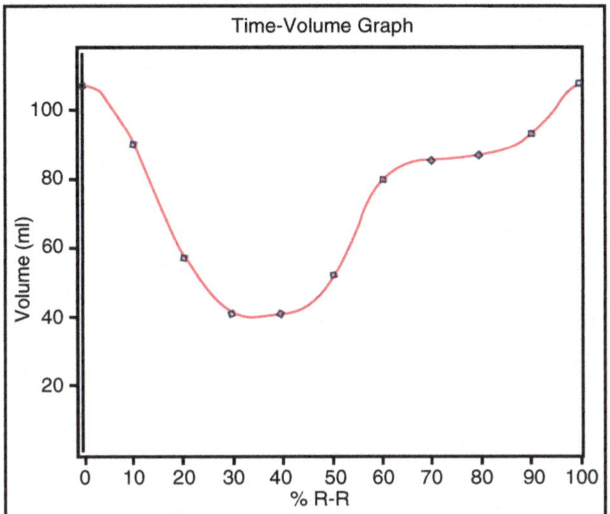

FIGURE 10.2 - Time-volume graph with the R-R interval divided into 0–100 % on the x axis and the volume on the y-axis. Note that the volume does not change from ~65 % to ~75 %, coinciding with diastole and the optimal time in the cardiac cycle to obtain images

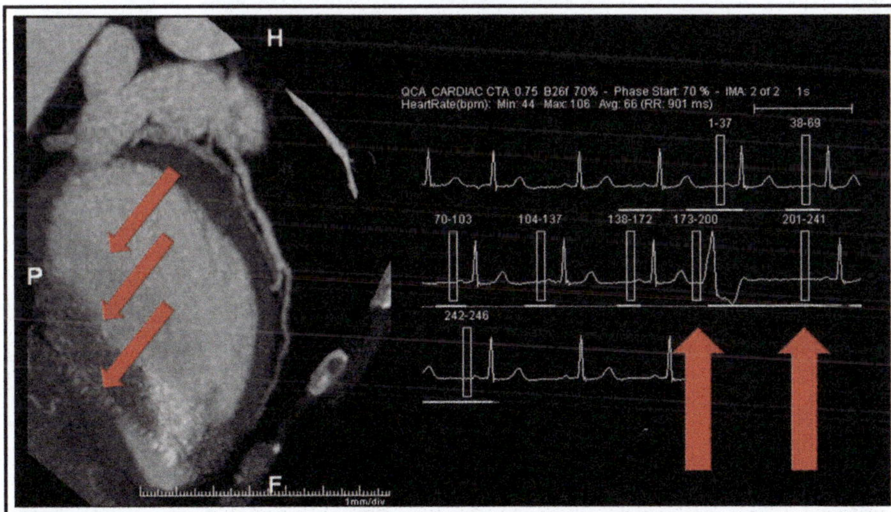

FIGURE 10.3 - In this image from a cardiac CTA scan, it is noted on the image to the *right* that acquisition times (*the rectangular boxes*) are all appropriate except in the region of the PVC (*arrows*). That corresponds to the imaging artifact noted on the image to the *left* (*smaller arrows*)

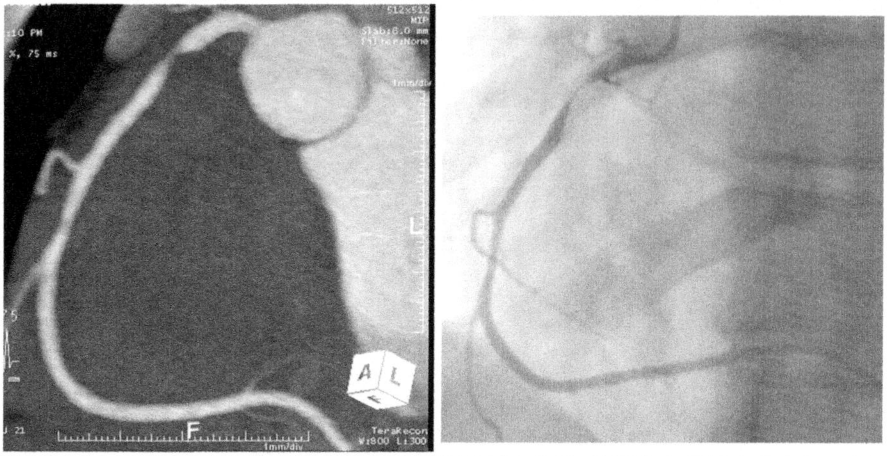

FIGURE 10.4 - Coronary CTA of the RCA (image on the *left*) and the subsequent cardiac catheterization image of the same segment (image on the *right*). There is strong correlation between the images

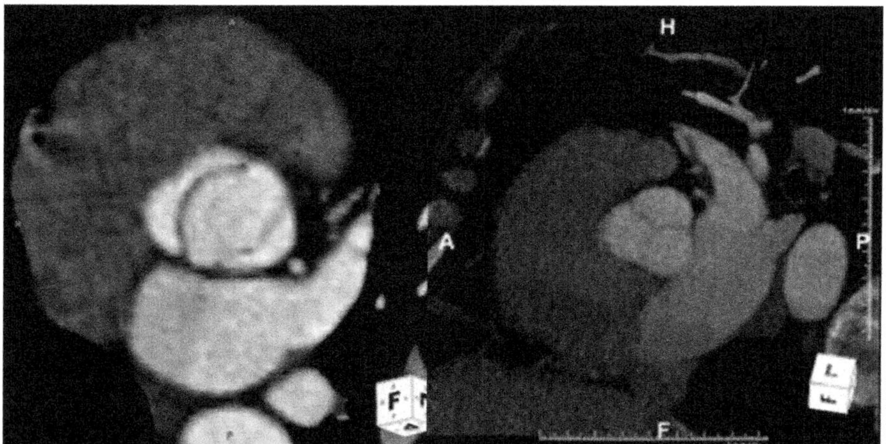

FIGURE 10.5 - En face images of the aortic valve in a patient with a bicuspid aortic valve (image on the *left*) and a patient with a normal, tricuspid aortic valve (image on the *right*)

Although the other indications for cardiac CTA are beyond the scope of this textbook, one indication for the use of cardiac CTA is the structural evaluation of the cardiac structures, such as the aortic valve (Fig. 10.5).

11 Lateral Chest Radiograph

Objectives:

1. Learn to use a systematic method for review of the left lateral chest radiograph.
2. Identify major structures (heart, aorta, central airways, pulmonary arteries, and hemidiaphragms) and recognize normal areas of lucency on the lateral view.
3. State how the silhouette sign and magnification can be used to differentiate the left and right hemidiaphragms on the lateral view.

Lateral View: Systemic Approach

Begin by reviewing the systematic approach to the left lateral chest radiograph in Fig. 11.1.

Start by reviewing the major structures, including the heart, aorta, pulmonary arteries at the hilum central airways, and the right and left hemidiaphragms. Follow this with a review of the areas of lucency in the retrosternal region, retrotracheal triangle, the large rectangular area extending inferiorly from the retrotracheal triangle to the diaphragms (with a gradual gradation of density from lighter to darker as one moves inferiorly), and the costophrenic angles. If you proceed in this manner on each x-ray, you will develop a consistent method for detecting abnormalities. This takes considerable practice.

The importance of the lateral view cannot be underestimated. Without a lateral view, the position of any abnormality projected over the lungs cannot be determined with certainty, in most cases. Figure 11.2 is a schematic of a skin lesion arising from the soft tissues of the back that is projected over the right lung on the frontal view.

H. Singh et al. (eds.), *Radiology Fundamentals: Introduction to Imaging & Technology*, DOI 10.1007/978-3-319-10362-4_11

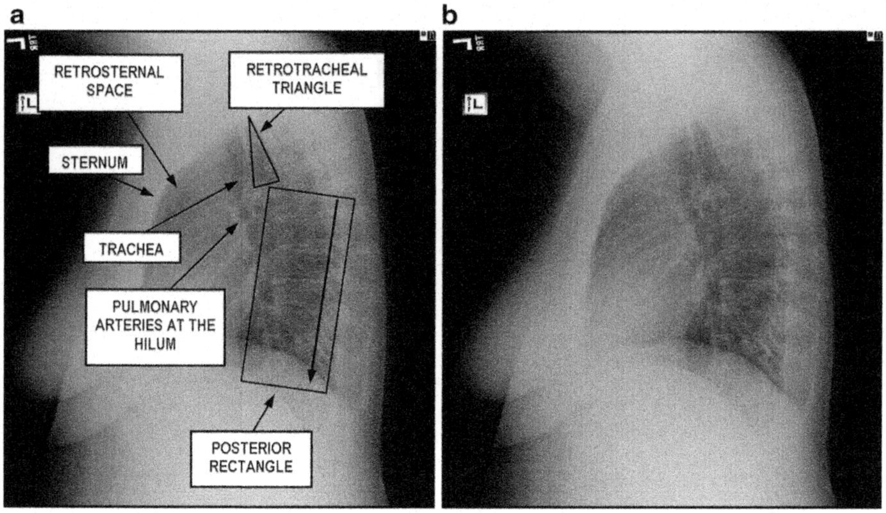

FIGURE 11.1 - THE LATERAL CHEST
(**a**) Normal lateral view. Use this image to identify structures and spaces on image (**b**)

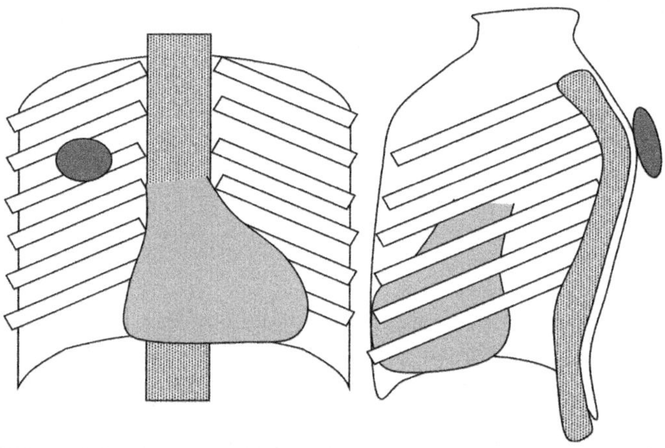

FIGURE 11.2 - THE LATERAL CHEST PROJECTION
Note that the lesion projected over the chest on the PA projection, assumed to be an intrathoracic mass, is actually in the soft tissues of the back

The lateral view can be useful in ascertaining whether a structure lies within or outside the patient. Figure 11.3 demonstrates frontal and lateral views of a patient with suspected bilateral pleural effusions. The bilateral pleural effusions are clearly evident on the lateral projection as curved menisci. However, the costophrenic

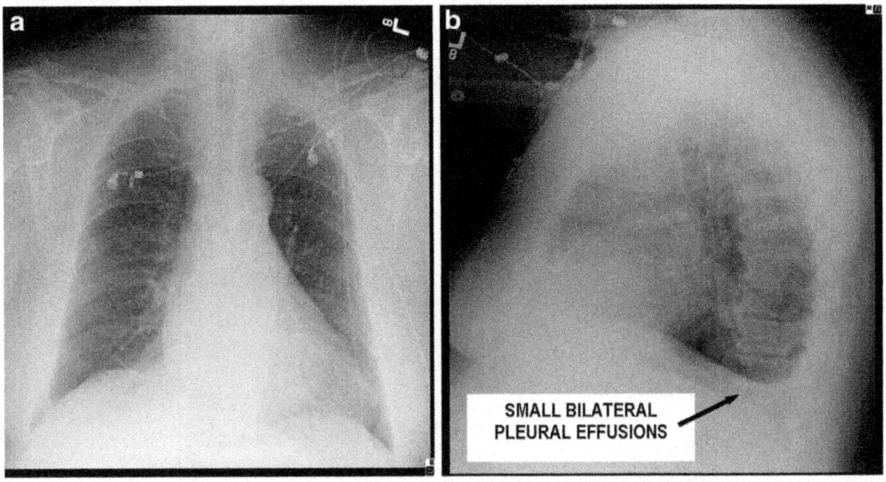

FIGURE 11.3 - BILATERAL PLEURAL EFFUSIONS
Frontal and lateral views of a patient with suspected bilateral pleural effusions. Note that although bilateral pleural effusions are clearly evident on the lateral projection (**b**), the costophrenic angles are clear and sharp on the frontal view (**a**)

angles are clear and sharp on the frontal view. This is a good example of how small pleural fluid accumulations that may be of clinical significance can be overlooked if one relies only on the frontal (AP or PA) projections. Similarly, patients with small areas of consolidation or nodules in the lower lobes may not be correctly diagnosed if one does not carefully review the lateral projection, as a portion of the lower lobes are obscured by the hemidiaphragms on the frontal view.

Hemidiaphragms

There are several ways to determine which hemidiaphragm and which costophrenic angle is the left versus the right on the lateral view (see Fig. 11.4 for correlation):

1. Since the anterior portion of the left hemidiaphragm comes into contact with the inferior aspect of the heart, it is often obscured or silhouetted anteriorly – another example of the silhouette sign. For this reason, the left hemidiaphragm cannot usually be traced as far anteriorly as the right hemidiaphragm.
2. Lateral chest radiographs are usually performed as left laterals. This means the patient's left side is placed against the cassette, and the beam traverses the patient from right to left. This is noted by an "L" marker somewhere on the radiograph. You will recall that objects that are further from the radiograph are magnified more.

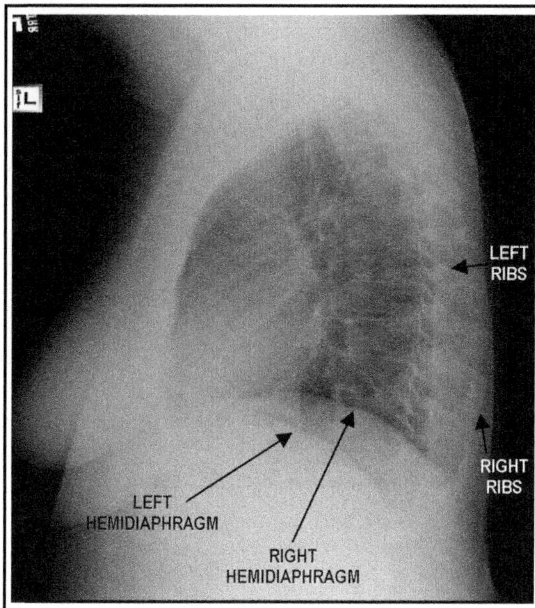

FIGURE 11.4 - HEMIDIAPHRAGMS
Lateral chest with well-visualized hemidiaphragms

If one looks at the posterior portion of the left lateral chest radiograph, two sets of ribs, a large set and a corresponding smaller set, can be seen. One can reason that the larger set of ribs must be located further from the radiograph and must represent the right ribs. The hemidiaphragm that can be traced to this set of ribs must be the right hemidiaphragm. This also allows separating the right and left costophrenic angles.

3. Since the left hemidiaphragm lies directly above the stomach, the left hemidiaphragm can be seen to have the stomach beneath it on the lateral view, if the left hemidiaphragm is slightly higher than the right in this region.
4. By correlating the height of the hemidiaphragm on the frontal projection with the highest point of the hemidiaphragm on the lateral projection, one may be able to distinguish left from right on the lateral view.

Think about these relationships since they represent a recapitulation of two important principles presented earlier – the silhouette sign and the principle of magnification.

Hilar Enlargement

Review Fig. 11.5a. The arrows on this PA view indicate the right and left interlobar pulmonary arteries. On the right side, there is increased density overlying the vessel. On the lateral view (Fig. 11.5b), one can clearly separate the right and left pulmonary arteries from an irregular mass. This was a lung adenocarcinoma. The lateral view may be useful in distinguishing hilar enlargement from enlarged pulmonary arteries (due to pulmonary hypertension) from hilar adenopathy.

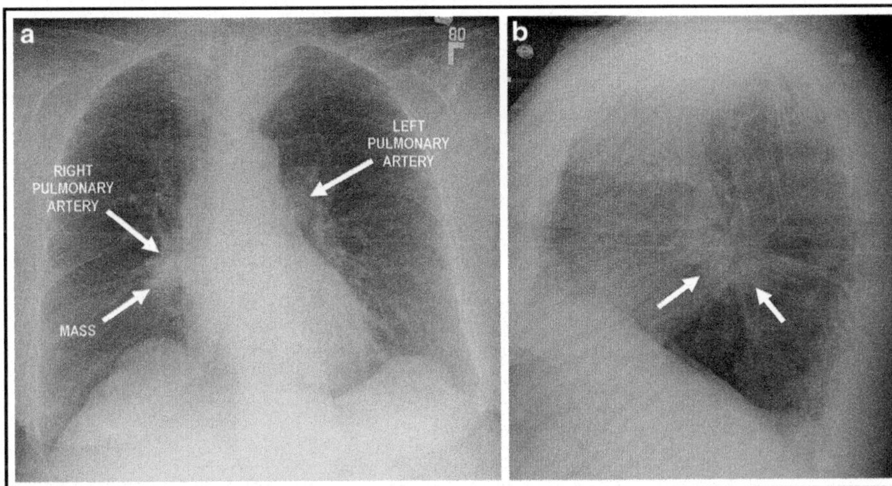

FIGURE 11.5 - HILAR MASS
PA (**a**) and lateral (**b**) chest radiographs show a patient with a right hilar mass. *Arrows* seen on the lateral (**b**) radiograph indicate the margins of the mass

12 Pulmonary Nodules or Masses

Objectives:

1. When evaluating a possible pulmonary nodule or mass on a chest radiograph, remember to assess the following characteristics of the lesion: size, location, margin characteristics, involvement of contiguous structures, calcification or cavitation, solitary versus multiple, time course of growth from old radiographs, and other chest radiograph findings.
2. List four differential diagnoses for a solitary pulmonary nodule.
3. Discuss the significance of calcification within a pulmonary nodule or mass.
4. Know the terms "round pneumonia" and "pseudotumor."

A pulmonary nodule is a well-circumscribed opacity measuring up to or equal to 3 cm in diameter. A mass is a lesion more than 3 cm in diameter. The principles of evaluation are the same for nodules and masses, and for the rest of this chapter, the term nodule is used.

Nodules within the lung are commonly suspected and/or appreciated on the conventional chest radiograph. There are several criteria which must be used to arrive at a list of potential differential diagnoses for a lung nodule.

H. Singh et al. (eds.), *Radiology Fundamentals: Introduction to Imaging & Technology*, DOI 10.1007/978-3-319-10362-4_12

Evaluation of a Pulmonary Nodule

1. *Is it pulmonary?* Make sure the nodule is in the lung and not a superimposed structure related to the chest wall, as would be the case in a patient with a skin or breast lesion or other external density (Fig. 12.1 below, and Fig. 11.2 from Chap. 11). Healing rib fractures can also simulate lung nodules.
2. Compare with old studies: The "cancer" you have just diagnosed may be a benign nodule which has been present for many years. If old studies are not available at your institution, you should check with the referring clinician or patient if old studies are available. A nodule that is new compared with a recent radiograph (from one to a few weeks earlier) is more likely to be infectious or inflammatory.
3. *Size*: Larger lesions are more likely to be malignant; however, bigger lesions are not always malignant, and smaller lesions are not always benign.
4. *Location*: Assess the location of the nodule with respect to the pulmonary lobes and pulmonary segments (if possible). This requires PA and lateral views. Computerized tomography (CT) is used to more accurately characterize and localize a nodule.
5. *Margin characteristics*: Assess whether the margins of the lesion are smooth or irregular. Obviously, the more irregular the margins of the mass, the more suspicious we are that we are dealing with a malignant process. Keep in mind, though, that many infectious or inflammatory lesions have quite irregular margins.

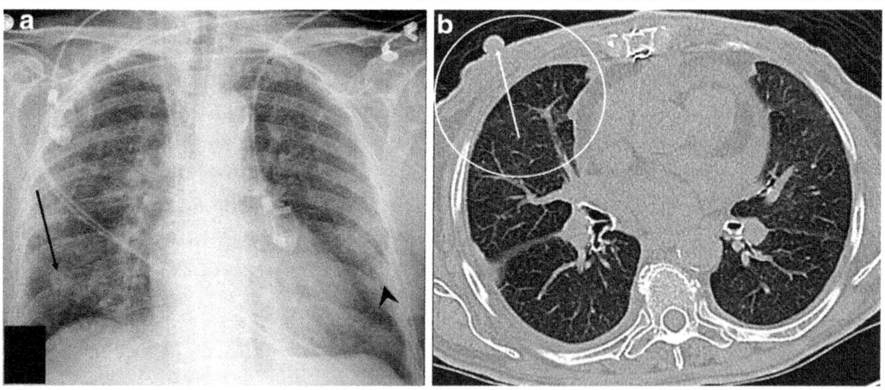

FIGURE 12.1 - NIPPLE SHADOWS
Image (**a**) depicts what appears to be a right lower lung nodule on a frontal chest x-ray (*black arrow*). The *arrowhead* shows a similar "nodule" on the left side indicating these represent the nipples. Note the appearance on the corresponding CT slice, image (**b**), (*arrow* inside of *circle*)

This should be correlated with the patient's symptoms. If there are clinical features of infection, a follow-up radiograph after treatment should be considered. Metastatic lesions may be very smoothly demarcated. Although the contours of a lesion should be evaluated, they are not absolute indicators of a benign versus malignant lesion.

6. *Involvement of contiguous structures*: This may be an important indicator of the etiology of the lesion. A mass that is close to the chest wall and destroys a rib is very likely to be a malignant process.
7. *Presence or absence of cavitation or calcification*: Cavitation may be seen in malignant and benign processes. Calcification, although once thought to indicate that a lesion was benign, is now known to be seen in both malignant and benign processes. Calcification that is diffuse or laminated is generally benign. Central, dense calcification occupying a significant portion of the nodule is also often benign.
8. *Solitary or multiple lesions*: Multiple pulmonary nodules often have a different connotation and differential diagnosis than a solitary lesion. For this reason, when one pulmonary nodule is seen, a careful search for other nodules should be made. Computerized tomography, because of its sensitivity for detection of nodules, is useful in this regard.
9. *Other findings*: Once you have found a nodule, do not stop your search for other abnormalities; "satisfaction of search" is a common problem. Additional findings such as mediastinal adenopathy, hilar adenopathy, or destructive rib lesions suggest malignancy and warrant early CT evaluation.

In addition to these findings, take into account the age and clinical history to guide your recommendations. Assess the temporal evolution, if prior imaging is available. The differential diagnosis of a solitary pulmonary nodule includes granulomatous disease (such as old tuberculous and histoplasma infection), primary lung malignancy, and post-inflammatory parenchymal scarring. Other less common causes of solitary pulmonary nodules include hamartoma, solitary metastasis, carcinoid tumors, round pneumonia, arteriovenous malformations, and cysts.

Cases to Review

The following series of radiographs depict various causes of pulmonary nodules or masses. Try to describe each in terms of the criteria provided and arrive at a brief differential diagnosis.

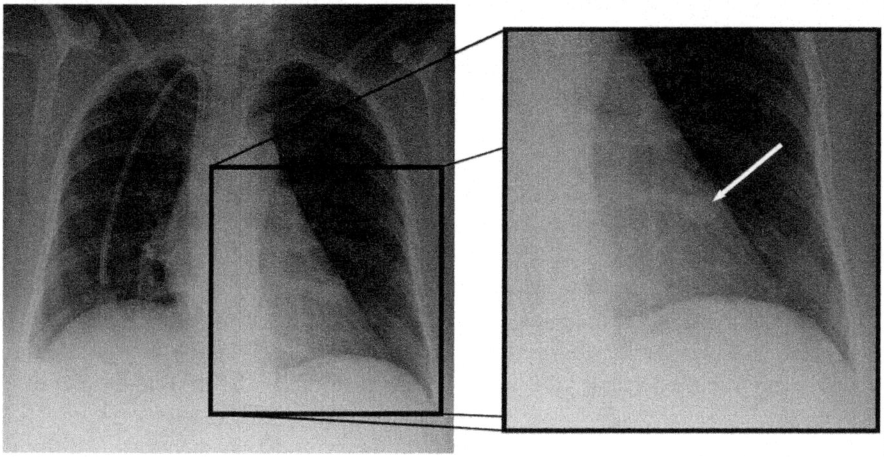

FIGURE 12.2 - COIN LESION
Always remember that this lesion is actually a three dimensional sphere

As always, the point is not to memorize the numerous possible diagnoses for each abnormality. You should however be fastidious in employing these criteria and remembering the pitfalls for all cases of pulmonary mass lesions.

Case 1: Figure 12.1 demonstrates an approximately 1 cm, soft tissue nodular opacity projected over the lower right chest. While this may be confused with a pulmonary nodule, its smooth margins (it is unusually well outlined because it is surrounded by air), classic position, and the presence of a corresponding similar density on the left side indicate that this represents the nipple. When a questionable nodule is suspected to be a nipple shadow, a repeat study with small metallic markers taped to the nipples may be performed for confirmation.

Case 2: Figure 12.2 demonstrates a solitary pulmonary nodule in the left lower lung behind the heart. This is the so-called coin lesion, even though it is a three-dimensional sphere. This lesion turned out to be a granuloma, but there are no distinguishing characteristics on the radiograph that would allow you to make this diagnosis. A biopsy was necessary to make this diagnosis.

Case 3: Figure 12.3 demonstrates a large smoothly marginated solitary lesion without evidence of cavitation in the left paracardiac region. Mottled densities may be seen within the mass representing "popcorn"-like calcifications. Although calcification within a lesion does not guarantee that it is of benign etiology, this pattern of calcification is nearly always associated with a particular benign neoplasm of the lung, a hamartoma. Of course, comparison with old studies also showed the mass to be unchanged in size. In this case, detection of this pattern of calcification and stability compared with prior imaging made surgical removal for diagnosis unnecessary.

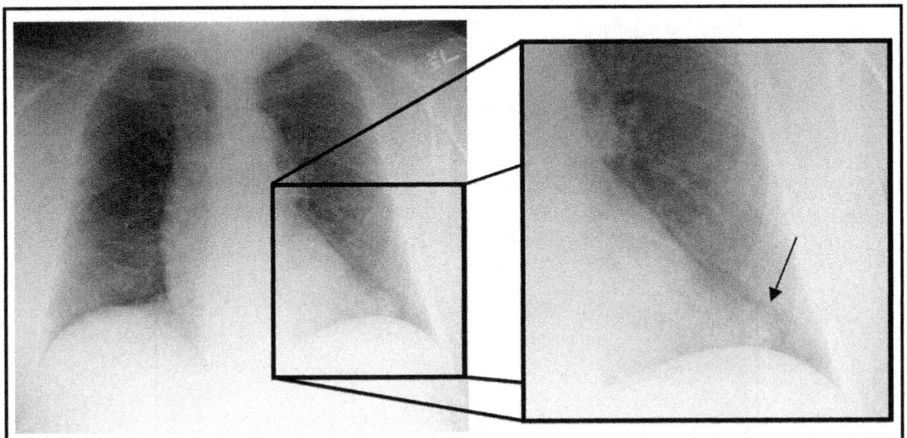

FIGURE 12.3 - HAMARTOMA
Hamartoma in the left lower lobe. Note the typical "popcorn" calcification within the lesion

Case 4: Figure 12.4 was obtained from a 60-year-old man with a history of heavy smoking who now presents with weight loss and hemoptysis. The left mid-lung mass demonstrates obvious cavitation. It is also contiguous to the left lateral chest wall, but it does not erode or destroy the ribs and does not produce a pleural effusion on this view. The hilum on the left side has a relatively normal appearance without definite evidence of lymphadenopathy. Again, as in so many disease processes of the chest, CT scans would better evaluate lymphadenopathy. The differential diagnosis of this cavitary lesion includes a primary lung neoplasm. Cavitation is most common in the squamous cell type of primary lung carcinoma. A lung abscess could give a similar appearance if the patient's symptoms related more to an inflammatory process than this patient's obviously malignant symptomatology. Cavitation may be artifactually simulated by a number of conditions, and before cavitation is accepted as a finding, it must be clearly present. Often debris or soft tissue density will be seen within a cavity. This can represent clotted blood, a "fungus ball" (due to an aspergilloma), or necrotic debris from the inner wall of the neoplasm. This lesion was a squamous cell carcinoma on biopsy.

Case 5: Figure 12.5 demonstrates multiple pulmonary nodules in both lungs that are highly suspicious for metastases. It is their size and multiplicity, which strongly suggests their etiology, and for this reason any time one nodule is found, others must be looked for carefully. Because metastases to the lungs are essentially an embolic process, metastases are more common in the lower lobes because of the normally increased blood flow to this region. Also, metastases are often initially detected in the subpleural, peripheral portion of the lung, since this is where the smaller blood vessels are, which are more prone to embolization. Computerized tomography (CT) is the most sensitive test for detecting early metastatic disease. Other processes such as granulomatous disease can also demonstrate multiple nodules.

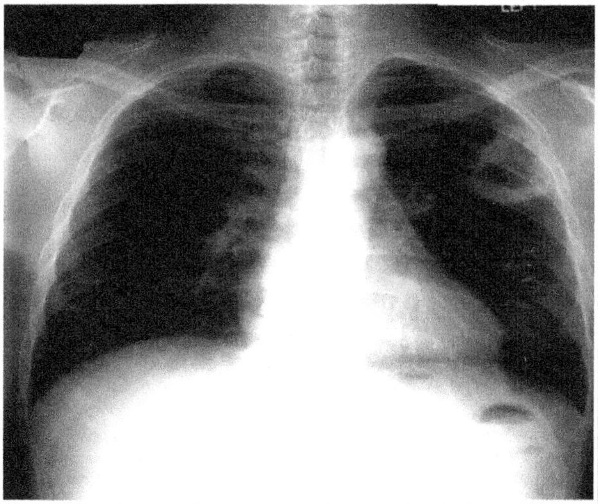

FIGURE 12.4 - CAVITARY LESION
Note the area of decreased density within the well-defined left upper lung mass

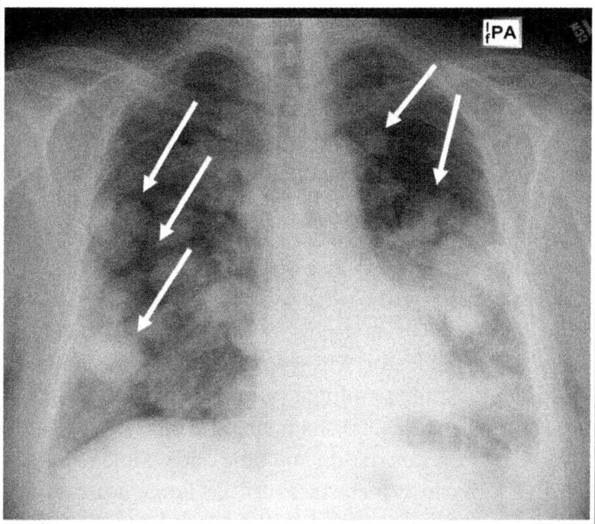

FIGURE 12.5 - PULMONARY NODULES
PA chest radiograph demonstrating numerous pulmonary nodules throughout both lungs

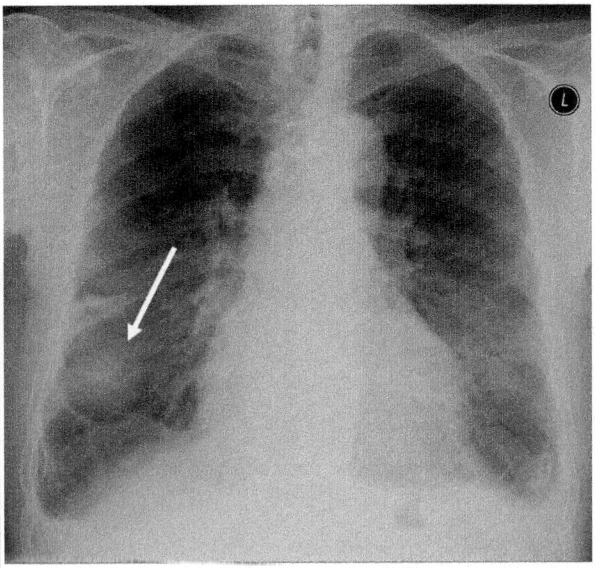

FIGURE 12.6 - ROUND PNEUMONIA
Round pneumonia in the right lower lung (*arrow*)

Case 6: Figure 12.6 is a frontal chest radiograph of a patient with a small amount of blood-tinged sputum and a fever of 101°. Obviously, the presence of the fairly well-marginated mass lesion in the right mid-lung is of concern for possible malignancy. However, because this patient's symptoms were primarily those of someone with pneumonia, a trial of antibiotics for 2 weeks was performed. A follow-up radiograph at that time showed some improvement. This is an example of "round pneumonia." Although more commonly seen in children, round pneumonia can also occur in adults, as in this case. Inflammatory exudate spreads from alveolar unit to alveolar unit through the pores of Kohn, opacifying the lung in an ever-expanding manner from a central focus. In certain cases, the pattern of expansion and flow of exudate can be very well defined and simulate a mass lesion. This case demonstrates the importance of paying attention to the clinical presentation of the patient in addition to the radiographic findings when evaluating a potential pulmonary mass.

Case 7: Figure 12.7a demonstrates a well-defined density projected over the right mid-lung. The lateral view (Figure 12.7b) demonstrates that this density has a lentiform (or lens-like) configuration and lies within the right major fissure. This density represents the so-called pseudotumor, caused by fluid loculated within a fissure. Clues to the diagnosis include location in the area of the fissure, ovoid shape with long axis in the plane of the fissure, and association with a pleural effusion either on the same radiograph or on prior studies.

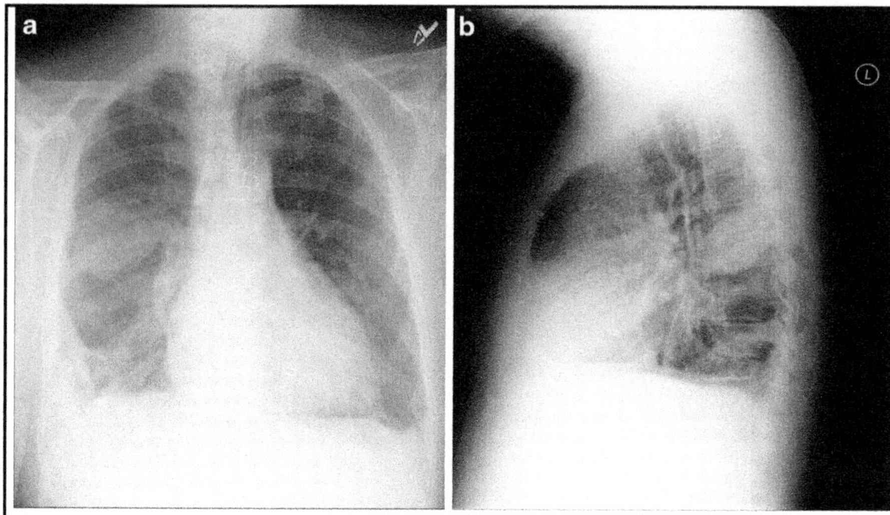

FIGURE 12.7 - PSEUDOTUMOR
Frontal (**a**) and lateral (**b**) chest radiographs demonstrating a pseudotumor in the right mid-lung along the right major fissure

In summary, the differential diagnosis of solitary or multiple pulmonary nodules is long. There is considerable overlap between the appearance of benign and malignant conditions. Time and expense may be saved through careful observation and analysis of the plain radiographs, comparisons with old radiographs, as well as correlation with the patient's clinical presentation. If the abnormality is not clearly benign or acute, then chest CT is often the next step in evaluation.

13 Airspace Disease

Objectives:

1. Describe the radiographic finding characteristic of airspace disease.
2. List the major differential diagnostic categories for acute airspace disease.
3. List two causes of chronic airspace disease.

The purpose of this chapter is to demonstrate the appearance of airspace disease in the lungs. The pulmonary acinus is the basic structural unit of the lung involved in gas exchange (Fig. 13.1). It is the structural unit of lung distal to the terminal bronchiole, is supplied by respiratory bronchioles, and is 6–10 mm in diameter. It contains alveolar ducts and alveoli. The terminal bronchiole is the most peripheral airway that is purely conductive in function with no gas exchange capability. A pulmonary lobule (or secondary pulmonary lobule) is the smallest unit of lung surrounded by connective tissue septa. One lobule contains between 3 and 25 acini. Recall the four densities seen on a radiograph – air, soft tissue, fat, and bone. Disease within the airspace is manifest on the radiograph as soft tissue density. Disease may involve numerous acini or spread from one acinar unit to another. The opacified acini become confluent, producing a fluffy, homogeneous radiographic pattern characteristic of airspace disease as seen in Fig. 13.2.

Since disease, which primarily affects the airspace, often spares the larger conductive airways, these airways become visible as tubular, branching, air-filled structures surrounded by the fluid-filled acini. These air-filled structures are normally surrounded by air-filled lung and are not normally distinguished on the chest radiograph. These air-filled bronchi surrounded by opacified airspace are called air bronchograms. Air bronchograms are the radiographic hallmark of airspace disease. Figure 13.3 is an excellent example of air bronchograms in a patient with pneumonia. The distribution of airspace disease and time course of development may be useful in determining its etiology.

H. Singh et al. (eds.), *Radiology Fundamentals: Introduction to Imaging & Technology*, DOI 10.1007/978-3-319-10362-4_13

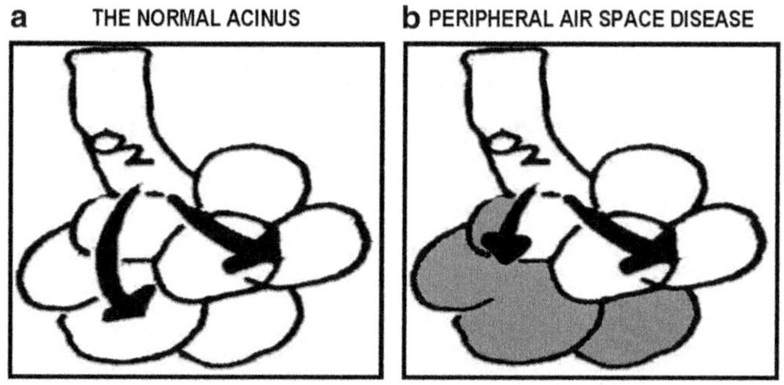

FIGURE 13.1 - LUNG ACINUS
(**a**) The normal acinus is approximately 8 mm in diameter. (**b**) In the picture on the *right*, volume is unaffected and the airways remain patent

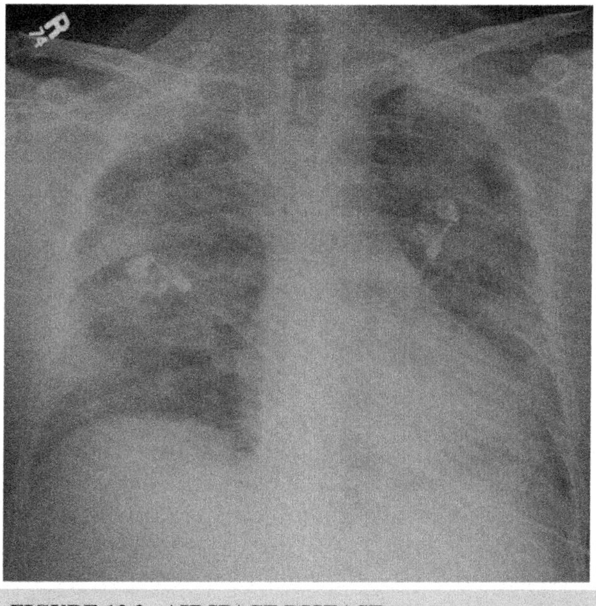

FIGURE 13.2 - AIRSPACE DISEASE
Frontal chest radiograph demonstrating perihilar predominant airspace disease, due to pulmonary edema. The radiograph 24 h after diuresis was normal

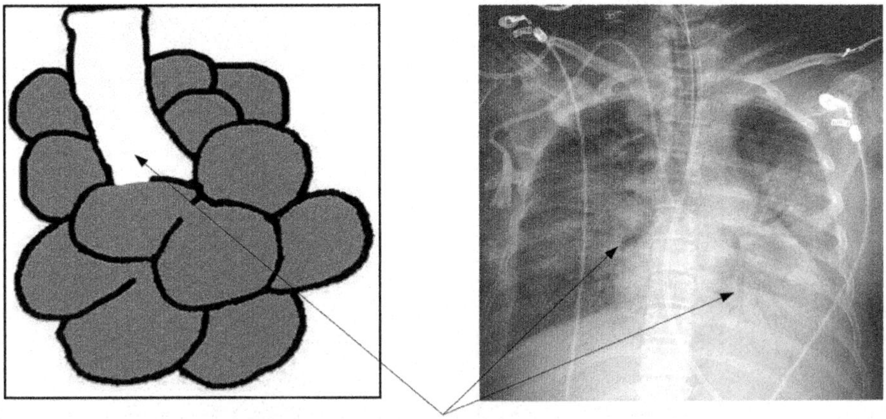

FIGURE 13.3 - AIR BRONCHOGRAMS
Schematic and radiograph of an air bronchogram. Note that the bronchi are usually not seen peripherally on a normal chest radiograph. With the acini surrounding the bronchus filled with fluid, the bronchus is outlined

Figure 13.4 demonstrates airspace disease in the right lower lung. In a patient with cough and fever, this would be consistent with pneumonia. The right dome of diaphragm and right heart border are preserved. A lateral view is necessary to localize this to the right middle or lower lobes.

Consider the common differentials for acute airspace disease:

1. Pulmonary edema: transudate fills the alveoli.
2. Infection: pneumonic exudate fills the alveoli.
3. Hemorrhage: blood fills the alveoli.

Within each of these major categories, however, multiple pathologies may be included:

1. Pulmonary edema – cardiogenic (CHF) or noncardiogenic (ARDS).
2. Infection – numerous organisms may cause pneumonia.
3. Hemorrhage – may be produced by many causes including pulmonary contusion, pulmonary infarcts, Goodpasture syndrome, and diseases that produce vasculitis.

This list is certainly not inclusive of all possibilities. Clinical information must be coordinated with old studies to narrow the diagnostic possibilities. Fever would suggest pneumonia, while hemoptysis would suggest pulmonary hemorrhage. The distribution and pattern of evolution of the abnormality may also help. Cardiogenic edema tends to be bilateral and associated with other findings (enlarged heart, pleural effusions). Pneumonia is classically more focal.

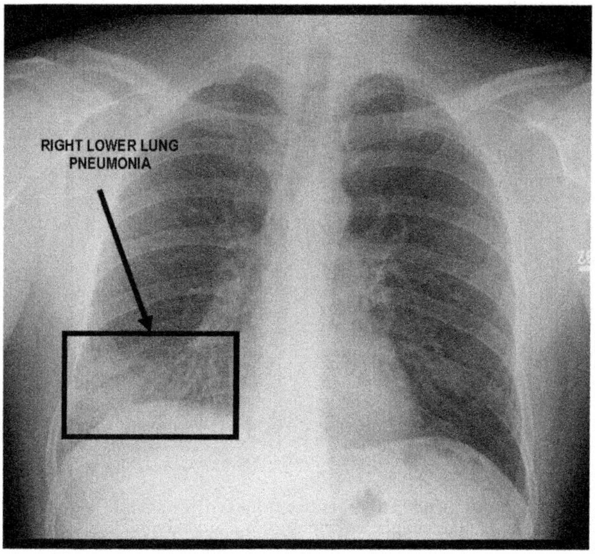

FIGURE 13.4 - PNEUMONIA
Patchy airspace disease in the right lower lung consistent with pneumonia

Pathologic processes involving the airspace (alveoli) can be further subdivided into acute and chronic in nature. The time course of appearance and regression of airspace disease is useful. Edema can come and go quickly (regression can occur within hours). Pneumonia regresses more slowly. Nonresolving airspace opacity may require evaluation for other processes such as neoplasms (including some types of adenocarcinoma and pulmonary lymphoma), hypersensitivity pneumonitis, alveolar sarcoidosis, and alveolar proteinosis.

14 Interstitial Disease

Objectives:

1. Know the radiologic appearance and anatomic location of interstitial disease associated with Kerley lines, peribronchial cuffing, subpleural thickening, a reticular or reticulonodular pattern.
2. List three common causes of interstitial lung disease.
3. Understand the significance of the broad classification of chest radiographic abnormalities into interstitial and airspace disease.

Introduction

The alveoli, conductive airways, and blood vessels of the lung are surrounded by the pulmonary interstitium. Figure 14.1 shows the anatomy of several secondary pulmonary lobules (or lobule). Recall that each lobule contains 3–25 acini. Notice that the interlobular septum defines the secondary pulmonary lobule. The peribronchovascular interstitium surrounds the pulmonary artery and accompanying bronchiole. The subpleural interstitium lines the inner aspect of the pleura. The interstitium is a continuum of dense elastic tissue and collagen throughout the lung that merges into the elastic component of the alveolar walls. It is not normally separately defined on the plain radiograph and becomes visible when disease increases its volume and/or radiographic density.

The anatomic subdivisions of the interstitial space are useful since involvement of various subdivisions give rise to the specific radiographic findings associated with interstitial disease. These radiographic findings are Kerley lines, peribronchial thickening or cuffing, reticular or reticulonodular opacities, and subpleural thickening. Most disease processes involve the airspaces and the interstitium. Even diseases that are called "interstitial diseases" often have some airspace involvement. However, the

H. Singh et al. (eds.), *Radiology Fundamentals: Introduction to Imaging & Technology*, DOI 10.1007/978-3-319-10362-4_14

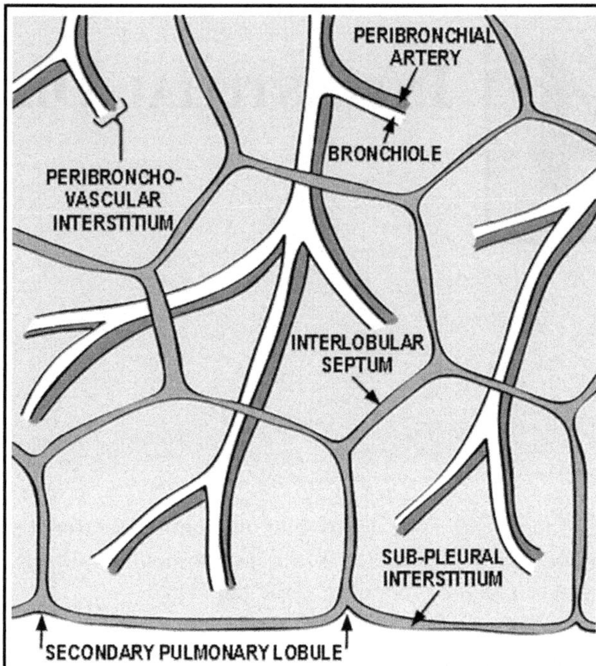

FIGURE 14.1 - SECONDARY PULMONARY LOBULES
Note the components of the interstitium and their relationship to the secondary pulmonary lobule

broad categorization into airspace or interstitial disease (based on the predominant pattern of involvement), in combination with the clinical presentation, allows a more accurate differential diagnosis.

Kerley Lines

The lung is subdivided into numerous secondary pulmonary lobules by connective tissue septa. It is the thickening of these septa that produces Kerley lines, identified by and named for Dr. Peter Kerley, an Irish radiologist. The septa contain lymphatics and pulmonary venules. The short, 1–2 cm horizontal lines in the inferolateral aspect of the lungs are called Kerley B lines (Fig. 14.2). These are typically described in congestive heart failure but can be seen in a number of other conditions. The less commonly seen 2–6 cm septa visualized radiating from the hila to the upper lobes cast shadows known as Kerley A lines when thickened. Kerley also described C lines that have no distinct anatomic correlate and are due to superimposition of A and B lines into a weblike pattern.

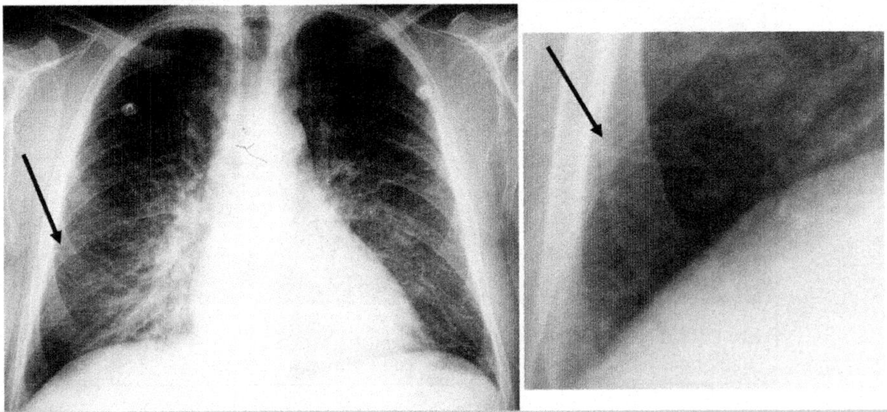

FIGURE 14.2 - KERLEY B LINES
Kerley B lines in a patient with congestive heart failure. Image on the right is a magnified view at the right CP angle

Peribronchial Cuffing

Bronchi, when seen on end, cast thin-walled ring shadows on the normal chest radiograph. These are usually seen in the perihilar region. Remember that the bronchus and pulmonary artery travel together and bifurcate to the terminal bronchial-pulmonary arterial level. When the peribronchovascular component of the interstitial space becomes thickened, the normally "paper thin" bronchial wall becomes more visible (Fig. 14.3). Causes of peribronchial thickening are varied and include CHF and infection. Diseases that thicken the bronchial wall on an inflammatory basis chronically, such as chronic bronchitis or cystic fibrosis, may also lead to thickened bronchial walls.

Reticular and Reticulonodular Patterns

Thickening or nodularity of the interstitium may result in increased linear and/or fine nodular opacities in the lungs (Fig. 14.4). In this situation, the descriptive terms reticular or, if there is a nodular component, reticulonodular may be employed to describe the findings. Common causes of reticular opacities include congestive heart failure and atypical infections. More chronic causes of reticular or reticulonodular opacities include sarcoidosis and interstitial fibrosis.

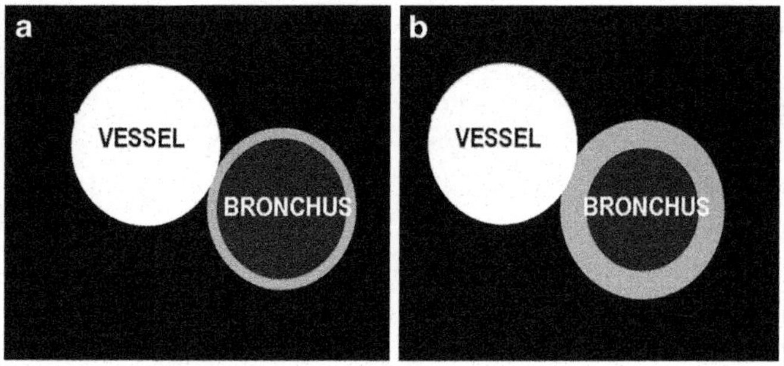

FIGURE 14.3 - PERIBRONCHIAL CUFFING
(**a**) Normal bronchovascular bundle. (**b**) Peribronchial cuffing

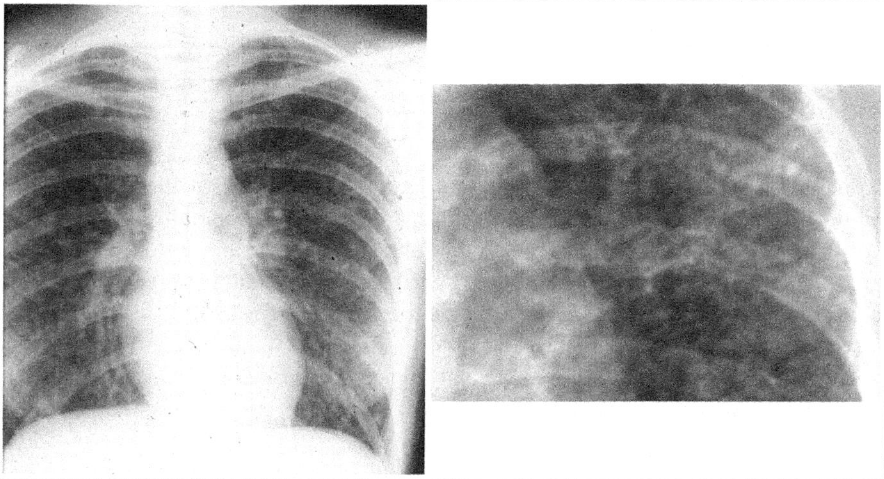

FIGURE 14.4 - RETICULONODULAR DISEASE
PA radiograph and close-up of the same patient showing the "lines and dots" of reticulonodular lung disease

Subpleural Thickening

When accumulation of fluid or thickening of the subpleural interstitial space occurs, increased radiographic density that outlines the fissures is produced. This occurs frequently in early pulmonary edema and is commonly attributed to "fluid within the fissure." Any process affecting the subpleural interstitial space will give this appearance of thickened fissures. Hence, thickening of the visceral pleural line can be seen in patients with early interstitial pneumonia or evolving interstitial disease from any cause.

Summary

There are many causes of interstitial disease. These include early CHF, atypical infections, sarcoidosis, fibrotic lung disease, occupational lung disease, and the distinctly interstitial form of metastatic disease seen in carcinoma of the lung, breast, and stomach called lymphangitic carcinomatosis. It is important to be able to recognize the radiographic findings of interstitial disease and correlate it with the clinical information for a differential diagnosis.

15 Atelectasis

Objectives:

1. Define "atelectasis."
2. Define and give examples of postobstructive atelectasis, cicatrization atelectasis, adhesive atelectasis, and passive atelectasis.
3. Explain why loss of lung volume does not always lead to increased radiographic density.
4. Learn the characteristic patterns of lobar atelectasis.

Introduction

You will find few chest radiographic reports that do not include the term atelectasis. Atelectasis means incomplete lung expansion. This term is frequently tossed about, and little thought is given to its significance. It is important to think about the underlying pathophysiology any time the term atelectasis is employed in describing a chest radiograph finding. Pneumonia and atelectasis are always considered in the differential diagnosis of airspace opacities. It can be difficult to differentiate between the two processes without examining the patient for signs of pneumonia (fever, elevated WBC, lung auscultation findings, etc.).

There are four basic mechanisms that lead to atelectasis or loss of lung volume. These can occur individually or in combination and are listed below:

1. Postobstructive atelectasis
2. Cicatrization atelectasis
3. Adhesive atelectasis
4. Passive atelectasis

H. Singh et al. (eds.), *Radiology Fundamentals: Introduction to Imaging & Technology*, DOI 10.1007/978-3-319-10362-4_15

Postobstructive Atelectasis

When a bronchus is obstructed, air within the alveoli and the bronchi distal to the obstruction is reabsorbed, leading to volume loss as depicted in Fig. 15.1. Extrinsic compression of a bronchus by a mass, endobronchial tumor, a foreign body, or a mucous plug can lead to postobstructive atelectasis.

In situations in which the inspired gas contains an elevated proportion of oxygen in comparison to room air, postobstructive atelectasis is more likely to occur. This is because alveoli will rapidly absorb gas that is rich in oxygen. Hence, postobstructive atelectasis, especially on the basis of mucous plugging, is a commonly observed phenomenon on portable radiographs obtained in the operating room or in the intensive care units where patients often breathe gas mixtures with a greater percentage of oxygen than found in room air.

Cicatrization Atelectasis

Cicatrix is a medical word for scar or replacement of normal tissue by fibrous tissue. This form of atelectasis occurs secondary to healing of inflammation from infection, radiation therapy, etc. It is characterized by marked perialveolar fibrosis with resultant loss of volume as noted in Fig. 15.2.

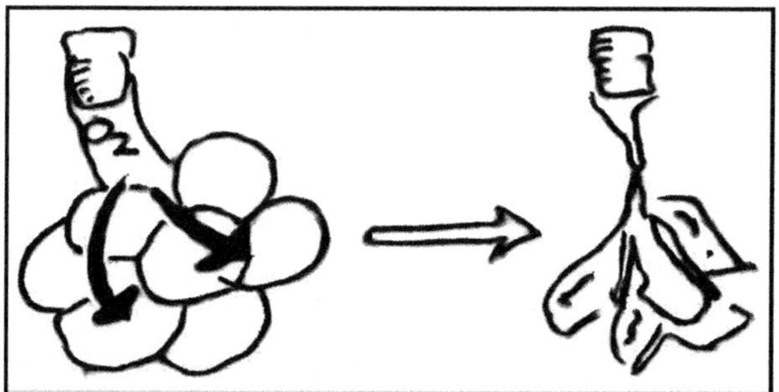

FIGURE 15.1 - POSTOBSTRUCTIVE ATELECTASIS
An airway obstruction results in collapse (incomplete expansion) of the airway and airspaces distal to the obstruction

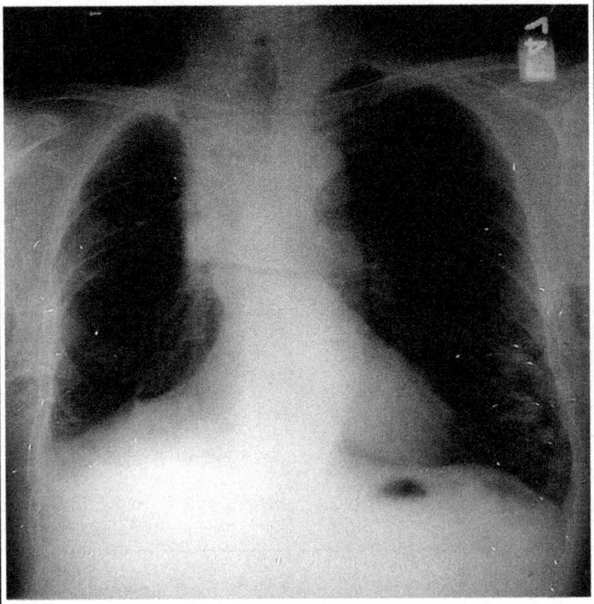

FIGURE 15.2 - CICATRIZATION
Replacement of normal tissue by fibrous tissue in the right middle lobe

Adhesive Atelectasis

When type II pneumocytes lining the alveolus decrease their surfactant production, the alveolus can no longer remain inflated, and adhesive atelectasis occurs. Collapse results, according to the law of Laplace. Laplace's law states that the pressure (P) required to keep an alveolus open is directly proportional to the wall tension (T) and inversely proportional to its radius (r). Hence, for any given tension, the smaller the radius, the larger the pressure required to keep that alveolus open. Surfactant decreases the surface tension, helping reduce the pressure required to keep small alveoli open (and maintain smaller alveoli open at a lower pressure) (Fig. 15.3).

The prototype of adhesive atelectasis is the respiratory distress syndrome of prematurity, which occurs in infants whose type II pneumocytes have not matured enough to produce surfactant. Adhesive atelectasis may also be seen commonly following cardiac surgery. The cooling of the heart performed to decrease the heart's metabolic requirements while on bypass also decreases the metabolic rate of type II pneumocytes in the adjacent lung. The most common location for this is in the left lower lobe.

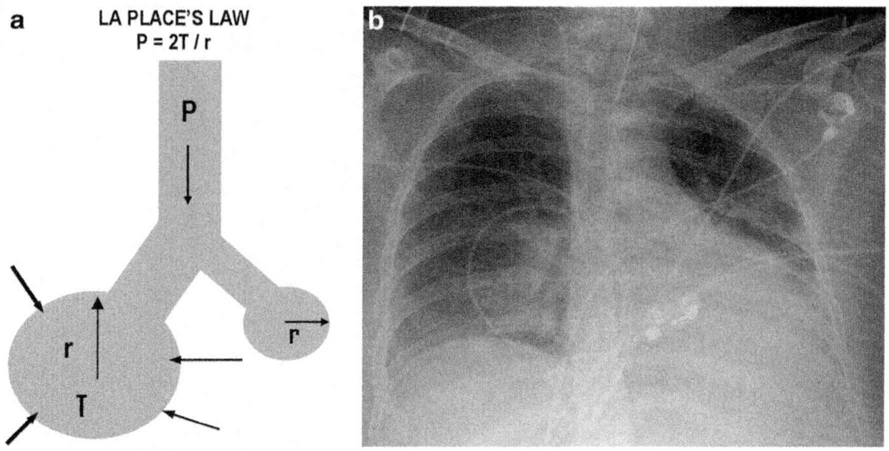

FIGURE 15.3 - ADHESIVE ATELECTASIS
(**a**) Figure illustrating Laplace's law. (**b**) AP chest x-ray showing left lower lobe adhesive atelectasis

Passive Atelectasis

The lung is highly elastic and normally exists at a volume "greater than it desires to be." The chest wall is also elastic and exists at a volume slightly "less than it desires to be." The equilibrium between the lung and chest wall establishes these relative volumes as you may recall from physiology. When something is introduced to change the equilibrium, the lung and chest wall also change volume in a predictable manner.

Anytime the lung loses volume due to a manifestation of its propensity for elastic recoil, this is termed passive atelectasis. The most obvious example of this is a pneumothorax, but similar changes occur when fluid is introduced into the pleural space as in a pleural effusion (Fig. 15.4).

Radiographic Opacity

Finally, it is important to remember that loss of volume does not imply increase radiographic opacity. Normal lung is so transparent to x-rays that it does not increase in opacity until it has lost 90–95 % of its volume. Hence the small areas of atelectasis seen on chest radiographs represent small foci of lung parenchyma, which have lost nearly all of their air.

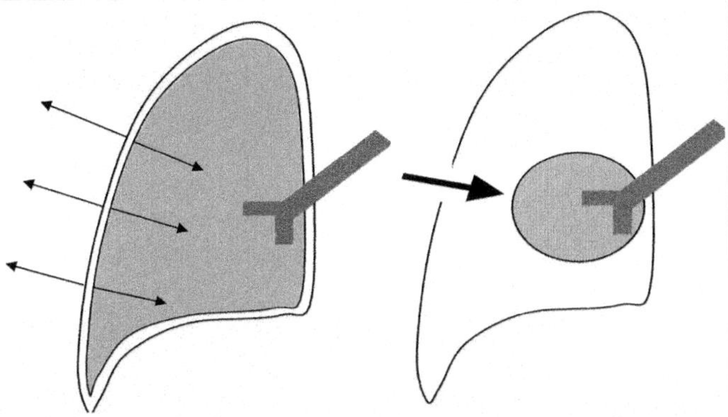

FIGURE 15.4 - NORMAL AND ABNORMAL FORCES ON THE LUNG
The normal elastic forces between the chest wall and the lung oppose each other, resulting in an equilibrium as noted in the picture on the *left*. With a pneumothorax, as seen on the *right*, when the chest wall is compromised, air enters the thorax, allowing the lung to collapse

Lobar Atelectasis

Atelectasis may involve an entire lung. It can also be lobar, segmental, or subsegmental. Lobar atelectasis (or lobar collapse) causes specific appearances. Lobar collapse usually results from bronchial obstruction. The atelectatic lobe usually appears as a triangle or pyramid with its apex pointing to the hilum.

With right upper lobe atelectasis (Fig. 15.5), the frontal view shows an ill-defined opacity in the right upper hemithorax, apparent right upper mediastinal widening, and superior displacement of the minor fissure. The lateral view shows superior displacement of the minor fissure as well as anterior displacement of the right major fissure.

With left upper lobe atelectasis (Fig. 15.6a,b), the frontal view shows an ill-defined opacity in the left hemithorax and a crescent of air between the aortic arch and the ill-defined opacity. The lateral view shows increased opacity adjacent to and parallel to the anterior chest wall, as well as anterior displacement of the left major fissure.

Right middle lobe atelectasis (Fig. 15.7a,b) will cause silhouetting of the right heart border, disappearance of the minor fissure, and increased right lower lung opacity on the frontal view. The lateral view will show a wedge of increased opacity between the inferiorly displaced minor fissure and the anteriorly displaced right major fissure.

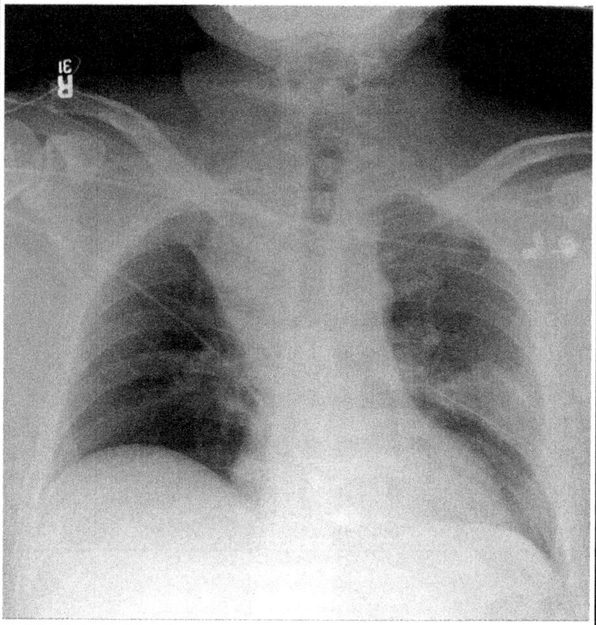

FIGURE 15.5 - RIGHT UPPER LOBE COLLAPSE
AP radiograph. Note the opacity in the right upper hemithorax, apparent right upper mediastinal widening, and superior displacement of the minor fissure

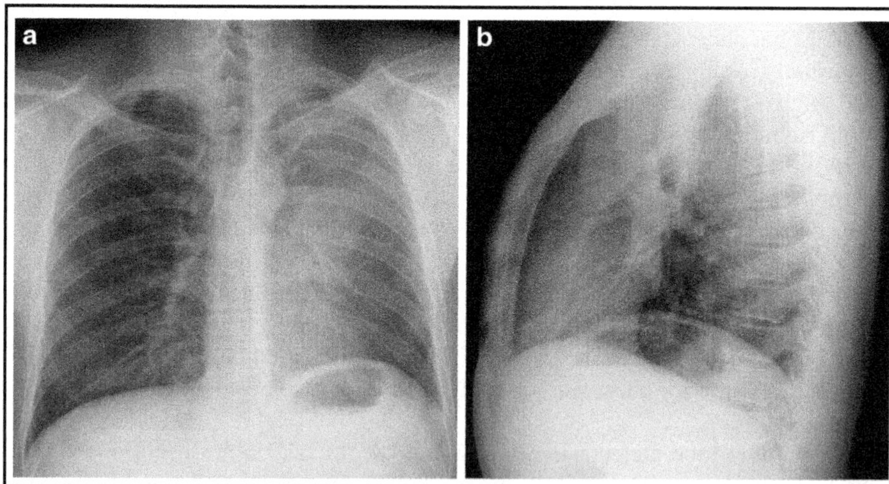

FIGURE 15.6 - LEFT UPPER LOBE COLLAPSE
(**a**) PA radiograph. Note the ill-defined opacity in the left hemithorax and a crescent of air between the aortic arch and the ill-defined opacity. (**b**) Lateral radiograph. Note the increased opacity adjacent to and parallel to the anterior chest wall

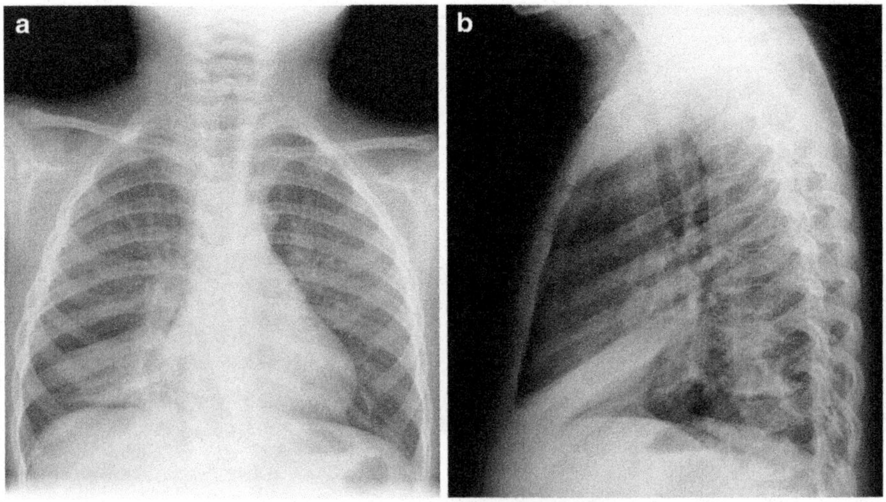

FIGURE 15.7 - RIGHT MIDDLE LOBE COLLAPSE
(**a**) PA radiograph. Note the right lower lung opacity causing silhouetting of the right heart border. (**b**) Lateral radiograph. Note the wedge of increased opacity between the inferiorly displaced minor fissure and the anteriorly displaced right major fissure

Lower lobe atelectasis (Fig. 15.8a–c) shows in the frontal view as an inferomedial triangular opacity silhouetting the diaphragm of the affected side. The lateral view will show increased opacity overlying the inferior spine and posterior bowing of the corresponding major fissure.

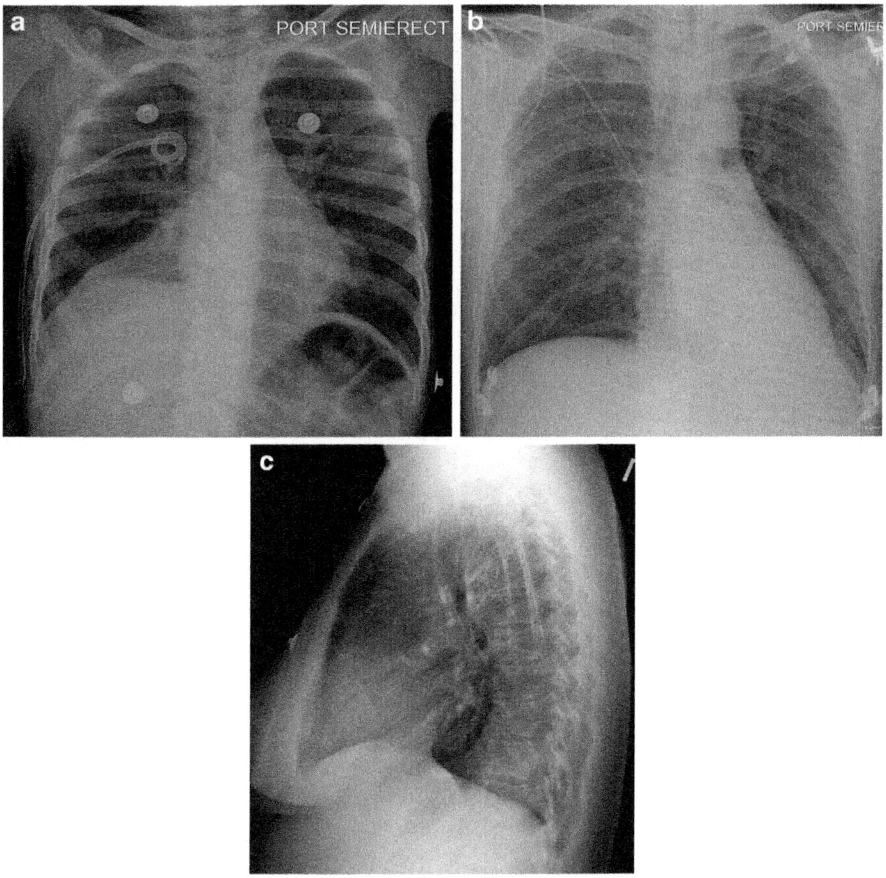

FIGURE 15.8 - LOWER LOBE COLLAPSE
(**a**) AP radiograph of right lower lobe collapse. Note the right lower lung triangular opacity silhouetting the right hemidiaphragm. (**b**) AP radiograph of left lower lobe collapse. Note the subtle triangular opacity overlying the heart, with silhouetting the left hemidiaphragm. (**c**) Lateral radiograph of left lower lobe collapse (different patient). Note the increased opacity overlying the inferior spine and posterior bowing of the left major fissure

16 Pulmonary Vasculature

Objectives:

1. Give three examples of technical factors that may make pulmonary vessels look more prominent.
2. Describe the physiology in pulmonary perfusion between the cephalad and more caudad portions of the lung in an upright patient.
3. Be able to distinguish pulmonary veins from pulmonary arteries in a PA chest x-ray and provide two criteria for differentiation.
4. Give two criteria for distinguishing a vessel on end from a pulmonary nodule.
5. List the components of the hilar shadow on a conventional chest radiograph.
6. State which hilum is usually higher on the upright chest radiograph.
7. List three physiological states in which the pulmonary vasculature is abnormal on the chest radiograph and give specific radiographic criteria for distinguishing them from one other.

Pulmonary Vessel Distribution in the Lung

We have already seen how inspiration and expiration can affect the appearance of the pulmonary vessels. Other technical factors such as underpenetration and supine positioning can also make the vessels look artifactually prominent.

In Fig. 16.1, note the difference in the number and size of blood vessels within the lung as one moves from the lung apex to the lung base. The vessels are larger and more numerous in the lung base because the force of gravity augments the hydrostatic force generated by the right ventricle. In the apices, the hydrostatic force generated

H. Singh et al. (eds.), *Radiology Fundamentals: Introduction to Imaging & Technology*, DOI 10.1007/978-3-319-10362-4_16

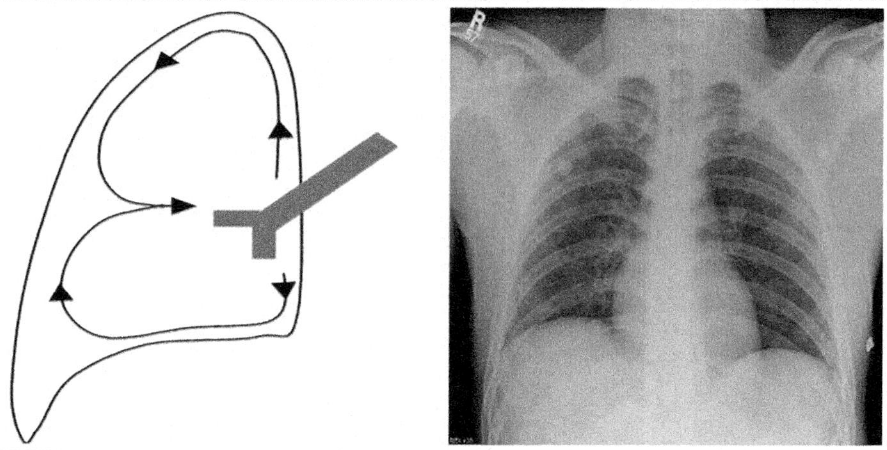

FIGURE 16.1 - PULMONARY VASCULAR FLOW
Pulmonary arteries tend to run in a vertical fashion, while pulmonary veins are more horizontal. Note the difference in number and size of blood vessel within the lung from apex to base

by the right ventricle is diminished by gravity. In effect, the right ventricle is pumping "uphill" to the apices of the lung. Of course, when the patient changes position, this relationship is also changed.

In general, the greatest perfusion will be to the portion of the lung that is most dependent. Certain pathologic situations can change this normal perfusion gradient, as we will see later in this section.

Identifying Pulmonary Vessels

To identify pulmonary vasculature, look for the round, well-defined nodular shadows most easily noted centrally, close to the hilum. These are vessels on end (an artery or vein running in a plane perpendicular to the detector). Vessels can be confused with pulmonary nodules in some patients. However, they can often be distinguished from a true nodule by two criteria:

1. Since bronchi and pulmonary arteries travel together, look for a bronchus that is on end adjacent to the suspected vessel on end. A bronchus is air filled and thus will have a black center, while the vessel will be uniform in opacity (Fig. 16.2).
2. A true nodule is spherical and should appear round on both PA and lateral views. A vessel on end will only have a round ("on end") appearance on one view, having the tubular appearance of a vessel on the other projection.

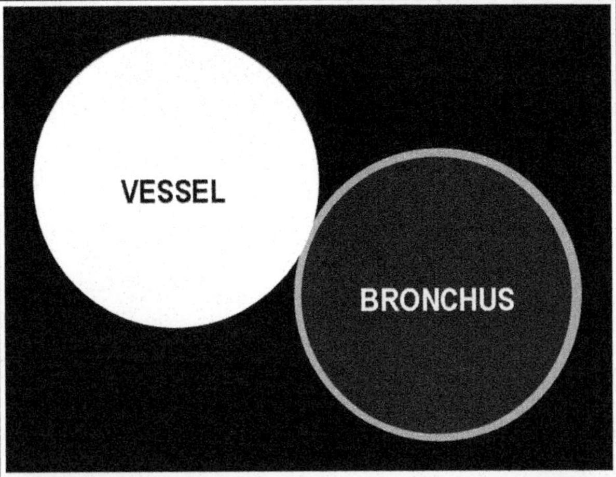

FIGURE 16.2 - VESSEL AND BRONCHUS
Note that the pulmonary artery and accompanying bronchus should be of relatively equal size and that the bronchial wall should be thin and sharp

Another way to identify vessels is by noting the hila. The hila are composed mainly of the shadow of the pulmonary arteries although there is a slight contribution from the bronchial structures. The left hilum is normally higher than the right in approximately 97 % of patients. This is because the left pulmonary artery must pass over the left main bronchus in its proximal course, while the right pulmonary artery travels adjacent but not over the right main bronchus. In 3 % of patients, the hila are of equal height. "The right hilum is never higher than the left in a normal patient."

Pulmonary Artery Hypertension

Figure 16.3 shows the radiographic appearance of pulmonary arterial hypertension. Note the enlargement of the main and central pulmonary arteries. Note also the rapid tapering of the pulmonary arteries peripherally causing the lungs to have a relatively oligemic (hypovascular) appearance.

Pulmonary arterial hypertension may occur as an idiopathic condition in young females or be related to a number of other causes, including acute or chronic pulmonary embolism, severe pulmonary lung disease either as a primary process (interstitial fibrosis, COPD, diseases associated with vasculitis) or on the basis of restriction related to the chest wall (severe kyphoscoliosis, morbid obesity, chronic fibrothorax, neurologic disorders that may impair the respiratory muscles, or chronic upper airway obstruction). Pulmonary arterial hypertension may also be the result of

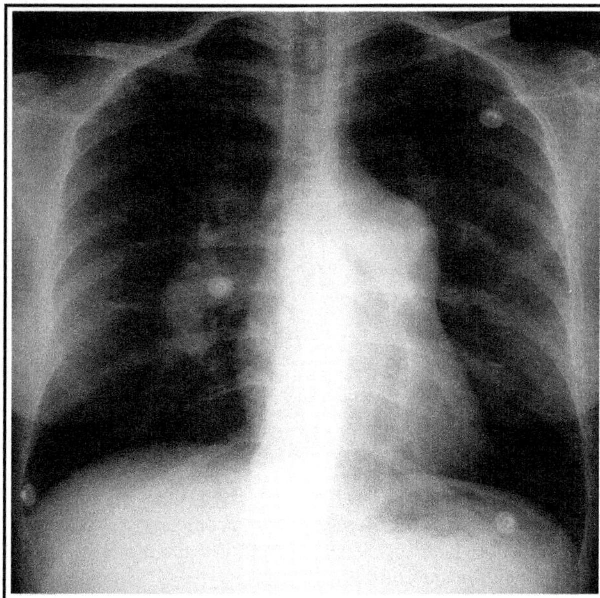

FIGURE 16.3 - PULMONARY ARTERIAL HYPERTENSION
Note the enlarged central pulmonary arteries with "pruning" of the vessels more peripherally

chronic left to right intracardiac shunts (such as atrial septal defects or ventricular septal defects) or extracardiac shunts, which can produce changes in the pulmonary vasculature resulting in elevated pulmonary arterial pressure. Finally, pulmonary arterial hypertension may be produced from long-standing pulmonary venous or precapillary hypertension such as may be seen in chronic left ventricular failure.

Shunt Vascularity

Figure 16.4 may at first appear identical to the radiograph on the previous patient. The enlargement of the hilar and main pulmonary artery segments is similar. However, note that the pulmonary vasculature is much more prominent in the periphery of the lung than on the previous study.

This patient has a large atrial septal defect producing a left to right intracardiac shunt, thereby increasing pulmonary blood flow. Other left to right shunts (ventricular septal defect, patent ductus arteriosus) could give a similar appearance although both would be considerably less likely in an adult.

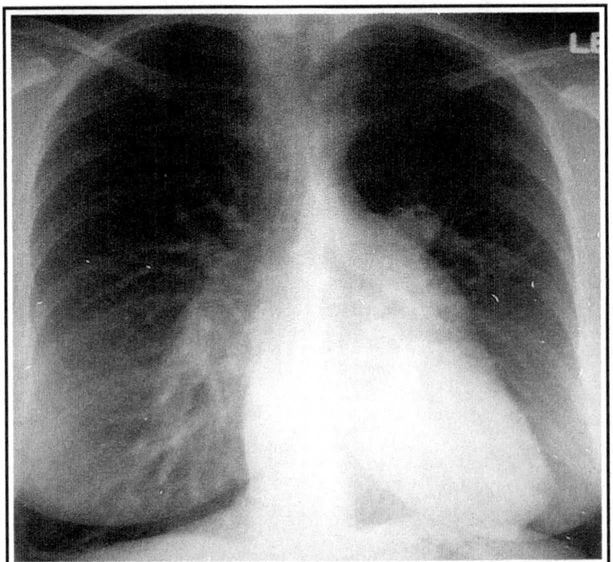

FIGURE 16.4 - SHUNT VASCULARITY
Note the prominence of the central hilar vessels as well as the more peripheral vessels, a pattern consistent with shunt vascularity

Pulmonary Venous Hypertension

Figure 16.5 is from a patient with pulmonary venous hypertension. Although the central pulmonary vasculature is prominent, it is not nearly as prominent as in pulmonary arterial hypertension or as in patients with left to right shunts. There is a convexity along the left cardiac border, which is similar to that seen in the previous two examples; however, it is located slightly more inferior with respect to the aortic arch. This represents a dilated left atrial appendage. The left atrium is not normally a border forming structure on the frontal radiograph; however, with dilation due to increased left atrial pressure, it may become visible. There is prominence of the upper lobe vasculature relative to the lower lobes (cephalization) representing redistribution of blood flow to the upper lobes. There may also be Kerley B lines and peribronchial cuffing as well as thickening of the fissures on the lateral view. All of the latter findings should sound familiar to you as radiographic components of interstitial disease. The interstitial findings relate to the increased pulmonary venous pressure that leads to transudation of fluid into the interstitium.

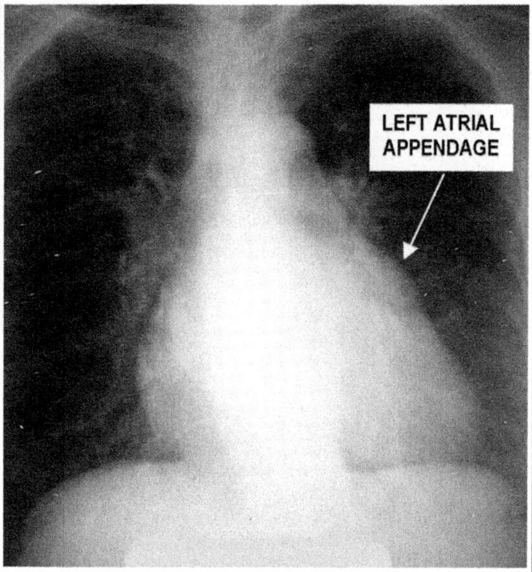

FIGURE 16.5 - PULMONARY VENOUS HYPERTENSION
Frontal and lateral radiographs showing pulmonary venous hypertension

Any obstructive lesion on the left side of the heart (where blood coming from the lungs is headed) can produce this appearance. Hence, processes that cause left ventricular failure, mitral stenosis, or obstruction to flow of blood into or out of the left atrium such as left atrial myxoma could produce the findings of pulmonary venous hypertension.

On a statistical basis, findings of pulmonary venous hypertension are much more common than the other two categories described since left ventricular failure is such a common clinical problem. The chest radiograph is useful in distinguishing the less common, but by no means rare, causes of increased pulmonary vascularity (Fig. 16.6).

Vascular Pattern	PULMONARY VESSELS: CENTRAL	PULMONARY VESSELS: PERIPHERAL
SHUNT VASCULARITY (OVERCIRCULATION)	INCREASED (Caliber)	INCREASED
PULMONARY ARTERIAL HYPERTENSION	LARGE	SMALL, DECREASED
PULMONARY VENOUS HYPERTENSION	INCREASED	INCREASED

FIGURE 16.6 - RADIOGRAPHIC DIFFERENCES BETWEEN SHUNT VASCULARITY, PULMONARY ARTERIAL HYPERTENSION AND PULMONARY VENOUS HYPERTENSION

By examining the caliber of the central and peripheral pulmonary vessels, one can determine the vascular pattern

17 PULMONARY EDEMA

Objectives:

1. State the chest radiograph findings of left ventricular failure.
2. Identify one pulmonary disease that may alter the radiographic distribution of pulmonary edema.

Pulmonary edema secondary to left ventricular failure is one of the more common problems encountered in clinical medicine. The term congestive heart failure (CHF) is often applied both clinically and radiographically. Technically, CHF is a clinical diagnosis with a constellation of findings, some of which are radiographic. Nevertheless, the terms cardiogenic pulmonary edema, left ventricular failure, and CHF are often used synonymously in informal discussion.

The chest radiograph is an excellent tool for the early diagnosis of pulmonary edema and for assessing the effectiveness of treatment. This is because the chest radiograph is very reflective of minute-to-minute changes in cardiopulmonary function and circulating blood volume. A detailed description of the physiologic aspects of chest radiographic interpretation is beyond the scope of this discussion. We will emphasize the changes in radiographic appearance on the chest x-ray only (Fig. 17.1).

Blood Flow Redistribution (Cephalization)

Figure 17.2 shows a normal and abnormal appearance of the pulmonary vasculature. As discussed in Chap. 16, the upper lobe vessels are normally smaller than those in the lower lobes due to the effect of gravity on the pulmonary circulation. The first abnormality detected in patients with early stages of left ventricular failure

H. Singh et al. (eds.), *Radiology Fundamentals: Introduction to Imaging & Technology*, DOI 10.1007/978-3-319-10362-4_17

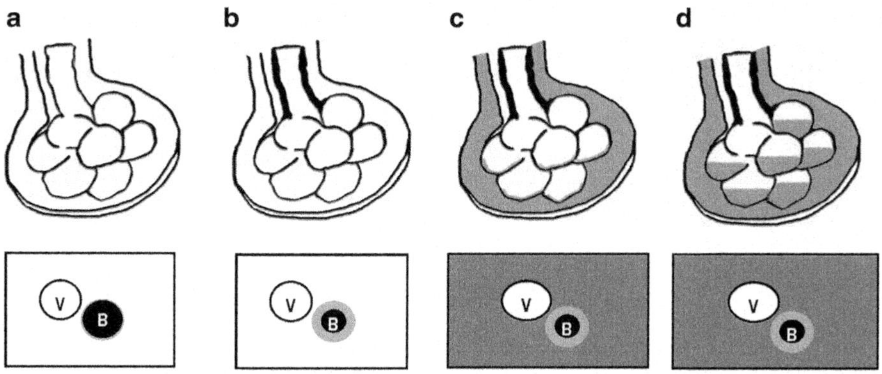

FIGURE 17.1 - PULMONARY EDEMA
In (**a**), the normal alveolus and vessel/bronchus relationship is noted. (**b**) Shows peribronchial cuffing. In (**c**), as the edema worsens, fluid starts to spill into the alveoli. (**d**) Shows the alveoli filled with fluid, markedly interfering with gas exchange

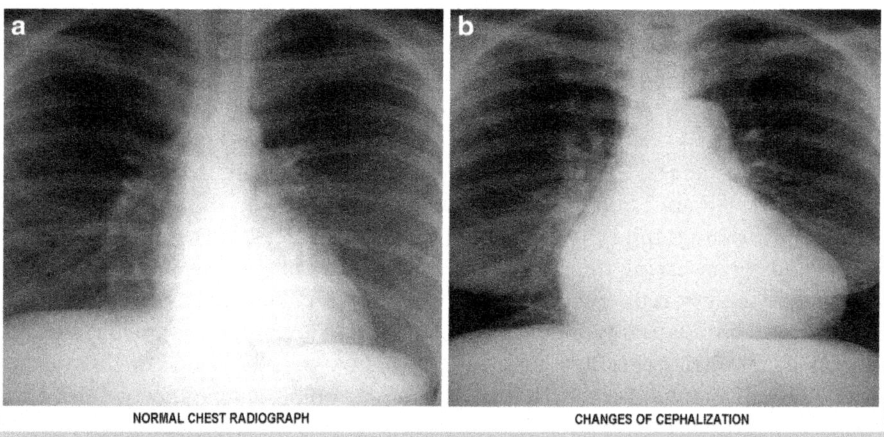

FIGURE 17.2 - REDISTRIBUTION OF VASCULAR FLOW (CEPHALIZATION)
Comparison of a normal chest radiograph and one with cephalization. Note the distribution of the pulmonary vasculature in the normal radiograph. Look carefully at the right suprahilar region and compare the vessels in this region to the vessels in the right lower lung. Now look at the radiograph showing cephalization. Note the prominence of the suprahilar vessels compared to those of the right lower lobe in the case of cephalization

is redistribution of pulmonary blood flow to the upper lung zones, so-called cephalization. With cephalization, the upper lobe vessels become engorged and larger than the lower lobe vessels. Cephalization may be a subtle finding for those not used to scrutinizing the pulmonary vasculature closely. Remember that in the supine patient, the normal craniocaudal gradation of perfusion due to gravity will no longer be present. Hence, cephalization will not be present on supine radiographs and therefore is lost as a useful diagnostic sign. This is another reason for obtaining an upright radiograph of the chest whenever possible.

Interstitial Edema

The next observable abnormality is the accumulation of fluid within the lung interstitium. This is the earliest stage at which there is radiographically detectable "extravascular lung water." Because this fluid is confined to the interstitium, it does not seriously compromise gas exchange. The findings (peribronchial cuffing, Kerley A and B lines, and subpleural interstitial thickening) are also seen in other forms of interstitial disease.

The transition from cephalization to interstitial edema to airspace edema may be quite rapid in many circumstances, and all of the described phases may not be discreetly observed. These changes correlate with pulmonary capillary wedge pressures measured with a pulmonary artery (Swan-Ganz) catheter (Fig. 17.3).

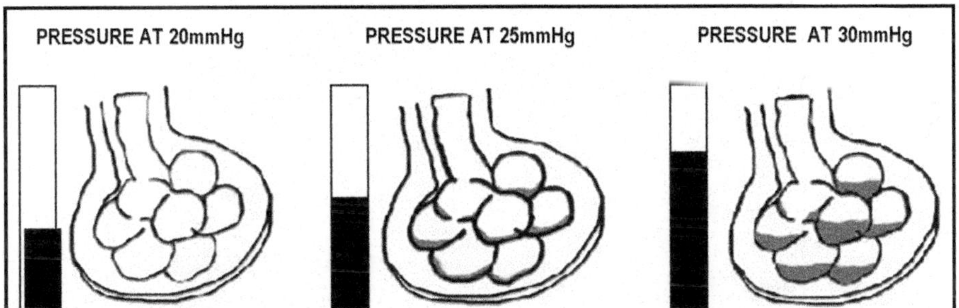

FIGURE 17.3 - PULMONARY EDEMA AND CAPILLARY WEDGE PRESSURE
Cephalization occurs when the pulmonary capillary wedge pressure is about 15–20 mm of mercury (mmHg). Between 20 and 25 mmHg, one will observe predominantly interstitial edema. Alveolar edema occurs at capillary wedge pressures greater than 25 mmHg

Alveolar Edema

Figure 17.4 shows the most severe form of pulmonary edema. This is airspace or alveolar edema. Fluid spills into the alveoli, forming a barrier to gas exchange causing clinically evident respiratory impairment. The radiographic findings will be those of airspace disease with air bronchogram and confluent acinar shadows producing a fluffy white appearance.

Figure 17.5 shows a patient with pulmonary edema predominantly in the upper lobes. This patient also has underlying chronic obstructive pulmonary disease (COPD). In COPD, the pulmonary capillary beds may be destroyed in certain regions of the lung (in this case, in the lower lobes) relegating pulmonary edema to an atypical distribution. One must always keep in mind that the appearance of pulmonary edema may be modified by the presence of severe COPD.

Pulmonary edema may be distinguishable from other forms of airspace disease radiographically by virtue of the fact that it is often bilateral and symmetric (as opposed to pneumonia or pulmonary hemorrhage, which are more commonly asymmetrically distributed within the lungs). Pulmonary edema may have a fairly rapid onset and resolution (in comparison to pneumonia, which usually develops and resolves more slowly). Of course, the diagnosis is best made by correlating the radiograph with an accurate medical history, physical examination, and appropriate laboratory data.

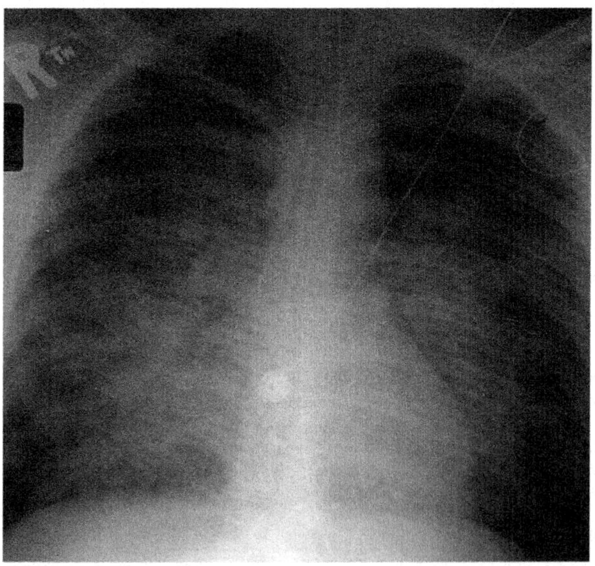

FIGURE 17.4 - AIRSPACE/ALVEOLAR EDEMA
Airspace with air bronchogram and confluent acinar opacities producing a fluffy white appearance

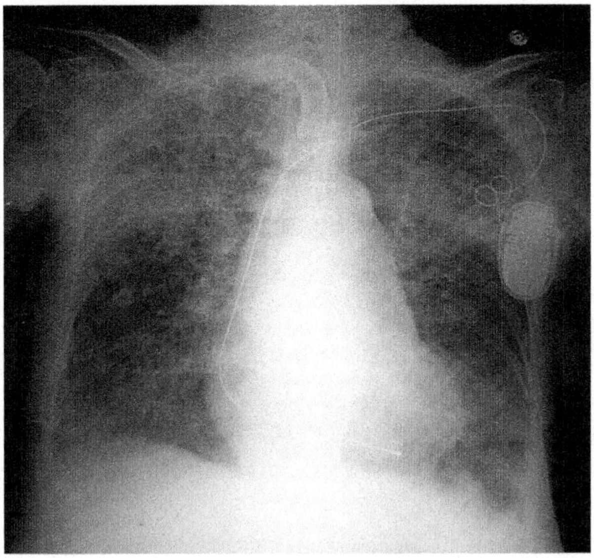

FIGURE 17.5 - PULMONARY EDEMA
Upper lobe predominant pulmonary edema in a patient with underlying COPD

Finally, noncardiogenic pulmonary edema, seen as a part of the adult respiratory distress syndrome (ARDS) is commonly seen in intensive care unit patients as the result of various etiologies such as sepsis and head trauma. Although the radiographic appearance of ARDS is similar to that of cardiogenic edema, the two are not totally identical, reflecting their very different physiological derangements. ARDS does not have the cardiomegaly or pleural effusions usually seen in CHF.

18 Pulmonary Embolism

> **Objective:**
> 1. Describe the chest radiograph findings in pulmonary embolus.

Pulmonary Embolus

Pulmonary embolus is seen as a complication of many surgical procedures, in patients with cancer, and those with some coagulation disorders. Pulmonary embolism has an increased incidence in hospitalized patients in general. The chest radiograph is normal or shows nonspecific findings (such as atelectasis and small pleural effusion) in most patients with pulmonary embolism. The primary purpose of a chest radiograph in suspected pulmonary embolism is to rule out other causes of chest symptoms. Rarely, patients with large or extensive pulmonary emboli will have decreased perfusion of the affected lung (relative oligemia) evident on CXR, a finding known as the Westermark sign, as seen in Fig. 18.1. Note also the enlarged right pulmonary artery (Fleischner sign) due to increased pressure proximal to the obstruction caused by the large embolus found in this patient.

Catheter pulmonary arteriography, performed in the Interventional Radiology Department, was the gold standard for diagnosing pulmonary emboli. For further information regarding pulmonary arteriography and IVC filter placement, refer to the CVIR section of this book.

Computed tomographic (CT) pulmonary arteriography has become the standard of care in the evaluation for pulmonary emboli, due to the less invasive nature of the test and the wide availability of multidetector CT scanners. To make the diagnosis of pulmonary embolism on a CT scan, IV contrast is administered, and the examination is timed in a way that maximizes the opacification of the pulmonary arteries.

H. Singh et al. (eds.), *Radiology Fundamentals: Introduction to Imaging & Technology*, DOI 10.1007/978-3-319-10362-4_18

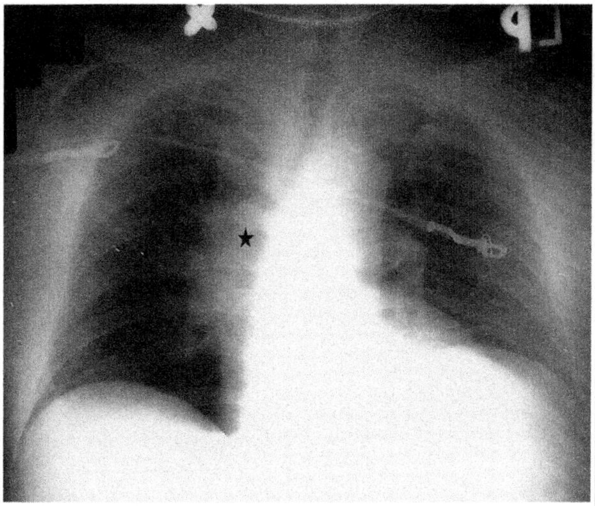

FIGURE 18.1 - WESTERMARK SIGN
Note the lucency of the right lung (Westermark sign) and the enlarged right pulmonary artery (*, Fleischner sign), due to increased pressure proximal to the obstruction caused by a large embolus found in this patient

The CT scan is then reviewed for filling defects (gray) within the opacified (white) pulmonary arteries (Fig. 18.2).

If a patient cannot receive IV contrast (most commonly due to renal insufficiency or allergy), the most widely accepted second line test is a lung ventilation/perfusion (VQ) scan, performed by the Nuclear Medicine Department. Refer to the pulmonary chapter in the Nuclear Medicine section of this book for a discussion on lung VQ scan.

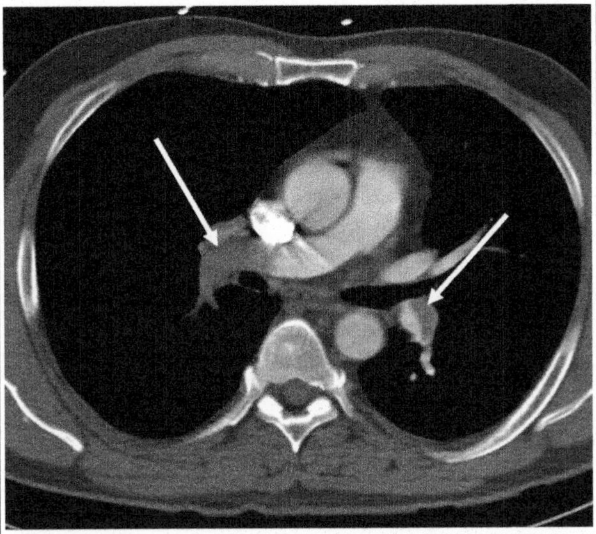

FIGURE 18.2 - PULMONARY EMBOLUS
Axial CT image showing large filling defects (*white arrows*) in both the right and left interlobar pulmonary arteries representing two distinct pulmonary emboli

19 PNEUMOTHORAX

Objectives:

1. Define "pneumothorax."
2. Learn to distinguish a pneumothorax from a skin fold overlying the chest.
3. Discuss the findings you would expect to see in a tension pneumothorax.
4. Discuss the most common location for a pneumothorax in an upright patient, supine patient, and patient in the decubitus position.

A diagnosis that seems to cause much confusion in the clinical situation is that of a pneumothorax, which is the presence of air in the pleural space. Air is not normally present in this space. The visceral and parietal pleura are in contact with each other except for a very thin layer of intervening fluid, which is not normally visible radiographically. The expected appearance of a pneumothorax can be anticipated by using the basic principles that have already been introduced (Fig. 19.1).

Radiographic Appearance of a Pneumothorax

Since a pneumothorax is composed of air, one would expect it to be less dense (darker) radiographically than the lung, which has a small soft tissue component in addition to its airspace component. Since air rises, the pneumothorax will occupy the least dependent (highest) position anatomically possible within the chest. This, of course, will vary depending on the patient's position. For example, in the upright patient, the highest point will be in the apex of the thorax (Fig. 19.2). In a lateral decubitus position, the lateral aspect of the higher hemithorax will be least dependent. However, if the pleural space is not normal (e.g., if the visceral and parietal

H. Singh et al. (eds.), *Radiology Fundamentals: Introduction to Imaging & Technology*, DOI 10.1007/978-3-319-10362-4_19

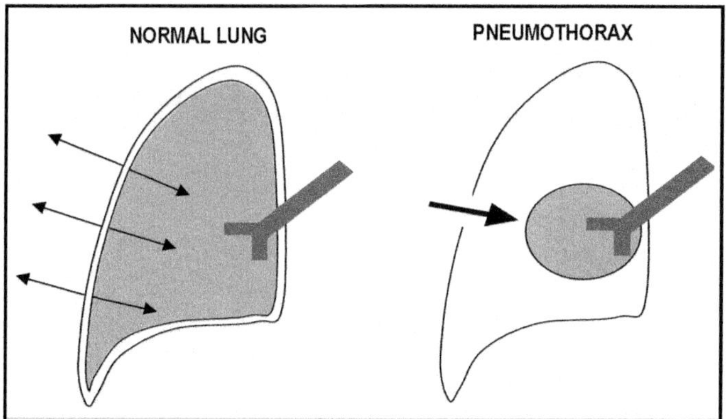

FIGURE 19.1 - NORMAL AND ABNORMAL FORCES ON THE LUNG
The normal elastic forces between the chest wall and the lung oppose each other, resulting in complete equilibrium as noted in the picture on the *left*. With a pneumothorax (as depicted on the *right*), the chest wall is compromised, allowing air to enter the thorax and the lung to collapse

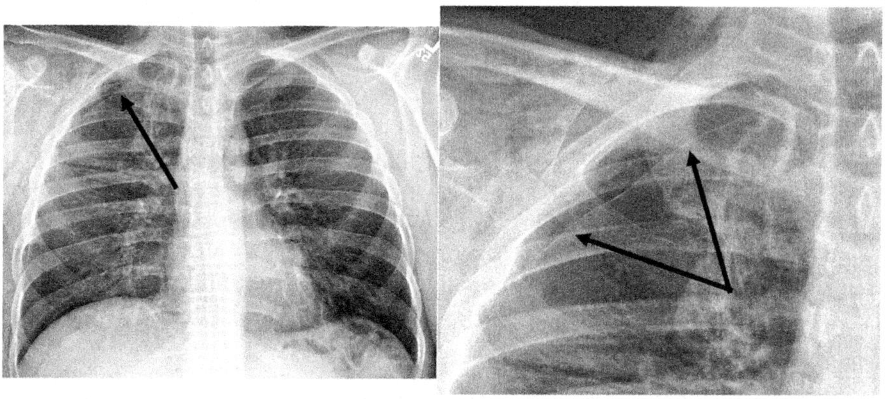

FIGURE 19.2 - PNEUMOTHORAX
Note how the edge of the right lung is delineated by a sharply demarcated thin white line (*arrows*), the visceral pleura, beyond which no pulmonary markings are identified (best seen on closeup image on *right*)

pleura are fused due to an old infection or trauma), then air may not be able to flow normally to the highest point in the chest. The term "loculated" is often applied to pleural air (or pleural fluid) that is constrained in such a manner. The compliance of the underlying lung may also affect the distribution of pleural air. In patients with rigid lungs (due to fibrosis, ARDS, pulmonary edema, etc.), the distribution of air in the surrounding pleural space may be altered.

Since the pleura have a small but detectable radiographic opacity, it will have the appearance of a thin white line at the edge of a pneumothorax in most cases. The pleura may become more easily visualized if it becomes thickened, in which case the white line will be more visible. The pleura will only be visualized in tangent as its density en face (head on) will not be great enough to produce a detectable shadow on the radiograph.

Indirect signs of a pneumothorax include sharp mediastinal or diaphragmatic borders and increased lucency, reflecting the location of the pneumothorax. Current digital radiographic technology allows for image manipulation that aids in the detection of a pneumothorax.

Tension Pneumothorax

In certain cases, air may be trapped in the pleural space on inspiration but not released on expiration, producing a collection of air capable of exerting positive pressure on surrounding structures.

Figure 19.3 shows such a collection, termed a "tension pneumothorax." This clinical situation is potentially life threatening since the increased intrathoracic pressure may shift the mediastinum enough to impair function of the contralateral

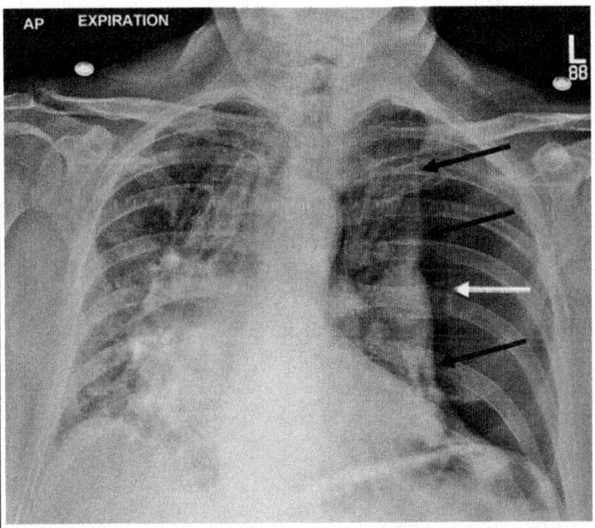

FIGURE 19.3 - TENSION PNEUMOTHORAX
Increased lucency of the left hemithorax with slight rightward mediastinal shift, widening of the left intercostal spaces, and inferior displacement of the left hemidiaphragm, consistent with a left tension pneumothorax

lung as well as to impair venous return to the heart. Signs indicating a tension pneumothorax include mediastinal shift away from the side with the pneumothorax and depression of the ipsilateral hemidiaphragm. Chest tubes (thoracostomy tubes and pleural tubes) are inserted to evacuate some pneumothoraces.

Deep Sulcus Sign

Figure 19.4 shows a radiograph obtained portably in a supine patient. One will notice a collection of air in the right costophrenic sulcus. When the patient is supine, this is often the least dependent position of the chest.

This finding constitutes what is called a "deep costophrenic sulcus sign." The deep costophrenic sulcus sign may be seen in supine patients who have a pneumothorax. The "deep sulcus sign" reflects the pneumothorax that is anterior and lateral. In this case, if one looks closely, the pleural line can be observed.

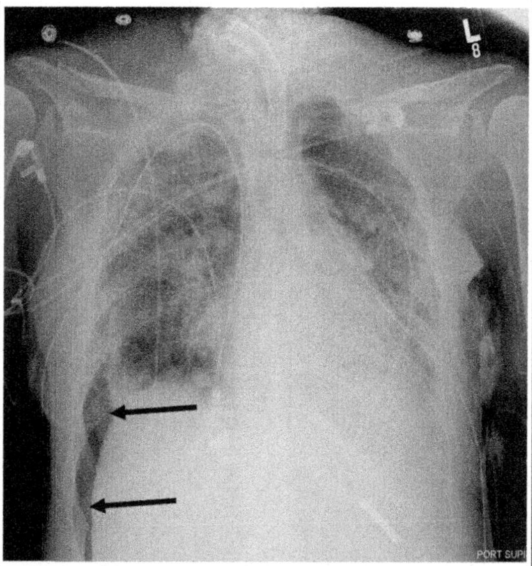

FIGURE 19.4 - DEEP SULCUS SIGN
Note the collection of air (*arrows*) in the right costophrenic sulcus

20 Miscellaneous Chest Conditions

Objectives:

1. Describe the radiologic appearance and etiology of calcific pericarditis.
2. Describe three distinct radiological appearances of intrathoracic tuberculosis.
3. Describe the appearance of two AIDS-defining pulmonary illnesses.
4. State the relationship between asbestos exposure and bronchogenic carcinoma of the lung.
5. List the differential diagnosis of an opacified hemithorax.

The following radiographs show examples of entities with diagnostic radiographic presentations. By seeing the "classic" examples of these entities, you will hopefully gain enough familiarity to make the diagnosis should you encounter them clinically.

Calcific Pericarditis

Fig. 20.1 shows a frontal radiograph and axial CT image of the chest in a patient with the diagnosis of calcific pericarditis. Note the rim of calcium surrounding the cardiac-pericardial silhouette on both the frontal and lateral views. In severe cases, this may cause decreased diastolic filling of the cardiac chambers and require surgical removal of the pericardium.

Currently, the most common etiology for calcific pericarditis is viral infection, often Coxsackie B virus. In the older population, granulomatous pericarditis secondary to tuberculosis is the most common cause of calcific pericarditis.

H. Singh et al. (eds.), *Radiology Fundamentals: Introduction to Imaging & Technology*, DOI 10.1007/978-3-319-10362-4_20

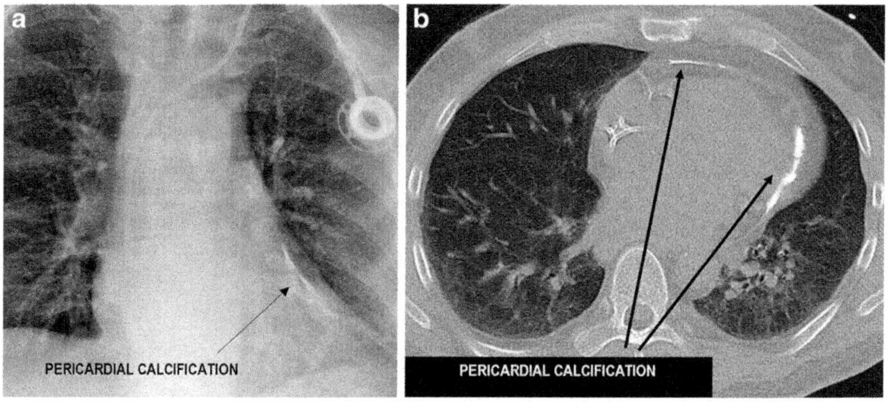

FIGURE 20.1 - CALCIFIC PERICARDITIS
Figure (**a**) is a cropped chest radiograph that shows a rim of calcium along the left heart border (*arrows*). Figure (**b**) is an axial CT slice from the same patient showing the rim of calcium along the left heart border. Also seen is a rim of calcium along the anterior heart border that was not seen on plain radiograph. In severe cases, this may cause decreased diastolic filling of the cardiac chambers and require surgical removal of the pericardium

Any cause of pericardial irritation (uremia, radiation) can eventually lead to calcific pericarditis. Approximately 50 % of these cases of calcific pericarditis will have radiographically visible calcification.

Tuberculosis

Fig. 20.2a shows a thick-walled cavitary lesion in the right upper lobe with surrounding areas of inhomogeneous parenchymal consolidation. In addition, there is airspace disease in the left mid lung. This is the appearance of cavitary tuberculosis with endobronchial spread. The air within the cavitary lesion comes from erosion of the initial focus of disease into the tracheal-bronchial tree of the right upper lobe. The necrotic caseous material within the consolidation is aspirated into the more dependent lingula, in this case, causing spread of disease. The differential diagnosis for a cavitary upper lobe lesion should always include tuberculosis, especially if the lesion involves primarily the apical or posterior segments.

Fig. 20.2b and c shows innumerable punctate nodular opacities distributed throughout both lungs on a chest radiograph and CT axial image, respectively. This is the appearance of a hematogenously disseminated infection to the lungs, in this case, miliary tuberculosis. This is an advanced case of this disease, and cavitation does not occur in this process. Healing, with proper therapy, will be complete with no radiographically visible residual abnormality within the lung.

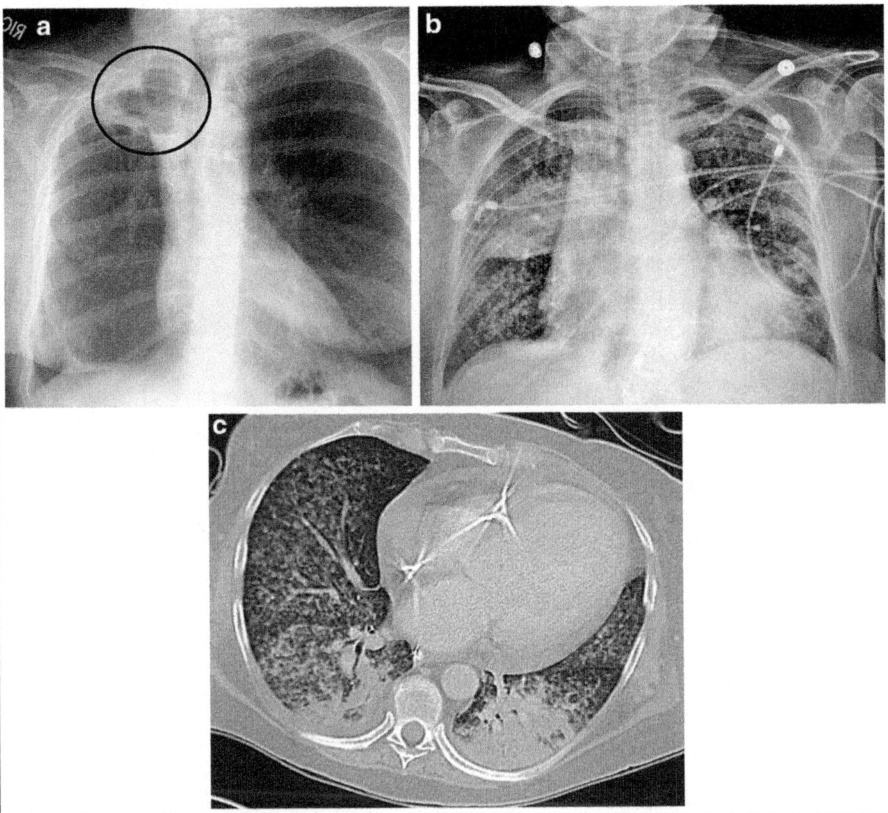

FIGURE 20.2 - TUBERCULOSIS
Figure (**a**) shows a cavitary lesion in the right upper lobe with surrounding areas of heterogeneous parenchymal consolidation from a patient with known tuberculosis. Miliary tuberculosis. Figures (**b**) and (**c**) are from the same patient with known miliary TB. The chest radiograph shows innumerable punctate nodular opacities distributed throughout both lungs and a focal area of consolidation in the right mid lung. The axial CT image also shows innumerable punctate nodular opacities in both lungs and areas of consolidation. Though this appearance is non-specific as it can be seen with miliary tumor metastasis, it is characteristic of hematogenously disseminated miliary tuberculosis

Mediastinal Lymphadenopathy

Fig. 20.3 shows widening of the superior mediastinum in both the right and left paratracheal regions extending down to the superior aspect of both hilar and subcarinal regions. This is the appearance of mediastinal lymphadenopathy. One cause of mediastinal lymphadenopathy is infection with *Mycobacterium avium-intracellulare* (MAI).

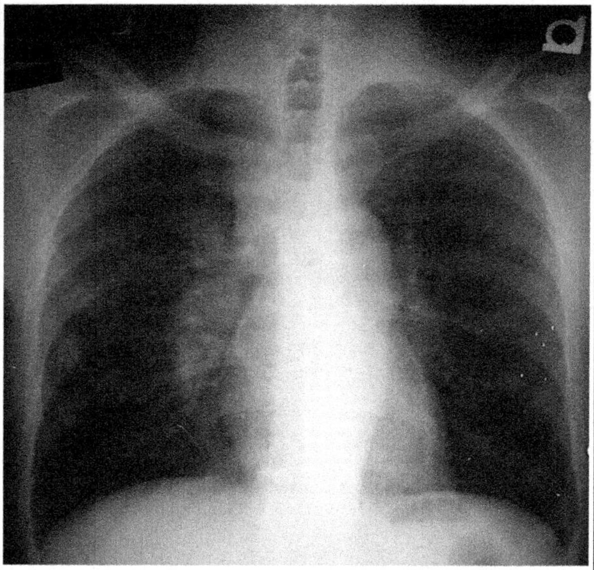

FIGURE 20.3 - LYMPHADENOPATHY
Widening of the superior mediastinum in both the right and left paratracheal regions extending down to both hilar and subcarinal regions, in a case of *Mycobacterium avium-intracellulare* (*MAI*) infection

MAI infections may present with minimal pulmonary findings and only mediastinal and hilar lymphadenopathy, as noted in this case. Fungal disease such as histoplasmosis may give a similar presentation. Of course, lymphoma and other malignant causes of lymphadenopathy and other nonmalignant causes, such as sarcoidosis, would be in the differential diagnosis. Patients who are HIV positive have a considerably elevated risk for the development of all forms of *Mycobacterium* infections.

Kaposi's Sarcoma

In an HIV-positive individual, a chest radiograph with many large nodules can have an extensive differential diagnosis. The differential diagnosis should include all forms of metastatic neoplasm as well as an unusual presentation of opportunistic infection such as fungal disease. It should also include Kaposi's sarcoma, an usually rare malignancy that is seen frequently in HIV-positive individuals. The radiographic manifestations of Kaposi's sarcoma in the chest are many. Multiple nodules are commonly seen (see Fig. 20.4). A slightly nodular, pneumonia-like appearance extending from the hilum into the mid and lower lungs is another presentation commonly seen in Kaposi's sarcoma.

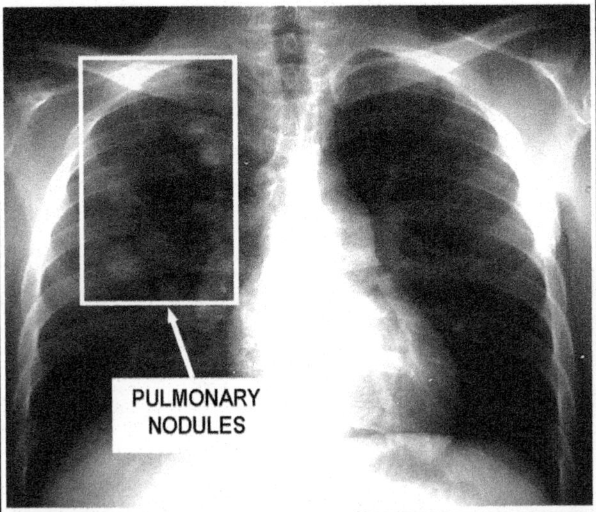

FIGURE 20.4 - KAPOSI'S SARCOMA
Numerous well-defined nodules primarily in the right upper and mid lung without evidence of calcification or cavitation

Pneumocystis carinii Pneumonia

Fig. 20.5 shows diffuse reticular disease distributed homogeneously throughout both lungs and associated with minimal volume loss in a young HIV-positive patient. Note that the patient is intubated, indicating that respiratory failure is present. This is a common presentation of *Pneumocystis carinii* pneumonia (PCP), a disease caused by the yeastlike fungus *Pneumocystis jirovecii* (an organism initially classified erroneously as a protozoan), seen almost exclusively in the HIV-positive population. Severe bullous disease as residua of PCP infection may predispose the patient to superinfection as well as pneumothorax. Pneumatoceles of smaller size and less extensive distribution may also be seen as residua of PCP infection.

Asbestos

Fig. 20.6 shows PA (a) and lateral (b) radiographs from a patient with numerous calcified and noncalcified bilateral pleural plaques. These are secondary to asbestos exposure. There is a long latent period between time of asbestos exposure and the development of the plaques, on the order of 10–15 years in most cases. The plaques are associated with the parietal pleura, unique to asbestos plaques. Calcified pleural

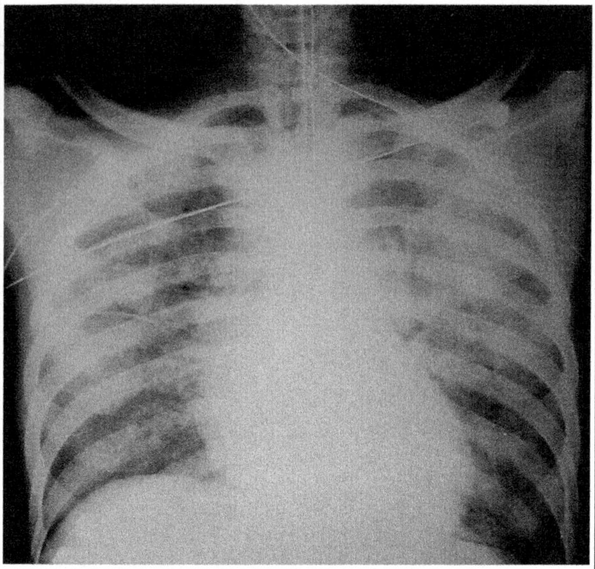

FIGURE 20.5 - PCP PNEUMONIA
Diffuse bilateral interstitial reticular opacities with minimal volume loss in a young HIV-positive patient

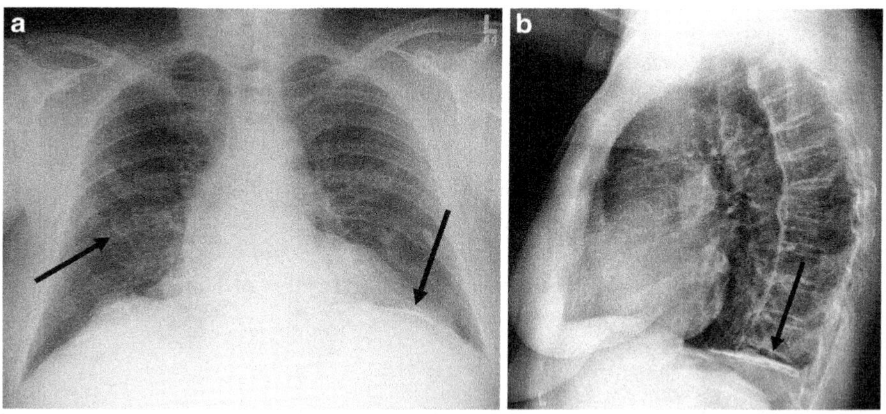

FIGURE 20.6 - PLEURAL PLAQUES
PA (**a**) and lateral (**b**) radiographs of two different patients showing calcified pleural plaques (*arrows*) secondary to asbestos exposure

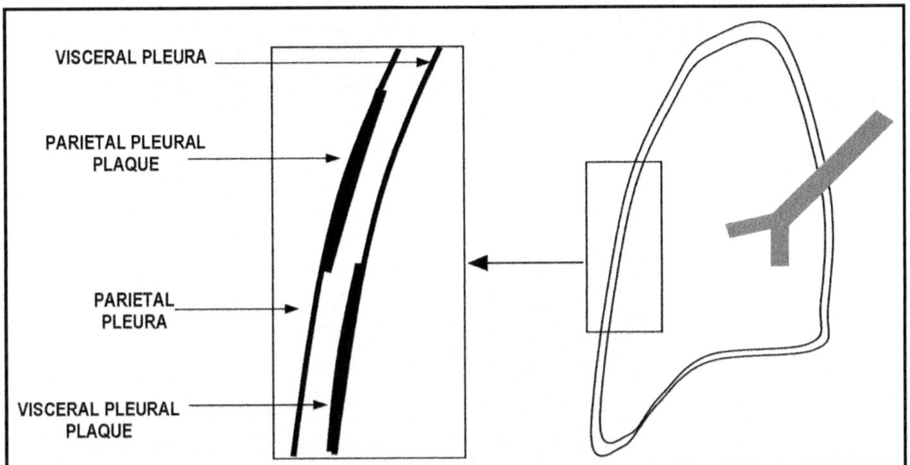

FIGURE 20.7 - PLEURAL PLAQUES
After a latent period of 10–15 years, asbestos exposure can result in parietal pleural plaques, a unique location related to the asbestos exposure. Patients with a history of empyema or hemothorax will have visceral pleural plaques

thickening may also be seen in patients with an old empyema or an old hemothorax. However, these characteristically primarily involve the visceral pleura and are often unilateral. Radiographically, you cannot tell between visceral and parietal pleural calcification, so clinical history is important (see Fig. 20.7).

Bronchogenic carcinoma is the most commonly associated malignancy in patients with a history of asbestos exposure. Mesothelioma, although more uniquely associated with asbestos exposure, is much less common. Patients with a history of asbestos exposure also have increased incidence of esophageal, gastric, and other gastrointestinal carcinomas because asbestos fibers are swallowed as well as inhaled. A patient with a history of asbestos exposure as well as significant smoking history has a very substantially increased risk of developing bronchogenic carcinoma.

Opacified Hemithorax

Fig. 20.8 shows a case of homogeneously increased opacity in the left hemithorax. Note that the mediastinum is shifted toward the left side so that the heart is not clearly distinguished, obscured by the surrounding increased opacity. This patient has undergone a left pneumonectomy, the post pneumonectomy space being filled with fluid. Note that there is still a small apical collection of air and therefore an air fluid level. Eventually, the whole hemithorax will be filled with fluid. The right lung has undergone compensatory hyperinflation.

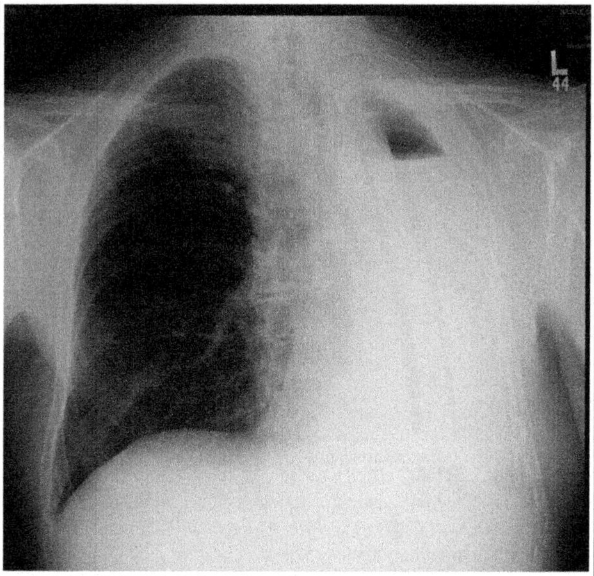

FIGURE 20.8 - OPACIFIED HEMITHORAX
Homogenously increased opacity in the left hemithorax. Note that the mediastinum is shifted toward the left and the heart is not clearly distinguished from the surrounding increased density

Other differential diagnoses in patients with a unilateral opacified hemithorax include a large pleural effusion, pneumonectomy, and total atelectasis of the lung. In a patient with a large pleural effusion, it would be expected that the mediastinum would be at least in the midline or, most likely, shifted to the opposite side of the opacified hemithorax due to the mass effect of fluid in the chest. Patients with complete atelectasis of the lung or pneumonectomy will have mediastinal shift to the same side as the opacified hemithorax. A quick history and physical examination should allow one to distinguish between atelectasis and pneumonectomy. Surgical scars on the chest wall will be present with the latter.

21 Tubes and Lines

Objective:

1. State the ideal positions for the endotracheal tube, central venous catheter, and nasogastric tube.

The main point of the following radiographs is to show normal and abnormal positions of various commonly seen tubes and catheters.

The Endotracheal (ET) Tube

Figure 21.1 shows proper positioning of an endotracheal tube terminating approximately 3 cm above the carina. The ideal position for an endotracheal tube is 3–4 cm above the carina. Portable radiographs, like this one, are commonly obtained to check endotracheal tube position.

The reason for positioning the ET tube 3–4 cm above the carina is that the tube moves within the trachea with changes in head position because the tube is fixed at its insertion point in the nose or the mouth. With flexion of the neck, the position of the tube moves inferiorly about 2 cm. With extension, the tube moves superiorly approximately 2 cm. Ideal positioning assures that the endotracheal tube tip or balloon cuff will not enter one of the main bronchi inferiorly or the larynx superiorly with changes in the patient's head position. The ET tube tip should be no higher than 7–8 cm above the carina and no lower than 2–3 cm above the carina. The balloon cuff should not dilate the trachea. Its diameter should be less than 3 cm in most patients.

H. Singh et al. (eds.), *Radiology Fundamentals: Introduction to Imaging & Technology*, DOI 10.1007/978-3-319-10362-4_21

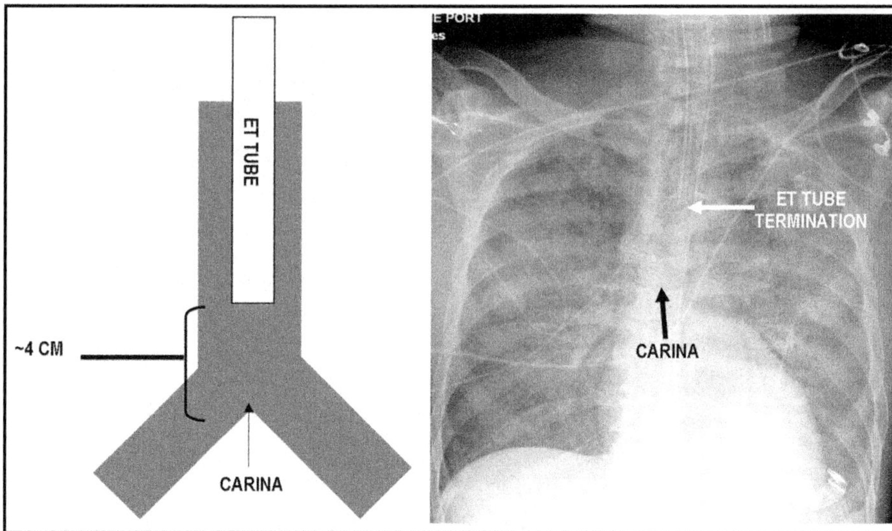

FIGURE 21.1 - PROPER ENDOTRACHEAL TUBE POSITIONING
The endotracheal tube tip should ideally be placed roughly 4 cm above the carina. The vertical radiopaque line represents a marker placed within the wall of the tube to make it visible on radiographs

Figure 21.2 shows an endotracheal tube with its tip positioned in the proximal right main bronchus. Atelectasis (collapse) of the left lung is seen. Atelectasis occurs because the left lung is not ventilated. This is a common complication related to misplacement of the ET tube, but it readily resolves when the ET tube is appropriately repositioned.

Central Venous Catheters

Figure 21.3 shows the pathways of central venous catheters. Catheters can be inserted via the subclavian vein or the internal jugular vein. They then traverse the brachiocephalic vein to get to the superior vena cava. If the line is a temporary venous access such as a peripherally introduced central catheter (PICC) or a permanent central venous access line such as an infusion catheter, the catheter tip will be at the superior cavoatrial junction (#1). If the line is an exchange or dialysis catheter, either temporary or permanent, the tip will be at the mid-right atrium (#2). If the line is a pulmonary artery catheter (aka Swan-Ganz catheter), the tip will be in either the main pulmonary artery or a central pulmonary artery branch (#3).

Figure 21.4 shows two central catheters. The first is a PICC inserted via the left basilic vein and terminating near the confluence of the brachiocephalic veins where

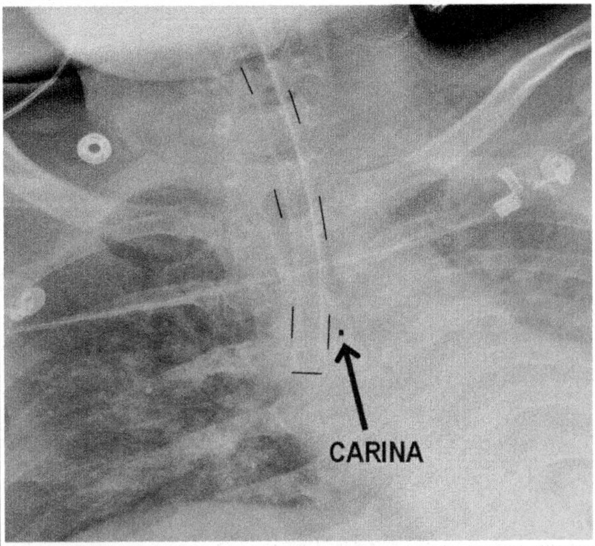

FIGURE 21.2 - RIGHT MAIN BRONCHUS INTUBATION
Endotracheal tube tip is in the right main bronchus. Diffusely increased opacity throughout the left lung is likely secondary to obstructive atelectasis, a common complication of improper endotracheal tube placement

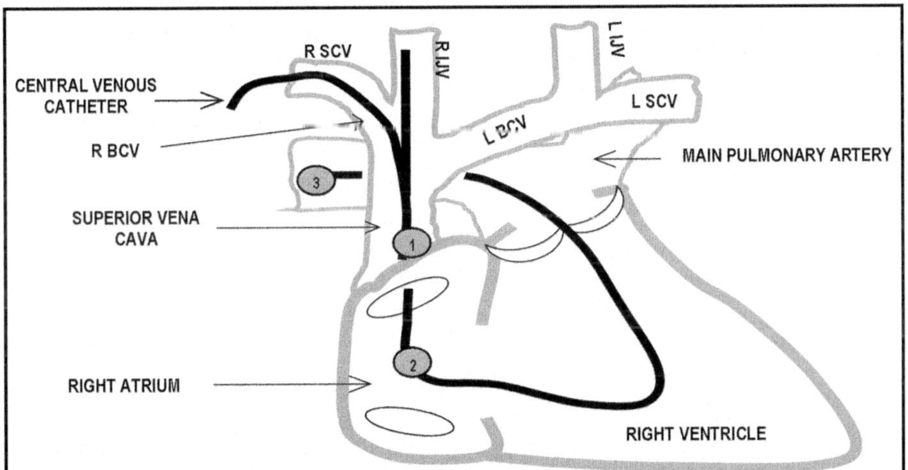

FIGURE 21.3 - COMMON PATHWAYS OF CENTRAL VENOUS CATHETERS
Nomenclature: *SCV* subclavian vein, *IJV* internal jugular vein, *BCV* brachiocephalic vein. The numbers denote the ideal tip placement for the following catheter types: *1* PICC, *2* dialysis catheter, *3* Swan-Ganz catheter

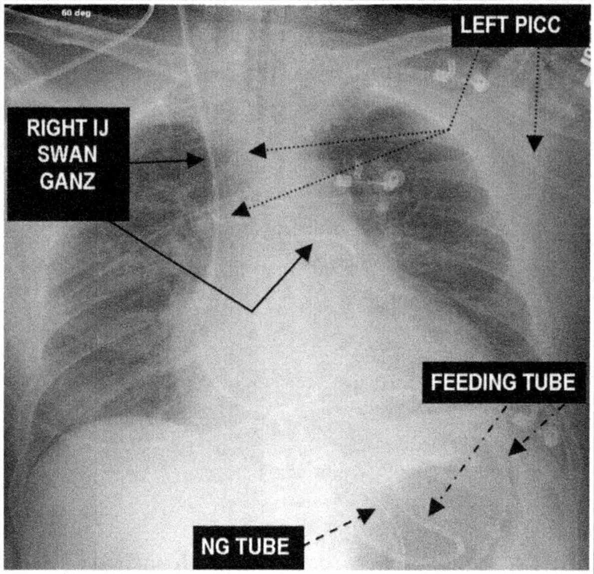

FIGURE 21.4 - CENTRAL CATHETERS
Note the Swan-Ganz catheter as it curves through the heart. The PICC terminates in the SVC appropriately. Also note the nasogastric tube and feeding tube coiled in the stomach

they converge to form the superior vena cava. The second is a Swan-Ganz catheter entering from a right internal jugular vein approach with the tip in the right pulmonary artery.

An uncommon complication of insertion of arterial or venous catheters in the subclavian region is pneumothorax since these vessels lie close to the apex of the lung. When venous access is attempted, the pleural space may be entered. For this reason, an upright radiograph should be obtained after line placement in these patients, as pneumothoraces will be more visible on an upright study.

Figure 21.5 shows an appropriately positioned PICC, with the tip in the superior vena cava. These catheters are of very weak radiopacity so that proper radiographic technique must be employed to visualize them. It is routine to obtain post line placement radiographs so that problems can be detected early.

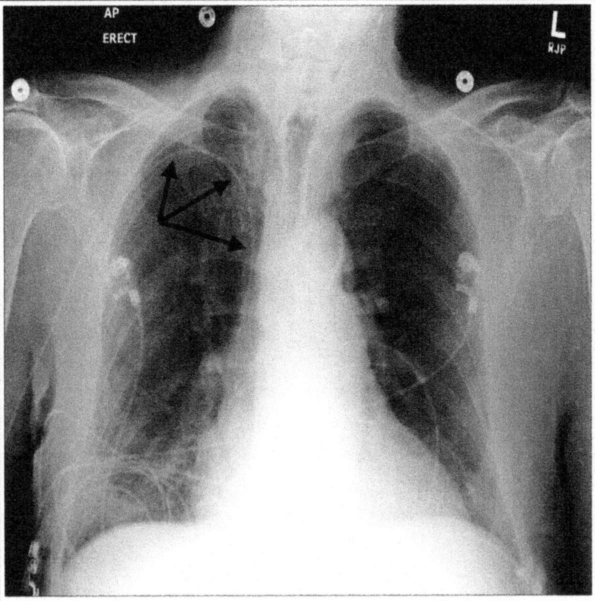

FIGURE 21.5 - PICC PLACEMENT
Right peripherally inserted central catheter (PICC) with tip appropriately positioned in the superior vena cava

The Nasogastric Tube

Figure 21.6 shows a normally positioned nasogastric tube. The tube tip should terminate in the stomach, which lies in the left upper quadrant of the abdomen. The radiopaque marker on the tube shows a single gap in the distal portion, approximately 8 cm from the tip, denoting the location of the side hole. The side hole should also be within the stomach.

Remember: You "must always" ensure that a line or tube is correctly placed before using it!

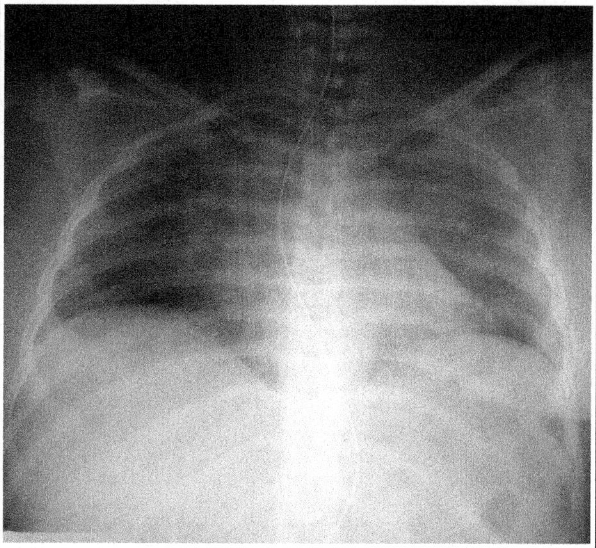

FIGURE 21.6 - NASOGASTRIC TUBE.
Nasogastric tube tip is below the diaphragm, excluded from the field of view, in satisfactory position

Part III
Women's Section

22 Breast Imaging

Objectives:

1. Understand the differences between a screening and diagnostic mammogram including the recommendations for screening mammography.
2. Describe additional imaging modalities used for evaluating the breast and the indications for each modality.
3. Understand the radiation dose of mammography in relation to other common imaging exams.
4. State the main radiographic criteria for detection of breast carcinoma.
5. Understand the BI-RADS classification system for communication of breast imaging results to clinicians.

Breast carcinoma is the most common neoplasm in women, with approximately 200,000 new cases each year, and the incidence of breast cancer increases with age. Risk factors are those primarily related to hormonal history and parity. Multiple randomized controlled trials have demonstrated a reduction in mortality in women who are routinely screened with mammography compared to women who are not screened. Although there has been some controversy regarding the benefits of screening women aged 40–49, currently the American Cancer Society, the American Medical Association, the American College of Radiology, and the American Society of Breast Surgeons all recommend routine screening of average-risk women beginning at age 40. The early detection of breast cancer through screening mammography has contributed to a decrease in mortality of up to 40 % (Duffy et al. 2002). Increased survival rates are likely due to both early detection of disease through mammography as well as improvements in the therapy for breast cancer with agents that target cancers based on their individual biology.

H. Singh et al. (eds.), *Radiology Fundamentals: Introduction to Imaging & Technology*, DOI 10.1007/978-3-319-10362-4_22

Table 22-1 The ACR guidelines for screening mammography

Risk	Qualifier	Age	Modality (annual)
Average	40–79 years (screening to continue until life expectancy is 5–7 years)	40	Mammogram
High	BrCA I or II mutation	30, not before 25	Mammogram and MRI
	>20 % lifetime risk	30, not before 25	Mammogram and MRI
	Chest irradiation between 10 and 30 years	8 years following Tx, not before 25	Mammogram and MRI
Moderately high	Personal history of breast cancer	Annually from diagnosis	Mammogram; consider supplemental MRI or US
Moderately high	High-risk histology: ADH, lobular neoplasia	From age of diagnosis, not before 25	Mammogram, consider MRI
Moderately high	Increased breast density	40, unless other risks present	Mammogram; consider US

The sensitivity of mammographic screening is in part based on breast density, with sensitivity increasing as breast density decreases (see Dense Fibroglandular Tissue below). However, early detection is also dependent on compliance with the recommendations for annual examinations. Annual screening increases the likelihood of detecting subtle changes on the mammogram, and this is particularly important in women with increased parenchymal breast tissue density. The American College of Radiology guidelines for screening mammography can be found in Table 22.1 (ACR BIRADS Lexicon). It is important to note the difference between screening and diagnostic mammography. Screening mammography is the annual routine examination performed in women who have no signs or symptoms of breast disease. Two views of each breast are obtained in the CC (craniocaudal) and MLO (mediolateral oblique) projections, described below. Diagnostic mammography is utilized to better characterize an abnormality that has been identified on a screening mammogram and is the appropriate first test for a patient over the age of 30 presenting with a breast symptom, such as a palpable lump. Diagnostic mammograms involve extra views in varied projections including specialized spot compression views of any symptomatic area and/or magnification views for the assessment of calcifications. Mammography is also the initial modality of choice in the evaluation of suspected male breast disease in patients over the age of 30.

The introduction of digital mammography has proven to be beneficial in women with dense breast tissue, premenopausal and younger women, and those at high risk for breast cancer (Pisano et al. 2005). Full-field digital mammography (FFDM) is a mammography system in which the x-ray film is replaced by solid-state detectors that convert x-rays into electrical signals. The electrical signals and unique breast-specific algorithms are used to produce images of the breast that can be viewed and manipulated on a computer workstation. This ability to manipulate the image by changing the contrast, combined with the use of specialized algorithms for displaying the mammographic images, results in a higher degree of sensitivity for digital mammography compared to analog or screen-film mammography. Results of the Digital Mammography Imaging Screening Trial (DMIST) suggest up to 30 % increase in sensitivity in the detection of occult malignancies (Pisano et al. 2005).

The purpose of the following section is to acquaint you with some basic aspects of breast imaging and the early detection of breast cancer.

Standard Mammography Views: CC and MLO

Figure 22.1 demonstrates the two standard views obtained during a routine mammogram.

The craniocaudal (CC) view is obtained by placing the x-ray tube overhead and the film cassette or digital detector beneath the breast so that the beam traverses the breast from a cranial to caudad direction.

A mediolateral oblique (MLO) view is obtained by placing the film cassette or digital detector in the axilla and allowing the x-ray beam to traverse the breast from the medial breast to the lateral breast and axilla.

The breast is compressed during mammography for the purpose of decreasing the amount of tissue the x-ray beam must traverse. Compression functions to stabilize the breast and reduce motion artifact as well as to spread out superimposed structures. Compression of the breast maximizes the mammogram image quality and decreases the radiation dose to the breast. This compression may be uncomfortable for some patients, but it is brief in duration and results in a mammogram with higher diagnostic quality.

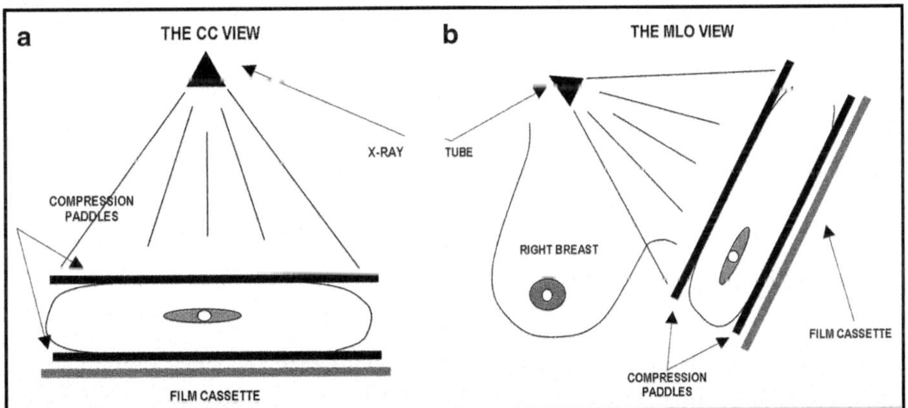

FIGURE 22.1 - THE CC AND MLO BREAST VIEWS
In the CC view, the breast is compressed between two radiolucent paddles to spread the tissue out, reducing tissue overlap and also decreasing dose. In the MLO view, the breast is compressed in an oblique fashion, with the tail of breast tissue that extends toward the axilla, included on the film

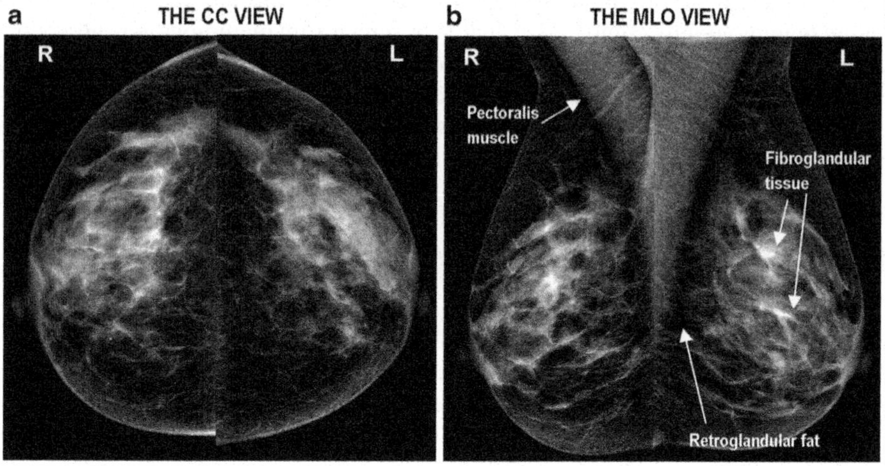

FIGURE 22.2 - THE CC AND MLO BREAST VIEWS
In the CC view, the breast is compressed between two radiolucent paddles to spread the tissue out, reducing tissue overlap and also decreasing dose. In the MLO view, the breast is compressed in an oblique fashion, with the tail of breast tissue that extends toward the axilla, included on the film

Figure 22.2 shows an example of a typical mammogram consisting of CC and MLO views. The darker, more lucent areas represent fat, while the whiter, less transparent areas are composed of fibroglandular tissue. Fibroglandular tissue is comprised of the glandular tissue of the breast as well as the underlying fibrous stromal elements that add support to the overall structure of the breast.

The fibroglandular tissue is generally distributed in a "cone" with the nipple at the apex and the base closer to the chest wall. Between the posterior aspect of the cone of fibroglandular tissue and the underlying pectoral muscle is the retroglandular fat. A well-positioned MLO view should contain the fibroglandular tissue in its entirety, the retroglandular fat and a good portion of the pectoralis muscle.

Dense Fibroglandular Breast Tissue

Figure 22.3 demonstrates a breast with a predominance of dense fibroglandular tissue. For comparison, Fig. 22.4 demonstrates breasts that are predominantly fatty tissue. Mammographic patterns showing mainly fatty breast tissue are typically found in older women, whereas younger, premenopausal women tend to have a greater percentage of dense fibroglandular tissue.

Detection of a small mass is more difficult when the background mammographic density is high. This must be kept in mind when reading a mammographic report. The

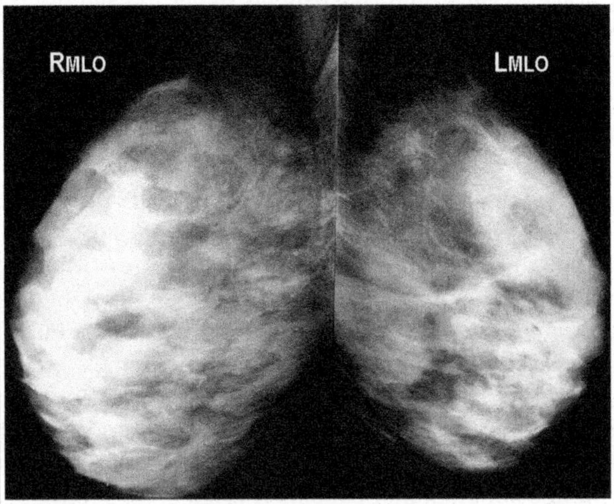

FIGURE 22.3 - DENSE BREAST TISSUE

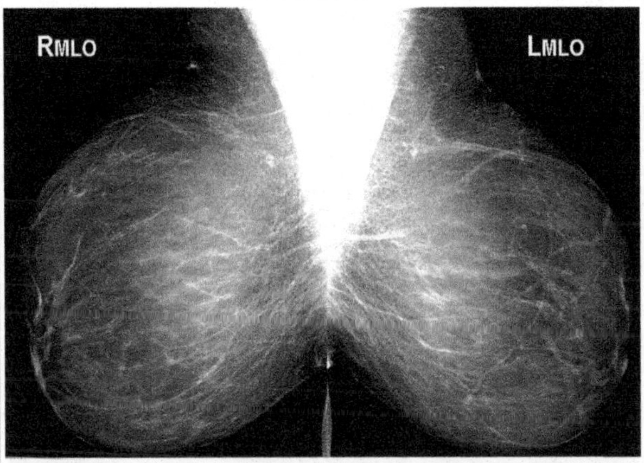

FIGURE 22.4 - FATTY BREAST TISSUE
An example of fatty breast tissue for comparison to the dense breast tissue in Fig. 22.3

current BIRADS lexicon includes the statement "increased mammographic density can lower the sensitivity of mammography" in the report to the woman's physician.

The young breast not only tends to be more dense but is also more sensitive to the potential carcinogenic effects of radiation. Therefore, unless the patient's personal risk factors indicate a higher than average risk of developing premenopausal breast cancer, screening for breast cancer should begin at age 40 (Maniero et al. 2013).

It is important, however, that high-risk patients under the age of 40 also be appropriately screened. Women with first-degree relatives with premenopausal breast cancer or with known genetic mutations should be screened annually, at an age 10 years younger than the age of the first-degree relative's cancer. Women who have had chest radiation for Hodgkin lymphoma are also considered high risk and should begin screening 8 years following the therapy, but not before age 25. Women under 40 years who have had biopsies showing certain pathologic findings (ductal or lobular atypia, etc.) are considered at increased risk and are advised to begin annual screening at the time of the diagnosis of high-risk histology (Maniero et al. 2013).

Increased breast density is associated with an increased risk of developing breast cancer, separate from the masking of small tumors that occurs. Published estimates suggest a five times risk of cancer in women with the highest breast density compared to those with lowest breast density (McCormack and dos Santos 2006). If possible, women with denser breasts should be screened using digital mammography technique as digital mammography has been shown to be superior to screen-film mammography in this population of patients (Pisano et al. 2005).

Breast Implants

Figure 22.5 demonstrates a very dense homogeneous opacity close to the chest wall. This is the appearance of a breast implant.

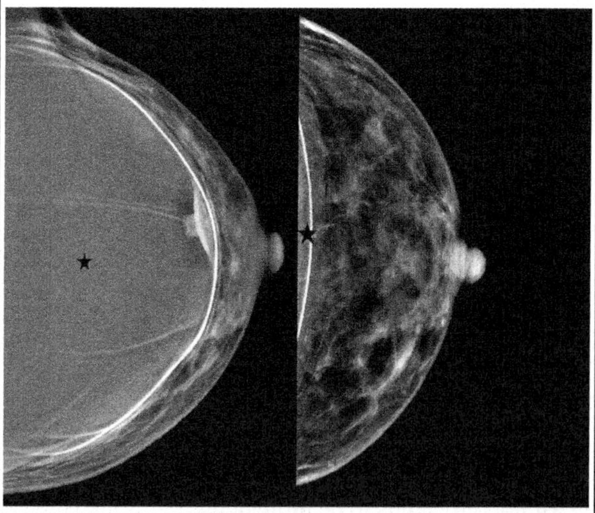

FIGURE 22.5 - BREAST IMPLANTS
The image on the *left* is a conventional CC view, while the one on the *right* is an implant (*) displaced CC view

Implants may be surgically located either anterior (prepectoral) or posterior to the pectoralis major muscle (retropectoral). When retropectoral, the muscle can be seen curving around the implant's anterior surface. On standard views, implants may obscure a considerable amount of breast parenchyma and can make detection of early carcinomas more difficult. For this reason, patients with breast implants undergoing mammography get four views of each breast, rather than two views. One set is the conventional type (MLO and CC), while the other set is taken with the implant displaced against the chest wall.

Mammographic Findings

To detect breast cancer at its earliest stage, radiologists evaluate the images for subtle changes in the density and architecture of the breast tissue, new asymmetries or masses, and new or suspicious microcalcifications. If an abnormality is detected on a standard screening exam, the more specialized diagnostic exam is ordered. The margins of masses are better characterized on spot compression views. Borders that are irregular or spiculated are suspicious for malignancy, while smoothly circumscribed margins favor benign disease. Calcifications must be evaluated with magnification technology before a final assessment is rendered.

Calcifications occur frequently in the breast, and when the calcifications are large and coarse, they can be confidently reported as benign. However, smaller calcifications (referred to as "microcalcifications") may require biopsy for definitive diagnosis. The following four figures provide examples of both benign and malignant calcifications (Figs. 22.6, 22.7, 22.8, and 22.9).

Figure 22.10 demonstrates two examples (a and b) of a well-circumscribed mass called fibroadenoma. In Fig. 22.10b, the mass contains coarse "popcorn" calcification characteristic of a degenerating fibroadenoma. Fibroadenomas are one of the most common benign tumors of the breast that may manifest as a mass on mammogram or breast ultrasound.

In contrast to the benign fibroadenomas above, Fig. 22.11a and b demonstrates a mass characteristic of carcinoma as seen on the standard two-view mammogram.

Radiation Dosage

Effective dose is the measurement of radiation that allows for the variable radiosensitivity of different tissues and for the quantification of the risk for future adverse outcomes related to the exposure. The effective radiation dose to the breast for a two-view examination (four total exposures) is approximately .2–3 mSv (200–300 millirads). The exposure is less for some digital imaging, measuring approximately 0.08–1.5 mSv (85–150 millirads). The federal limit for exposure during a mammogram is up to 0.3 mSv or 300 millirad per exposure.

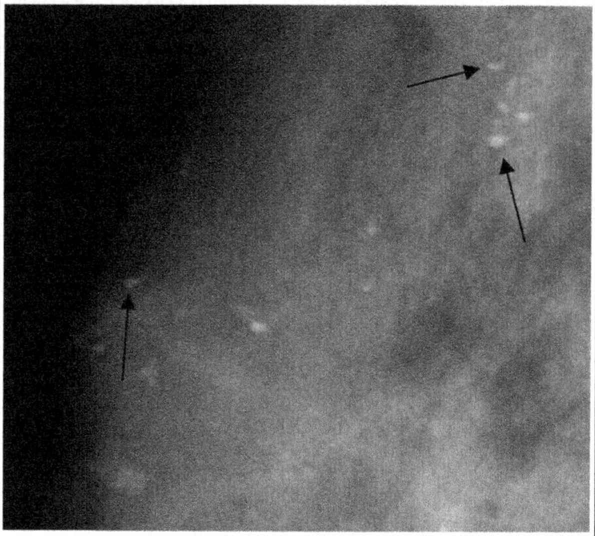

FIGURE 22.6 - BENIGN CALCIFICATIONS
Milk of calcium layering out in a gravity-dependent fashion, demonstrated with 90° positioning of the breast (*arrows*)

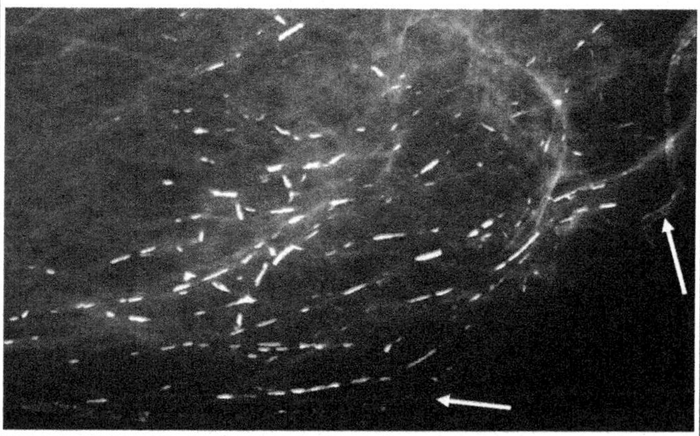

FIGURE 22.7 - BENIGN CALCIFICATIONS
Two examples of benign calcifications. First, the large, *rod*-shaped calcifications scattered throughout the breast. Second, vascular calcifications common with age (*arrows*)

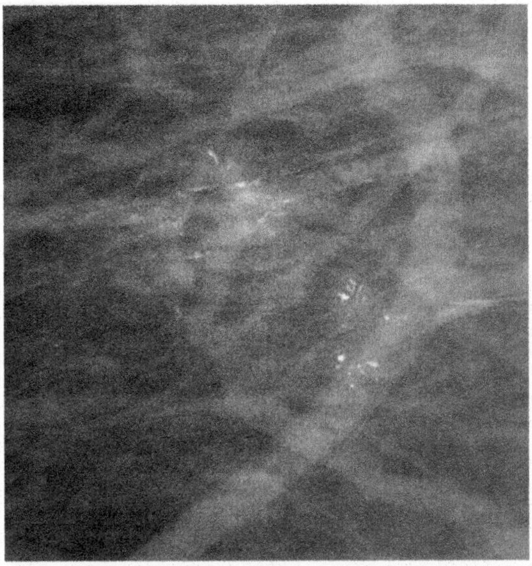

FIGURE 22.8 - MICROCALCIFICATIONS
Spot magnification compression views showing pleomorphic, fine branching microcalcifications related to DCIS

The normal background radiation is comprised predominantly of cosmic radiation and natural occurring radiation in the ground such as Radon. For a person living at sea level, the average background radiation is approximately 3 mSv per year. Therefore, a standard mammogram is the equivalent to approximately 7 weeks of normal background radiation

At the stated dose level, mammography carries the hypothetical risk for approximately one excess cancer case per year per million women examined. If one assumes 50 % breast cancer mortality, the hypothetical risk would be one excess death per two million women examined. The term hypothetical is used because, at such low increased risk, a large number of patients followed for a long period of time would be required to statistically demonstrate an effect. Because of the large population size needed for valid research, the actual research study has never been performed, and the statistics are extrapolations of patients exposed to higher dosage levels from other sources. Background radiation contributes more exposure to each of us each year, particularly those who fly frequently, due to the exposure to cosmic radiation. The airport scanners contribute little, with 100–200 backscatter scans equal to 1 day of natural background radiation exposure. It is important to keep these relationships in mind, since you will be asked frequently by patients about the safety of mammography (Wall and Hart 1997).

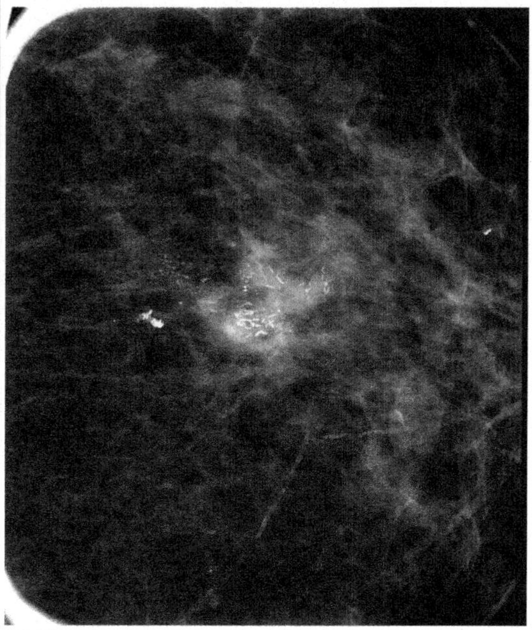

FIGURE 22.9 - MICROCALCIFICATIONS
Spot magnification compression views showing classic pleomorphic, linear branching calcifications associated with a spiculated mass in coexisting invasive ductal carcinoma and DCIS

The overall sensitivity of mammography for detecting breast carcinoma is approximately 90 %. However, this sensitivity can be diminished substantially and can be as low as 40 % in young patients with dense breasts.

Ultrasound Utilization in Breast Imaging

Breast ultrasound is advocated for focused evaluations of abnormalities on physical examination, focused evaluation of abnormal mammographic findings, and occasionally as a "second look" tool after an abnormal breast MRI. Ultrasound is also the modality of choice in the evaluation of masses in children and anyone (male or female) under the age of 30.

When a circumscribed (smoothly marginated) breast mass is discovered on mammography, the differential diagnosis includes breast carcinoma, benign tumor of the

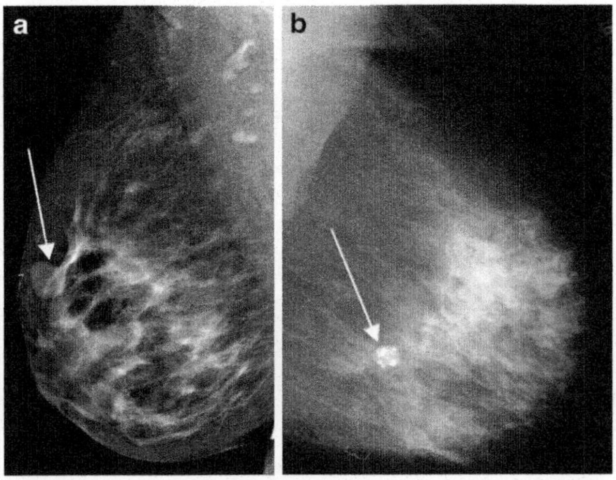

FIGURE 22.10 - FIBROADENOMA
Two different examples (**a** and **b**) of fibroadenomas. Both are smoothly marginated. Note how the one on the *right* contains coarse calcifications, which is characteristic of a degenerating fibroadenoma

breast such as fibroadenoma, and simple breast cyst. To avoid performing biopsies on women with breast cysts and other clearly benign lesions, ultrasound is employed to discriminate cystic from solid lesions and to characterize solid masses to determine the need for biopsy.

Figure 22.12 demonstrates a mammogram of a palpable mass highlighted by a triangular marker placed on the skin over the area of concern. This lesion was subsequently imaged by ultrasound and is depicted in Fig. 22.13. The ultrasound shows an oval lesion that is free of echoes (anechoic) and smoothly marginated. This corresponds in location to the opacity seen on the conventional mammogram depicted in Fig. 22.12. The sonographic characteristics are definitive for a simple fluid-filled cyst, and no further evaluation is required.

Whole breast ultrasound alone has not been proven to be sensitive or efficient enough to use as a screening test for breast cancer in lieu of mammography. However, screening breast ultrasound has been shown to increase the cancer detection rate in patients at elevated risk or in patients with dense breasts (Berg et al. 2008). Therefore, supplemental screening with US should be considered in high-risk women who are not eligible for MRI and in the intermediate-risk patient, particularly in the setting of dense breasts (http www acr org media ACR Documents AppCriteria Diagnostic BreastCancerScreening pdf).

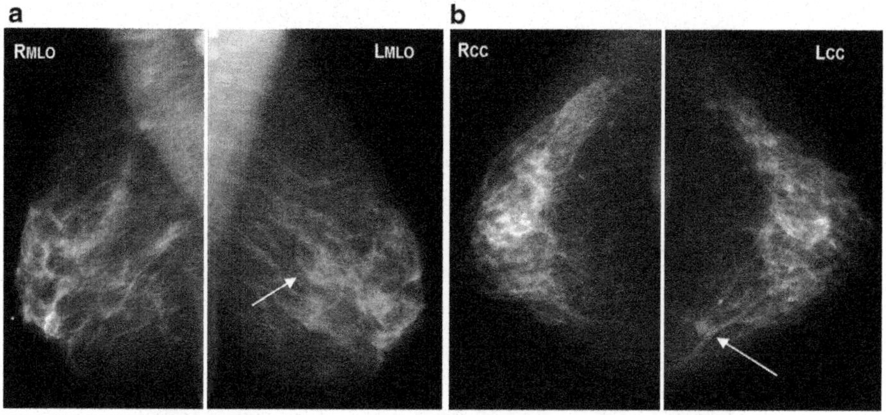

FIGURE 22.11 - (A) BREAST MASS MLO VIEWS
Mass in the left breast suspicious for carcinoma
(B) BREAST MASS CC VIEWS
Mass in the left breast suspicious for carcinoma

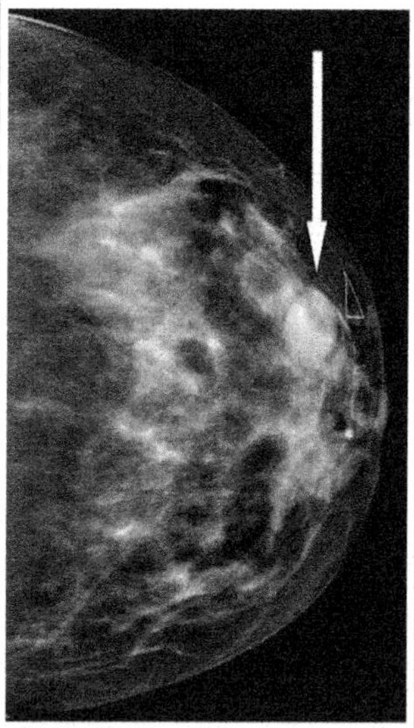

FIGURE 22.12 - PALPABLE MASS
Skin marker (the metallic triangle) used to indicate a palpable mass

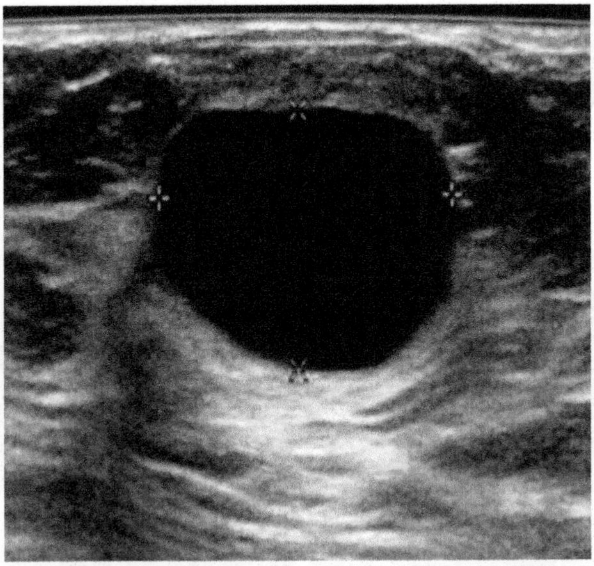

FIGURE 22.13 - SIMPLE BREAST CYST
A simple cyst is defined as anechoic, well-circumscribed, with well-defined borders, and posterior acoustic enhancement

Breast MRI

Breast MRI utilizes gadolinium contrast to highlight areas of increased vascularity in the breast. Therefore, MRI provides not only an anatomic evaluation of the breast but also a physiologic assessment of the vascularity of breast tissue. Because breast cancers are often associated with tumoral vascularity ("neovascularity"), and because differentiation of soft tissues is 10–100 times greater on MRI images than on conventional x-ray, MRI is a highly sensitive tool to detect breast cancer. However, though it is a highly sensitive tool (and more sensitive than mammography, ultrasound, and clinical exam combined), it is not a highly specific tool. Many benign, proliferative and inflammatory processes will show increased vascularity on gadolinium-enhanced MRI. This low specificity combined with the higher cost of MRI limits its use as a screening modality for average-risk women. However, the higher sensitivity outweighs the disadvantages of low specificity for screening high-risk women. Women with a National Cancer Institute (NCI) lifetime risk assessment of 20 % or greater, those with a known genetic mutation or a first-degree relative with a genetic mutation known to be associated with breast cancer, and those women who have undergone previous chest irradiation, usually for Hodgkin lymphoma, should be counseled on the benefits of supplemental MRI screening. MRI cannot

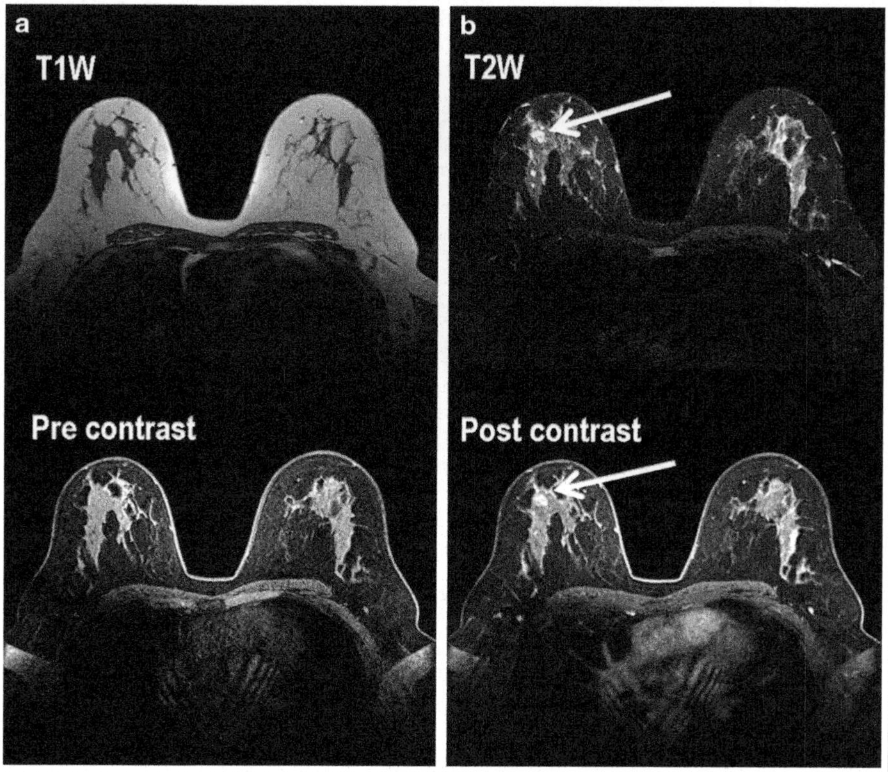

FIGURE 22.14 - BREAST MRI
A breast MRI showing enhancement in a breast cancer

detect the small calcifications that mammography can identify, and therefore, MRI screening is in addition to, not in place of, mammography. Some malignant lesions seen on MRI cannot be seen with any other imaging tool, even in retrospect. Therefore, any institution providing breast MRI services should have imaged guided biopsy capability, or a relationship with an institution that can provide this service.

MRI is indicated in any woman with a new diagnosis of breast cancer. Its primary strength is near 100 % sensitivity in the detection of invasive breast cancer. Therefore, it should be used as a tool to define extent of disease of a known malignancy and to exclude additional sites of disease in the same or opposite breast in the preoperative setting. Surgical planning also depends on accurate evaluation of skin, chest wall, and regional lymph nodes. MRI of the breast is also helpful in assessing tumor response following neoadjuvant chemotherapy, which is initiated prior to surgery to reduce tumor burden and increase the success of breast conservation (Fig. 22.14).

Image-Guided Biopsy

Suspicious findings identified by any imaging modality can be assessed with core needle biopsy under imaging guidance. Mammographic findings such as microcalcifications are best approached with stereotactic mammographic guidance. This method can also be used for the biopsy of mammographically detected masses when there is no ultrasound correlate. Images of the breast are obtained at 15° off center, and this "stereo pair" is used to calculate the x, y, and z coordinates of the location of the abnormality within the breast. After the administration of local anesthesia, a probe is then positioned at these coordinates for sampling. Lesions at the chest wall are difficult to reach with this method and may require other modalities to biopsy.

As mentioned above, ultrasound is often used to evaluate the site of a palpable mass or mammographic abnormality. It is also an ideal modality for image-guided biopsy. It is a more comfortable and cost-effective examination for the patient, and lesions in any part of the breast can usually be safely sampled under ultrasound guidance.

BI-RADS®

The following table shows the BI-RADS® classification used by breast radiologists to communicate findings to other clinicians in a standard and consistent form. BI-RADS stands for Breast Imaging-Reporting and Data System and is a quality

Category	Assessment	Explanation
0	Incomplete	Your mammogram or ultrasound did not give the radiologist enough information to make a diagnosis. Follow-up imaging is necessary
1	Negative	There is nothing to comment on; routine screening is recommended
2	Benign finding(s)	A definite benign finding; routine screening is recommended
3	Probably benign findings-initial short-interval follow-up suggested (findings with < 2 % risk of malignancy)	Findings that have a high probability of being benign (>98 %); 6 month short interval follow-up
4	Suspicious abnormality-biopsy should be considered	Not characteristic of breast cancer, but reasonable probability of being malignant (3–94 %); biopsy should be considered
5	Highly suspicious of malignancy-appropriate action should be taken (>95 % probability)	Lesion that has a high probability of being malignant (>95 %); take appropriate action
6	Known biopsy proven malignancy-appropriate action should be taken	Lesions known to be malignant that are being imaged prior to definitive treatment; assure that treatment is completed

assurance tool published by the American College of Radiology. At the end of every mammogram report, one of these numbers is listed.

BI-RADS® is a registered trademark of the American College of Radiology, Reston, VA.

References

ACR BIRADS Lexicon, American College of Radiology, Reston, VA.

Berg WA, Blume JD, Cormack JB, et al. Combined screening with ultrasound and mammography vs mammography alone in women at elevated risk of breast cancer. JAMA. 2008;299(18): 2151–63.

Duffy SW, Tabar L, Chen H, et al. The impact of organized mammography service screening on breast carcinoma mortality in seven Swedish counties. Cancer. 2002;95(3):458–68.

http://www.acr.org/~/media/ACR/Documents/AppCriteria/Diagnostic/BreastCancerScreening.pdf

ICRP Publication 103. The 2007 Recommendations of the International Commission on Radiologic Protection. Ann ICRP. 2007;37:2–4.

Maniero MB, Lourenco A, Mahoney MC, et al. ACR appropriateness criteria breast cancer screening. J Am Coll Radiol. 2013;10(1):11–4.

McCormack VA, dos Santos SI. Breast density and parenchymal patterns as markers of breast cancer risk: a meta-analysis. Cancer Epidemiol Biomarkers Prev. 2006;15(6):1159–69.

Pisano ED, Gatsonis C, Hendrick E, et al. Diagnostic performance of digital versus film mammography for breast-cancer screening – the results of the American College of Radiology Imaging Network (ACRIN) Digital Mammographic Imaging Screening Trial (DMIST). N Engl J Med. 2005;353(17):1773–83. [Published correction appears in N Engl J Med. 2006;355(17):1840.]

Wall BF, Hart D. Revised radiation doses for typical x-ray examinations. Brit J Radiol. 1997;70: 437–39

23 Women's Ultrasound

Objectives:
1. Understand how different imaging modalities contribute to evaluating conditions and diseases unique to women.
2. Name several causes of abnormal uterine bleeding and appreciate their ultrasound characteristics.
3. Name several masses seen in the ovary and appreciate their ultrasound characteristics.
4. List imaging modalities and applications in the evaluation of fertility and pregnancy.

Women's imaging is a subspecialty area of radiology devoted to the diagnosis and treatment of conditions and diseases that are unique to women. Women's imaging uses all imaging modalities to evaluate gynecologic and obstetrical conditions and breast health and contributes to urologic evaluations and overall health. Discussions about some of these modalities and applications are further addressed in specific chapters on breast imaging and women's health interventional procedures.

Ultrasound plays the primary role for much of women's imaging applications with fluoroscopy studies, CT, MRI, and nuclear medicine studies performed to assist in the subsequent evaluation. Ultrasound does not produce ionizing radiation, and examinations rarely require sedation, making it a desirable modality for women of all ages.

H. Singh et al. (eds.), *Radiology Fundamentals: Introduction to Imaging & Technology*, DOI 10.1007/978-3-319-10362-4_23

Evaluation of Premenstrual Females

Women's imaging can begin before puberty. Ultrasound is used to evaluate a variety of problems in girls. Indications include evaluation for congenital abnormalities of the uterus, vaginal bleeding, precocious puberty, and palpable pelvic masses. Ultrasound abnormalities often prompt further evaluation with laboratory information, CT, MRI, and sometimes direct visualization (surgery).

Evaluation of the Uterus and Uterine Bleeding

Abnormal uterine bleeding is bleeding unrelated to normal menstruation and can occur in women of any age. Organic causes of abnormal uterine bleeding include problems related to pregnancy, medication, benign and malignant masses, and systemic disease. Dysfunctional uterine bleeding (DUB) is defined as abnormal bleeding that does not have an organic cause and is commonly related to anovulation and abnormal function of the hypothalamic-pituitary-ovarian axis. Common dysfunctional uterine bleeding terms include menorrhagia (prolonged bleeding), metromenorrhagia (irregular bleeding), and spotting (intermenstrual bleeding).

Ultrasound is commonly used to begin the evaluation of abnormal uterine bleeding. Ultrasound may identify structural causes for the abnormal bleeding such as fibroids and polyps that extend into the endometrial cavity. Ultrasound can assess the thickness and contour of the endometrial lining and determine if the bleeding may be the result of a thin atrophic endometrium or a thick endometrium, which may reflect hypertrophy or cancer. Ultrasound may identity structural changes in the endometrium from drugs such as tamoxifen. Pelvic ultrasound can contribute to the evaluation of amenorrhea such as seen with polycystic ovarian syndrome and pregnancy (Figs. 23.1 and 23.2).

Transabdominal ultrasound is commonly performed first to evaluate the pelvis as it provides an "overview" of pelvic structures. The urine-filled urinary bladder is used as an acoustic window to best evaluate pelvic structures. Transvaginal ultrasound is performed with an ultrasound probe that is cleaned and covered with a sterile probe cover and inserted into the vagina; the transvaginal approach provides more detail of the uterus, the endometrium, and the ovaries. Transvaginal pelvic ultrasound evaluation is similar to a speculum pelvic examination, and the patient does not have the discomfort of maintaining a full bladder.

Additional imaging may be prompted by ultrasound findings. MRI may be performed to further evaluate the myometrium and endometrial-myometrial junction. MRI can be used to evaluate for adenomyosis, a process where endometrium is deposited into the endometrial myometrial junction and myometrium. CT may follow an ultrasound if a pelvic mass is identified and there is concern for more extensive disease; however, this does involve radiation. Diagnostic imaging does not always explain the cause of abnormal uterine bleeding but may direct the indication and location for biopsy, hysteroscopy, surgery, or follow-up.

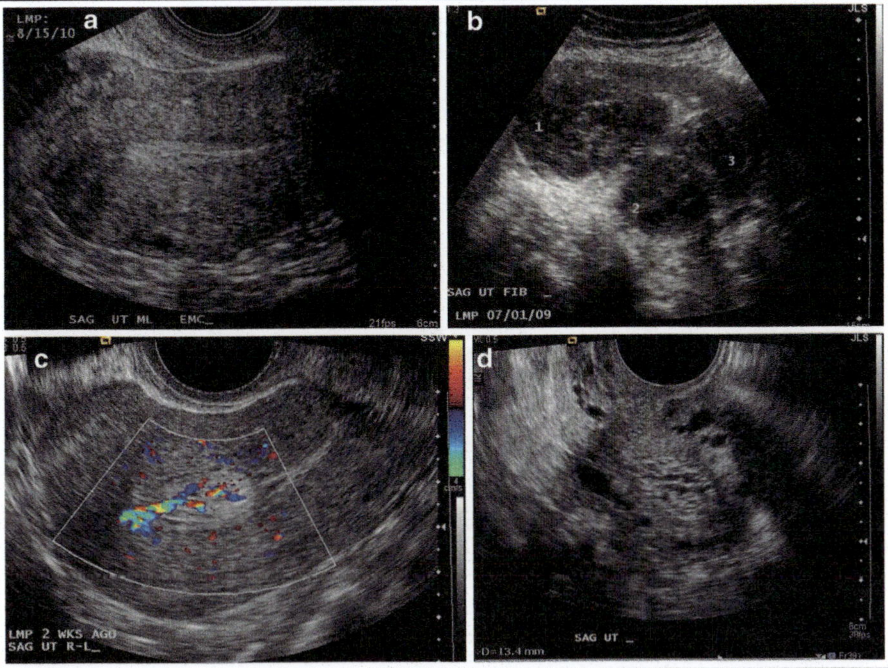

FIGURE 23.1 - TRANSVAGINAL ULTRASOUND. Examples of (**a**) normal endometrium, with bright walls and central cavity delineated by a white line (**b**) multiple hypoechoic fibroids, (**c**) echogenic polyp with central vascular stalk, and (**d**) cystic changes of endometrium from tamoxifen

Evaluation of the Ovaries

Imaging commonly is an adjunct to physical examination of the adnexa. It may be difficult to tell if a "full" adnexa is merely stool-filled bowel or pathology in the ovaries or in surrounding structures. Ultrasound commonly begins the evaluation. While there are some "classic" ultrasound findings of ovarian structures such as normal functional follicles, hemorrhagic cysts, and endometriomas, many ovarian masses have nonspecific findings. A complex cystic mass in the adnexa is particularly hard to manage because the differential diagnosis is extensive and includes benign and malignant cystic neoplasm, atypical cyst, endometrioma, dermoid, torsed ovary, abscess, hydro- and pyosalpinx, as well as nongynecologic masses such as mesenteric cysts and nongynecologic processes (Fig. 23.3). Clinical evaluation is essential to determine if the process needs immediate intervention such as antibiotics or surgery. If patient is not acutely ill, follow-up ultrasound in two to three menstrual cycles is commonly recommended and performed. If follow-up ultrasound remains concerning, MRI may further characterize the ovarian mass but

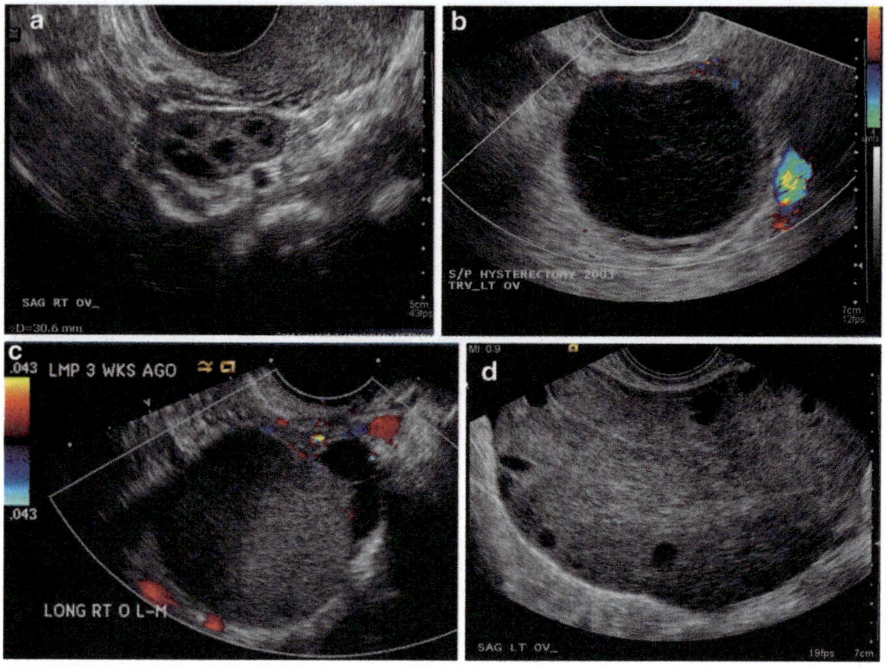

FIGURE 23.2 - TRANSVAGINAL ULTRASOUND. Examples of (**a**) normal ovary, (**b**) hemorrhagic cyst with reticulated mesh-like echoes, (**c**) endometrioma with homogeneous echoes, and (**d**) enlarged torsed ovary with peripheral follicles

the patient and her physician may elect to go to laparoscopy for visual and pathologic diagnosis. CT may be performed to determine extent of disease such as the presence of ascites or peritoneal metastases.

Pregnancy

An evaluation of pregnancy may begin with infertility. Fallopian tube patency can be assessed with hysterosalpingography in which contrast is instilled into the uterine cavity under fluoroscopy. If the fallopian tubes are patent, contrast will spill out of the tubes into the peritoneal cavity. Hysterosalpingography, ultrasound, and MRI can assess the contour of the cavity itself and look for problems that might affect pregnancy such as large fibroids, congenital anomalies, and scarring of the cavity. Fallopian tube blockage and its possible treatment are reviewed in the Women's Health Interventions chapter. The male partner may be evaluated for problems that may affect fertility such as varicoceles and testicular pathology with scrotal ultrasound.

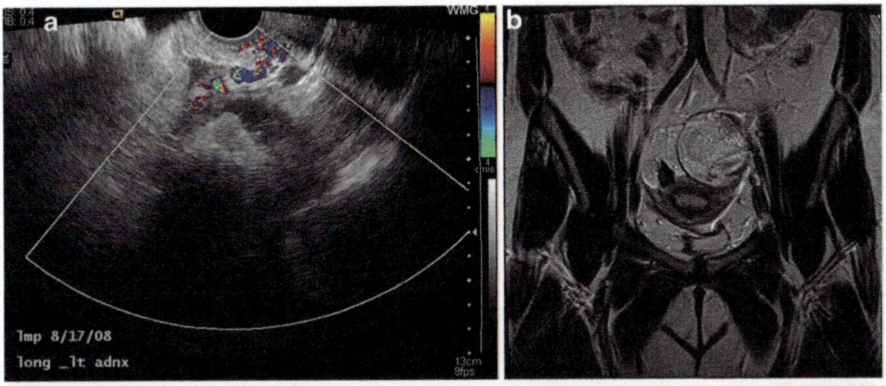

FIGURE 23.3 - OVARIAN DERMOID. "Tip of the iceberg" configuration of an ovarian dermoid (cystic teratoma) is noted on ultrasound (**a**); the multiple types of tissue that make up a dermoid such as hair, blood, fat, cartilage, and calcifications create an acoustic shadow, which blocks all sound waves and the mass is essentially obscured. The corresponding MRI (**b**) shows the extent and complex nature of the mass. Fat identified in an ovarian mass on CT or MRI is classic for dermoid

Ultrasound is used to assess for the presence of intrauterine pregnancy initially and then for appropriate fetal growth and well-being. Ultrasound is commonly used to assess for ectopic pregnancy when the patient has a positive pregnancy test and may have vaginal bleeding and/or pain. It is important to interpret the ultrasound results in conjunction with the patient's quantitative serum B-HCG levels. That is, sometimes the ultrasound is performed so early that an intrauterine pregnancy cannot be identified and the differential includes very early intrauterine pregnancy, ectopic pregnancy, and early pregnancy loss. Ultrasound is used in the evaluation of retained products of conception and gestational tropoblastic disease (Fig. 23.4).

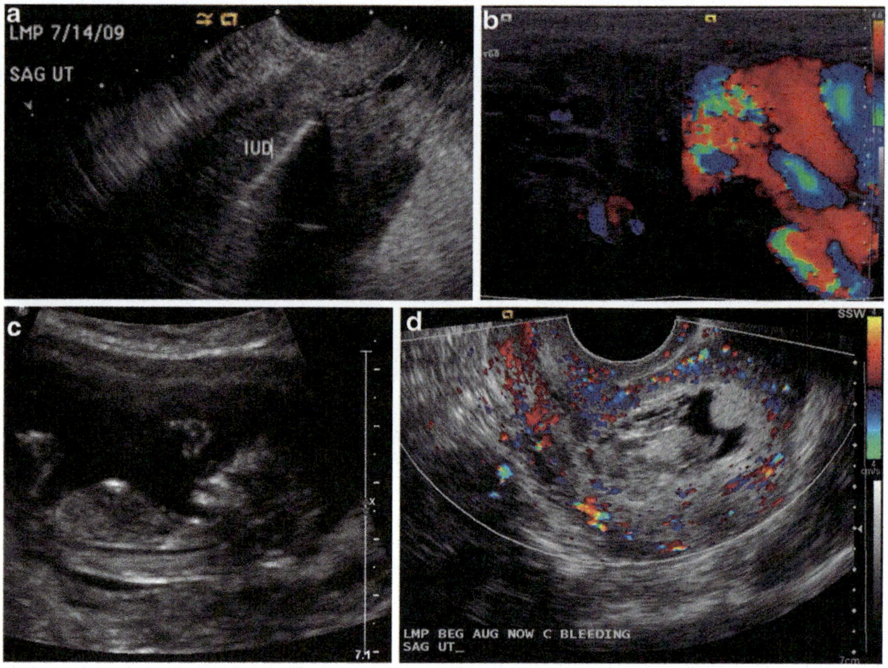

FIGURE 23.4 - Examples of (**a**) bright echogenic IUD in endometrial cavity, (**b**) hypervascular varicocele that increased in size and vascularity with Valsalva maneuver, (**c**) intrauterine fetus, and (**d**) irregular heterogeneous tissue with degeneration of gestational trophoblastic disease (molar pregnancy)

24 Women's Health Interventions

Objectives:
1. Describe which three interventional procedures are considered part of women's health interventions.
2. Understand the indications for each of the procedures.
3. Describe the basics of how each procedure is performed.

Introduction

"Women's health interventions" describes the group of interventional radiology procedures that are related to female pelvic structures and includes uterine artery embolization (or uterine fibroid embolization), ovarian vein embolization for pelvic congestion syndrome, and fallopian tube recanalization. Each procedure will be discussed separately.

Uterine Artery or Fibroid Embolization (UAE or UFE)

Of the approximately 600,000 hysterectomies performed in the US each year, about 200,000 are for symptomatic fibroids. Symptoms can include significant menorrhagia, dysmenorrhea, urinary frequency and/or urgency, constipation, back pain, lower extremity pain, and dyspareunia. There are many treatment methods for symptomatic fibroids including oral contraceptives, chemical menopause, myomectomy, and hysterectomy. UAE or UFE represents a specific method of treating symptomatic patients. The "ideal" patient is an approximately 45-year-old female

H. Singh et al. (eds.), *Radiology Fundamentals: Introduction to Imaging & Technology*, DOI 10.1007/978-3-319-10362-4_24

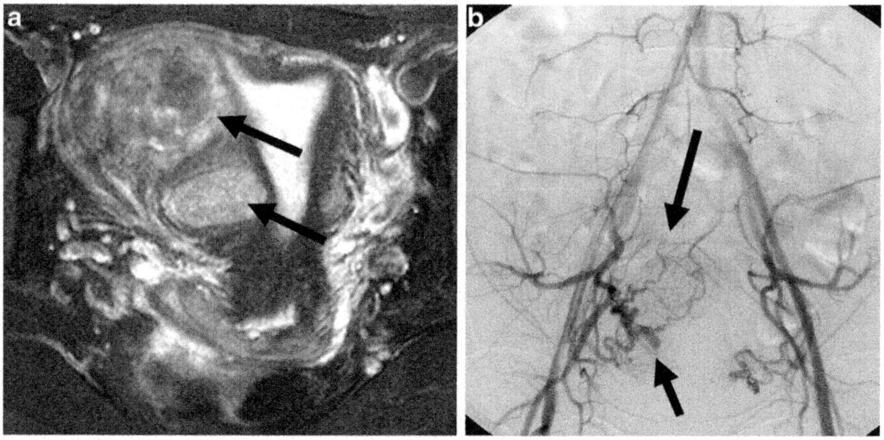

FIGURE 24.1 - UTERINE FIBROID EMBOLIZATION
On the axial image from a pelvic MRI (**a**), the fibroids (*arrows*) are seen in the right uterine wall. Note the uterine cavity appears as the white triangular shape in the midline. On the non-selective pelvic arteriogram (**b**), flow to the fibroids can easily be made out (*arrows*)

with multiple small fibroids who has completed child bearing and has severe menstrual symptoms. Contraindications include pedunculated subserosal fibroids and young patients still interested in future child bearing. Pelvic MRI is currently the standard of care for mapping the fibroids and identifying other possible causes of the patient's symptoms; of note, MRI alters the treatment algorithm approximately 20 % of the time. UFE is performed as an outpatient procedure using conscious sedation. Via arterial access, superselective uterine arteriography is performed on each side with embolization with PVA (polyvinyl alcohol particles) to occlude blood flow to the fibroid(s). This is performed on both left- and right-side vessels. The patients are then admitted for a short hospital stay (usually overnight) and have an overall recovery time of approximately 2 weeks, during which time the patients are fairly functional. Success rates are noted to be about 85 % for relief or marked improvement in symptoms. That number increases to greater than 90 % for bleeding symptoms and is about 75 % for bulk-related symptoms (Figs. 24.1 and 24.2).

Ovarian Vein Embolization and Pelvic Congestion Syndrome (PCS)

Chronic pelvic pain in women is a difficult entity to sort out because there are so many possible causes. These can include ovarian vein reflux, endometriosis, adhesions, atypical urological or menstrual pain, and irritable bowel syndrome. Although noninvasive diagnostic tests are used more and more, a thorough history

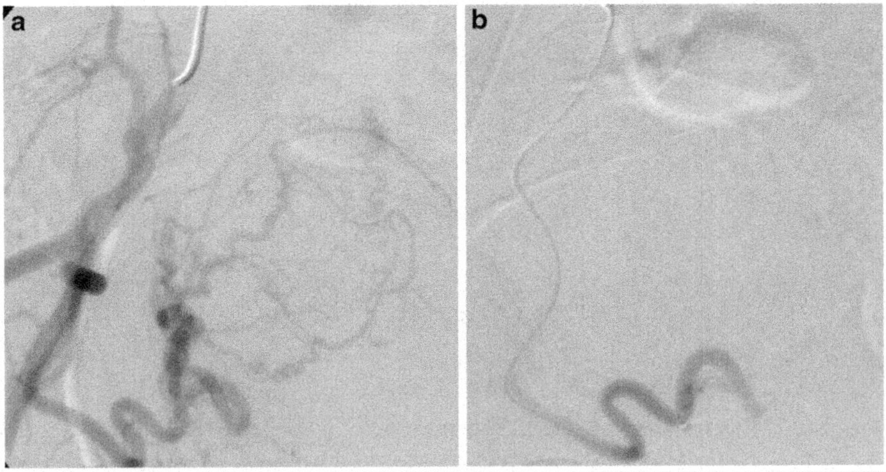

FIGURE 24.2 - UTERINE FIBROID EMBOLIZATION
Selective right uterine arteriogram showing successful embolization pre (**a**) and post (**b**) images

and physical examination can be very helpful. For pelvic congestion syndrome (PCS), which is a clinical diagnosis, patients relate a history of pelvic pressure that is not present first thing in the morning, gets worse as the day goes on, and can be associated with varicosities of the abdominal wall and upper thighs. Spectral (or duplex) ultrasound was the gold standard for diagnosis in the past, but now pelvic MRI is a more sensitive imaging modality. More recently, with multislice CT scanners, the diagnosis of a dilated gonadal vein can be made with exquisite spatial resolution.

Definitive diagnosis is made with a gonadal venogram. For this, the patient is admitted to a CVIR short-stay ward. Under conscious sedation, access to the right jugular vein is obtained, and a catheter is advanced to the left renal vein. Venography that demonstrates reflux of contrast to the level of the pelvis indicates venous valvular insufficiency and with that findings compatible with PCS. Treatment can be performed at the same time, which entails embolization of the gonadal vein (and all its tributaries) starting at the level of the pelvic brim. From here, the entire gonadal vein back to the renal vein is embolized to occlusion. The right gonadal vein, a direct branch of the IVC, needs to be evaluated as well. The procedure is performed as an outpatient procedure. Symptoms will take approximately 4 months to improve. Success rates are about 65 % and with concomitant or subsequent internal iliac vein embolization about 75 % (Fig. 24.3).

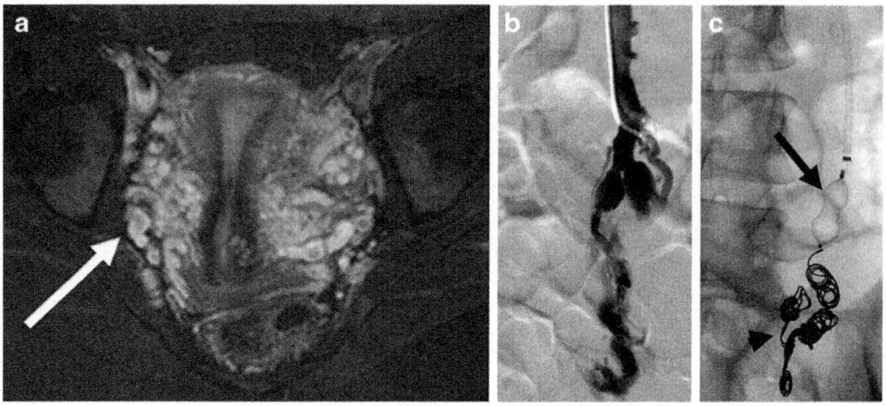

FIG. 24.3 - PELVIC CONGESTION SYNDROME
Axial image from a pelvic MRI (**a**) demonstrates markedly dilated veins (*white arrow*) on either side of the pelvis. Injection (**b**) and embolization (**c**) on a different patient, using a combination of coils (*arrowhead*) and Amplatzer plugs (*black arrow*)

Fallopian Tube Recanalization

Fallopian tube recanalization is performed to improve a women's ability to have a physiologic intrauterine pregnancy. Fallopian tube recanalization was first accomplished in 1849 by passing a whalebone bougie through the cervix out the cornu of the uterus and out the fallopian tube. In the 1980s, with the development of microcatheters, fallopian tube recanalization took a great leap forward and has changed little since that time. A thorough gynecological history including fallopian tube surgery and a preprocedural hysterosalpingogram are very useful for identifying the possible cause of the fallopian tube obstruction with a vast majority of patients suffering from blockage by menstrual debris. Patients with a history of pelvic inflammatory disease may have a partially successful outcome, while those with prior tubal ligation are the most difficult to recanalize. Patients are advised that the risk of the procedure is very low, but it does increase the risk of an ectopic pregnancy by 1–2 % overall.

The procedure is done as an outpatient. The patient is placed on the angiography table in the lithotomy position. The perineum is prepped as usual, and a speculum is placed. The cervical os is identified and cannulated with a wire and catheter. Over this combination, a 9Fr sheath is placed. Through the sheath, an angled catheter is advanced to the cornu, and contrast injection performed. This sometimes is enough to clear the debris and reopen the fallopian tube. If not, through the angled catheter,

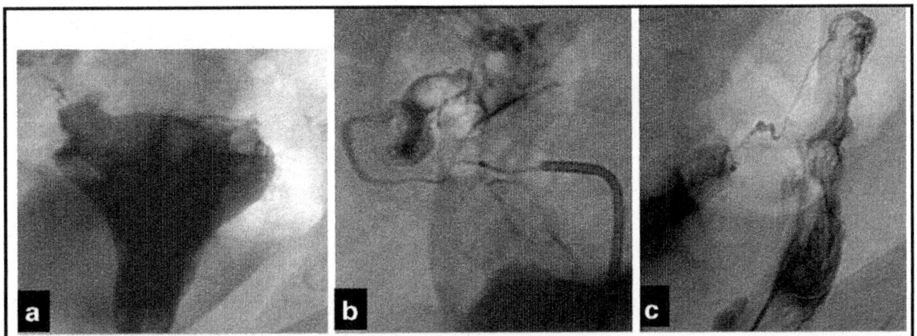

FIG. 24.4 - FALLOPIAN TUBE RECANALIZATION
On the initial hysterosalpingogram, there is no filling of the either fallopian tube (**a**). Selective cannulation of each fallopian tube (**b**) clears debris from each tube, the most common cause. Selective injection demonstrates patency of each tube with free spillage of contrast (**c**)

a microcatheter and wire are passed out the fallopian tube. The wire should pass to the fimbrial portion of the tube. The wire is then removed and contrast injected looking for free spillage (Fig. 24.4).

As devices become smaller and technology advances, patients will benefit from minimally invasive procedures. This is no more apparent than in the female patient.

Part IV
Abdominal Section

25 Abdominal Calcifications

Objectives:

1. Describe the patterns of calcification and their location on radiographs for the following: chronic pancreatitis, vascular structures, uterine fibroids, appendicolith, and renal calculi.
2. Describe the usefulness of an oblique view for assessing the localization of abdominal calcifications.
3. State what percentage of renal calculi are normally visible on the plain radiograph.

Calcifications are frequently seen on radiographs of the abdomen. The purpose of this section is to demonstrate the typical appearance of the more commonly occurring calcifications. Location and morphology are key characteristics to identify when evaluating abdominal and pelvic calcifications. For instance, gallstones are sometimes seen as round calcifications in the right upper quadrant. Knowing the typical appearance and location helps the diagnosis. What percentage of gallstones are radiopaque? Check out the Gallbladder chapter to find out.

Chronic Pancreatitis

Figure. 25.1 shows multiple calcifications of variable size in the mid upper abdomen and left upper quadrant. These are calcifications within the pancreas of a patient with chronic pancreatitis.

H. Singh et al. (eds.), *Radiology Fundamentals: Introduction to Imaging & Technology*, DOI 10.1007/978-3-319-10362-4_25

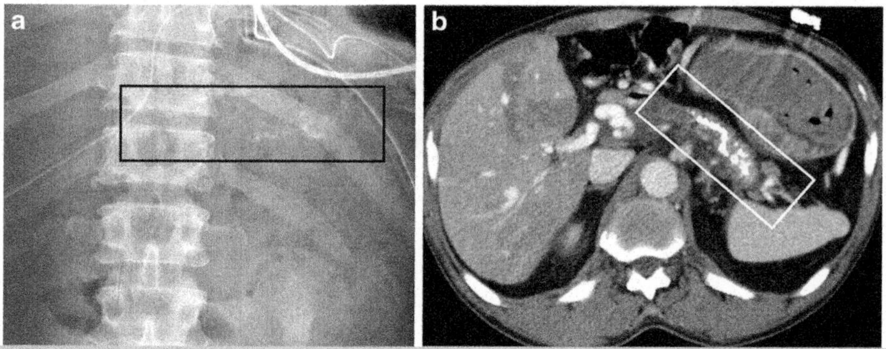

FIGURE 25.1 - CHRONIC PANCREATITIS
Supine radiograph collimated to the pancreatic bed (**a**) and corresponding axial CT slice (**b**) show pancreatic bed calcifications (*boxes*)

Vascular Calcifications

Vascular calcification takes several forms. In Fig. 25.2, numerous small, round, smoothly marginated calcifications are noted representing phleboliths within pelvic veins. Phleboliths are calcified venous thrombi. They often contain a central lucency that relates to recanalization of the occluded veins.

Figure. 25.3 shows calcification of the abdominal aorta. Sometimes the calcification is extensive enough to outline an abdominal aortic aneurysm, as in this case. Concerning calcifications on abdominal radiographs should prompt additional evaluation for abdominal aortic aneurysms with modalities such as ultrasound or CT.

Uterine Fibroids

Various tumors, both benign and malignant, may calcify. Figure. 25.4 demonstrates popcorn-like calcification noted in uterine fibroids, the most common tumor found in the pelvic region. Fibroids are "almost" universally benign.

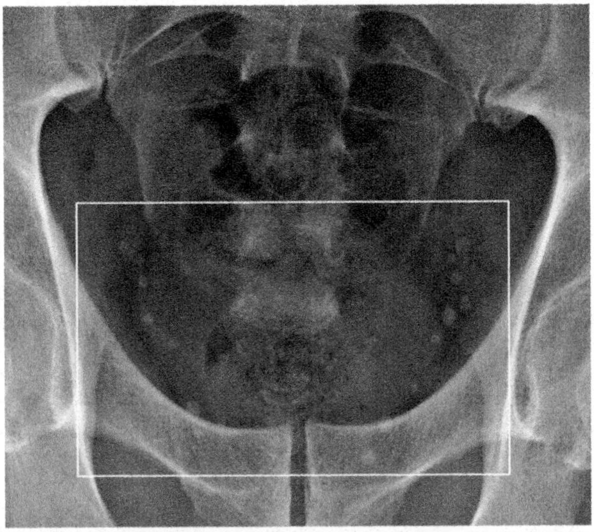

FIGURE 25.2 - PELVIC PHLEBOLITHS
Note the rounded calcifications in the pelvis with central lucency derived from calcified pelvic venous thrombi

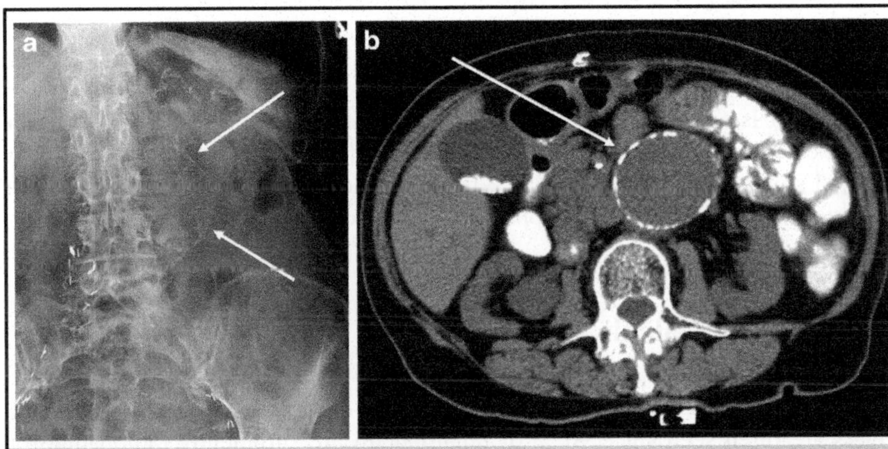

FIGURE 25.3 - AORTIC CALCIFICATION
Supine abdominal radiograph and corresponding axial CT slice showing a calcified aortic abdominal aneurysm (*arrows*)

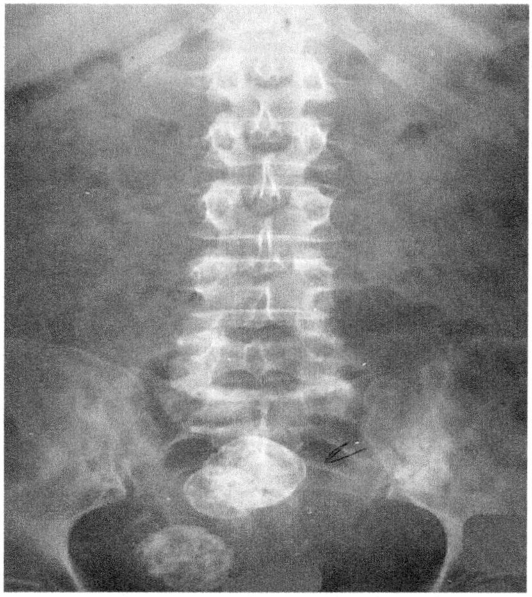

FIGURE 25.4 - CALCIFIED FIBROIDS

Appendicolith

Figure. 25.5 is an abdominal radiograph on a patient with right lower quadrant pain. A calcification is seen in the right lower quadrant. This is an appendicolith, a calcified stone within the appendix. When this finding is seen in association with acute right lower quadrant pain, appendicitis should be strongly considered.

Urinary Tract Calculi

Calcifications projected over the renal outlines or over the expected course of the ureters are often seen since 90 % of renal calculi are sufficiently radiopaque for visualization on the plain radiograph (Fig. 25.6). Certain calcifications may overlie the renal outline on a frontal projection but be displaced from the renal outline on oblique views because they are anterior or posterior to the kidneys. Their exact location can be surmised by knowing the obliquity of the radiograph and the direction in which the calcifications would be expected to move with rotation.

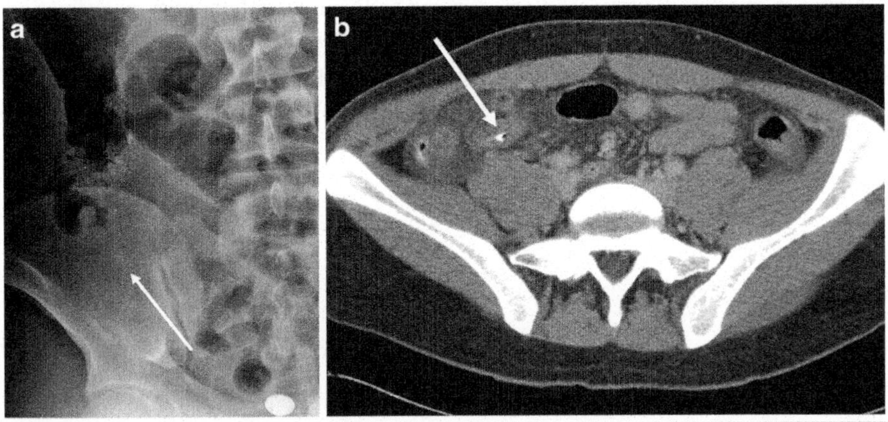

FIGURE 25.5 - APPENDICOLITH
Calcified appendicolith (*arrows*) on AP abdominal radiograph and axial CT image

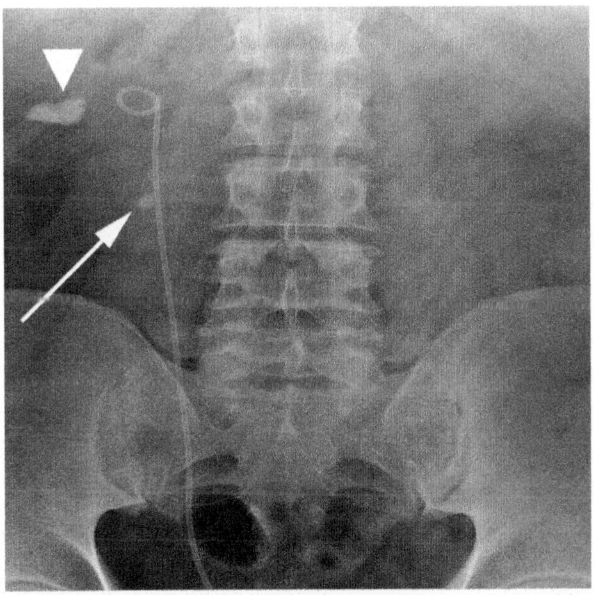

FIGURE 25.6 - RIGHT RENAL CALCULI
Calcified stone in the right renal pelvis (*arrowhead*) and proximal right ureter (*arrow*)

Now CT is often the first study performed to localize and quantify calcifications in the urinary tract. Calcium-containing stones such as calcium oxalate and calcium phosphate stones are radiopaque and usually seen on plain radiographs. Radiolucent stones such as uric acid, indinavir, and pure matrix stones are radiolucent and are not usually visualized on plain radiographs.

26 Abdominal Hardware and Tubes

Objectives:
1. Become familiar with common abdominal hardware and tubes.
2. State the desired location of nasogastric and enteric feeding tubes.

Surgical Clips

Many different types of clips are used in a variety of procedures performed in abdominal and pelvic surgery. The most common that are encountered radiographically are cholecystectomy clips. These are readily identified by their appearance and location in the right upper quadrant as seen in Fig. 26.1. Bowel surgery that results in resection and anastomosis will often involve a metal stapler that will leave a chain of small staples similar to those in Fig. 26.1. These staples can be helpful in both fluoroscopy and CT when trying to identify points of obstruction or leakage. Tubal ligation is a contraceptive procedure which occludes the fallopian tubes and can involve the use of clips that have a characteristic appearance located on both sides of the pelvis.

Gastrointestinal Tubes

It is necessary to be familiar with the appearance and desired location of gastrointestinal tubes. Nasogastric and enteric feeding tubes enter the abdomen via the esophagus. Typically the nasogastric (NG) tube will have its tip well within the stomach because most tubes have side holes that extend several centimeters back

H. Singh et al. (eds.), *Radiology Fundamentals: Introduction to Imaging & Technology*, DOI 10.1007/978-3-319-10362-4_26

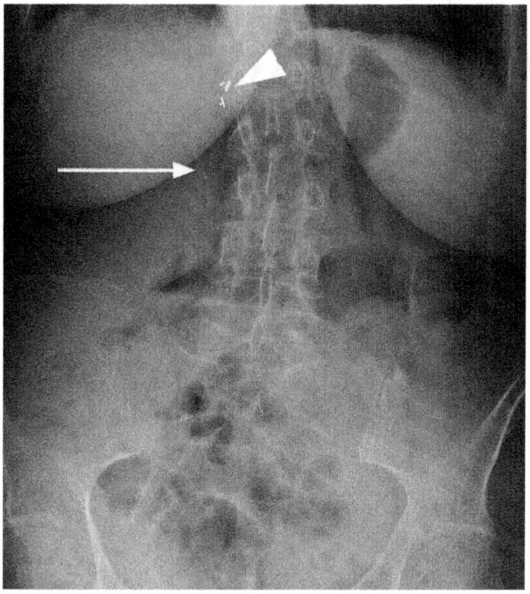

FIGURE 26.1 - TYPICAL POSTSURGICAL CLIPS
Radiograph of the abdomen showing metallic cholecystectomy clips (*arrowhead*) and a bowel resection staple line (*arrow*)

from the tip. In order to effectively decompress the stomach, the side holes should also be located below the diaphragm and not in the esophagus. Enteric feeding tubes are radiographically dense on both sides of the tube (unlike the NG tube) and often have a dense weighted tip. In many clinical settings, it is desirable to have the tip of the feeding tube beyond the ligament of Treitz well past the ampulla of Vater to prevent stimulation of biliary and pancreatic secretion. Therefore, the feeding tube should outline the expected course of the duodenum similar to Fig. 26.2. Gastrostomy tubes are another common type of GI tube that is frequently encountered during abdominal imaging. These tubes will have a balloon or flange near their tip which holds them in place in the gastric lumen.

Genitourinary Tubes

Abdominal radiographs can be used to help verify the location of urinary stents and catheters. Ureteral stents follow the expected course of the ureter from the renal fossa to the bladder and have a loop at each end to help hold them in place as

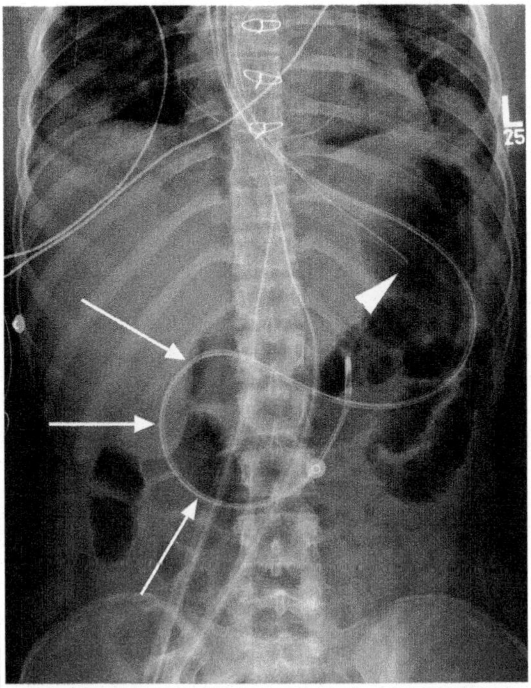

FIGURE 26.2 - UPPER GI TUBES
Radiograph of the abdomen and pelvis demonstrating a weighted-tip enteric feeding tube/NJ tube following the typical course duodenal C loop (*arrows*). The tip of an NG tube is seen near the air bubble of the gastric fundus (*arrowhead*). Additional lines, tubes, and sternotomy clips are seen in the lower chest

illustrated in Fig. 26.3. Prior to placing a ureteral stent, patients may have a nephrostomy tube placed to decompress an acutely obstructed kidney. The nephrostomy tube will have a single looped end located in the renal pelvis and then course externally, connected to a drainage bag.

There are additional hardware devices besides tubal ligation clips (Fig. 26.4) which are used for contraception. An intrauterine device (IUD) is normally seated in the uterine cavity in a characteristic T-shape with the short arms directed toward the cornua. The Essure® device comprises two separate flexible inserts that are placed within the lumen of the fallopian tubes to prevent pregnancy (Fig. 26.5).

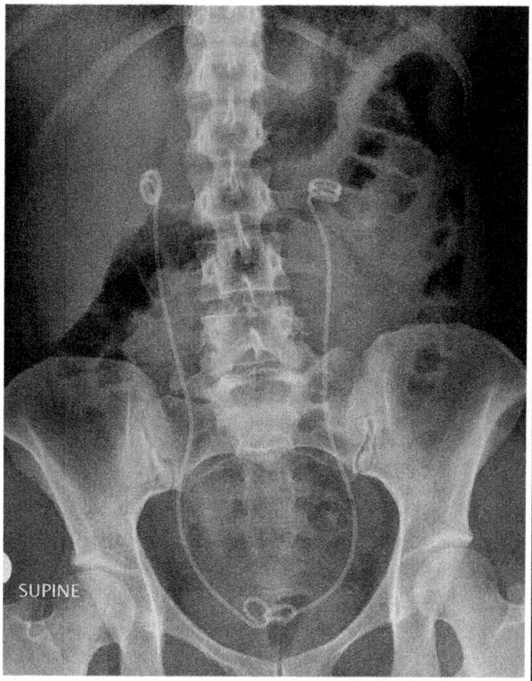

FIGURE 26.3 - URETERAL STENTS
Supine abdominal radiograph showing bilateral internal double-J ureteral stents with ends appropriately positioned in the renal pelvis and bladder

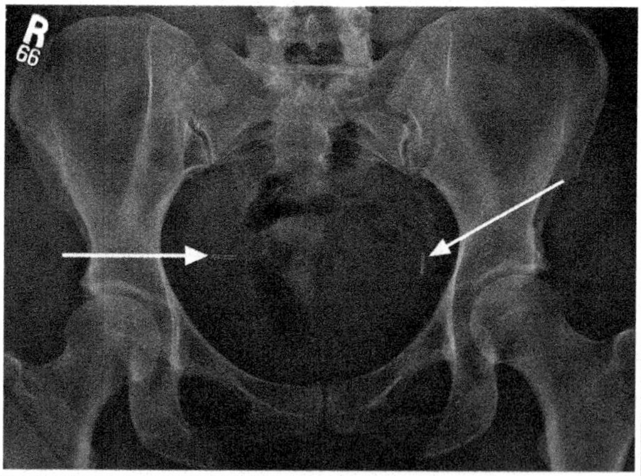

FIGURE 26.4 - TUBAL LIGATION CLIPS
AP view of the pelvis showing metallic bilateral tubal ligation clips (*arrows*) which close the Fallopian tubes

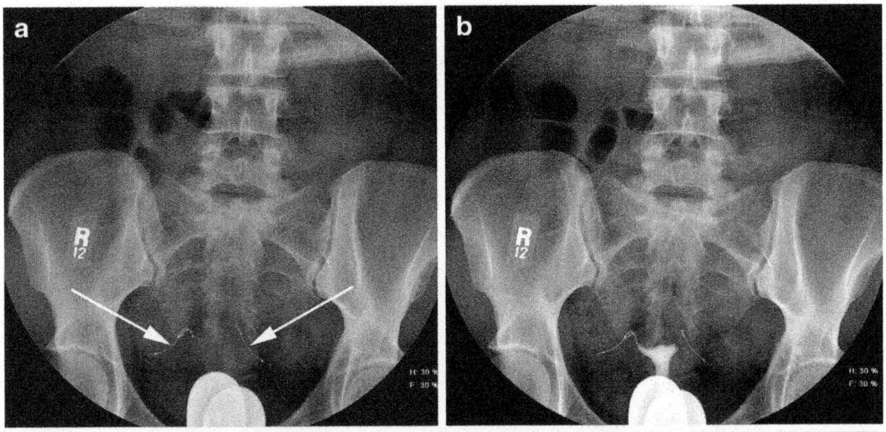

FIGURE 26.5 - ESSURE DEVICE
(**a**) Radiograph prior to hysterosalpingogram showing radio-opaque inserts (*arrows*) in both Fallopian tubes. Note the vaginal speculum in place along the inferior margin of the image. (**b**) Injection of dye through the cervical os demonstrating the uterine cavity and no flow or "free spillage" of contrast into the peritoneal space confirming the occlusion of the Fallopian tubes. Note a small air bubble in the left cornua

Vascular Hardware

Management of common vascular diseases will include the use of hardware devices. Abdominal aortic aneurysms can sometimes be treated with endovascular stent grafts. Fig. 26.6 shows an endograft along with an inferior vena cava (IVC) filter. IVC filters can be evaluated with radiography with careful attention to integrity and position (location and tilt). Arterial embolization can involve the use of metallic coils placed endovascularly which are designed to stop blood flow. Femoral arterial and venous catheters are placed much less frequently than subclavian or jugular catheters. In the neonatal population, vascular catheters are frequently seen on abdominal imaging.

Miscellaneous Hardware

Numerous other intra-abdominal devices are used and encountered during radiologic examination. Ventricular-peritoneal drainage catheters are designed to alleviate elevated intracranial pressure by draining cerebral spinal fluid (CSF) from the ventricles into the peritoneal space where it gets absorbed. A "shunt series" includes frontal and lateral radiographs of the skull, a chest x-ray, and an abdominal x-ray so

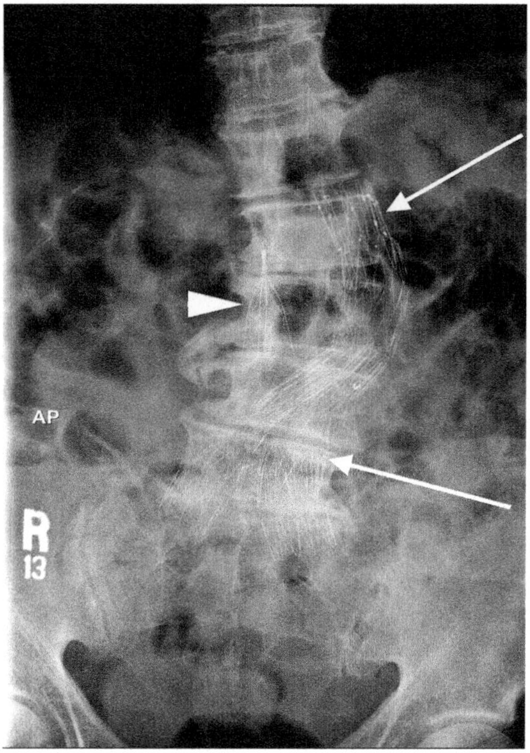

FIGURE 26.6 - TYPICAL VASCULAR HARDWARE Collimated AP radiograph of an aortoiliac endovascular stent (*arrows*) and an IVC filter (*arrowhead*). Note that the medial leg of the filter is inappropriately displaced toward the midline

that the entire course of the catheter can be scrutinized. In the abdomen, the catheter will typically coil randomly with the tip shifting its location over time. Surgical drainage catheters can be located anywhere in or around the abdomen. Drains are sometimes assessed fluoroscopically by injecting water-soluble contrast to identify the exact space that the tip is in.

Bibliography

Hunter TB, Taljanovic MS. Medical devices of the abdomen and pelvis. Radiographics. 2005; 25(2):503–23.

27 Abnormal Air Collections in the Abdomen

Objectives:
1. State the difference between an "interface" and a "line shadow."
2. State the expected radiographic findings in pneumoperitoneum in both a supine and upright patient.
3. Discuss the significance of intramural air within the bowel wall.

Pneumoperitoneum

When a hollow viscus ruptures, air (and bowel contents) is released into the abdominal cavity. "Free air" will collect in the least dependent (highest) portion of the peritoneum. Pneumoperitoneum has a broad range of etiologies from benign expected postoperative air to life-threatening hollow viscus rupture. Anytime a pneumoperitoneum is identified, it needs to be explained. Often the investigation of pneumoperitoneum begins with abdominal radiographs. If free air is noted, CT is often done to further delineate the extent of free air and determine the source.

In an upright patient, the air will collect just beneath the hemidiaphragms. In cases where a small amount of air is suspected, an upright chest radiograph, in addition to abdominal radiographs, may also be useful in detecting a pneumoperitoneum (Fig. 27.1). When the patient is not very mobile and/or there is a concern of subtle or loculated collection of "free" air outside the bowel lumen, CT is recommended.

In cases of pneumoperitoneum, the right hemidiaphragm is seen as a "line shadow." In other words, there is different radiographic density both superior and inferior to it, giving it the appearance of a line. In effect, if one was asked to measure the thickness of the right hemidiaphragm, this could be easily done when there is air beneath the hemidiaphragm. Normally, the right hemidiaphragm represents an

H. Singh et al. (eds.), *Radiology Fundamentals: Introduction to Imaging & Technology*, DOI 10.1007/978-3-319-10362-4_27

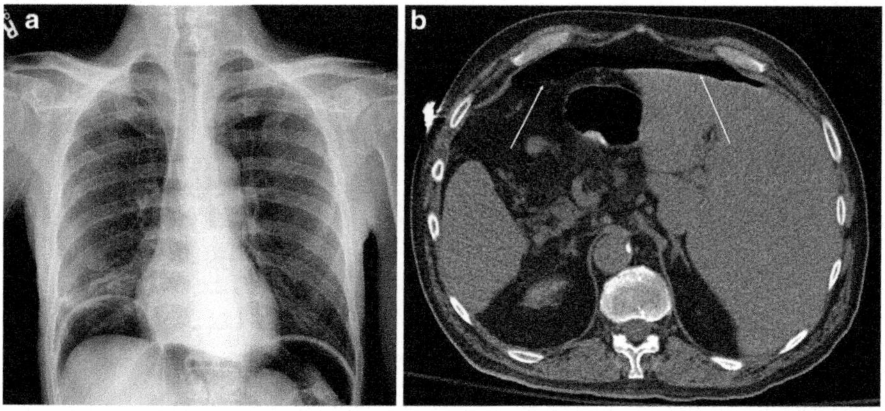

FIGURE 27.1 - PNEUMOPERITONEUM
(**a**) Note the intraperitoneal free air underneath the diaphragm on the PA chest radiograph. (**b**) Intraperitoneal free air collections (*arrows*) in a nondependent position following rupture of a hollow viscus

interface, not a line shadow. This means that only its superior margin is clearly defined by the air in the adjacent lung. Inferiorly, the soft tissue of the hemidiaphragm blends imperceptibly with the soft tissue of the dome of the liver (remember the silhouette sign). The change from interface to line shadow is often a useful finding in discerning the presence of abnormal air collections within the abdomen.

In an upright view of a patient's abdomen looking for a pneumoperitoneum, the bowel wall that is normally seen as an interface becomes visible as a line shadow due to the presence of air within the bowel lumen as well as free air within the peritoneum external to the bowel loop (known as Rigler's sign). Occasionally, intraperitoneal free air can be identified outlining the falciform ligament. In the supine position, air collects centrally within the abdomen since this, not the subdiaphragmatic region, is the highest point. For this reason, the radiographic presentation of pneumoperitoneum is different in the supine patient versus in the upright patient.

Pneumatosis Intestinalis

Sometimes air can be found within the wall of the bowel itself. This condition is referred to as pneumatosis intestinalis and can be seen in a variety of conditions from idiopathic to benign to vascular occlusion with bowel ischemia. Fig. 27.2 is an example of pneumatosis intestinalis in the cecum. Pneumatosis in infants may reflect necrotizing enterocolitis, with bowel wall ischemia, and infection.

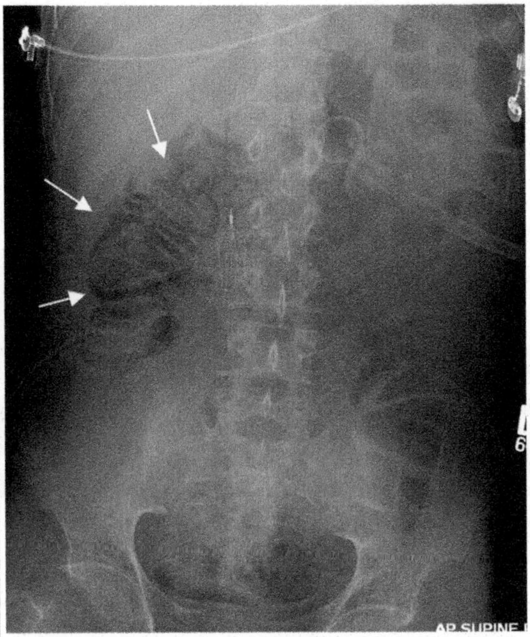

FIGURE 27.2 - PNEUMATOSIS INTESTINALIS

Portal Venous Gas

Portal venous gas is the result of dying or dead bowel and portends imminent patient demise. As the bowel necroses, gas is absorbed into the draining venous system (superior mesenteric vein and inferior mesenteric vein) and delivered to the liver via the portal vein. When this occurs, air is characteristically seen in the periphery of the liver as portal venous blood flows hepatopetaly (Fig. 27.3). Portal venous air must be differentiated from pneumobilia (air within the biliary system). Since bile flows out of the liver in the hepatofugal direction, pneumobilia is more centrally located in the liver (Fig. 27.4). Etiologies of pneumobilia are more often benign and related to prior procedures such as papillotomy. When air is peripherally located in the liver, portal venous gas must be suspected and urgently communicated to the clinical team.

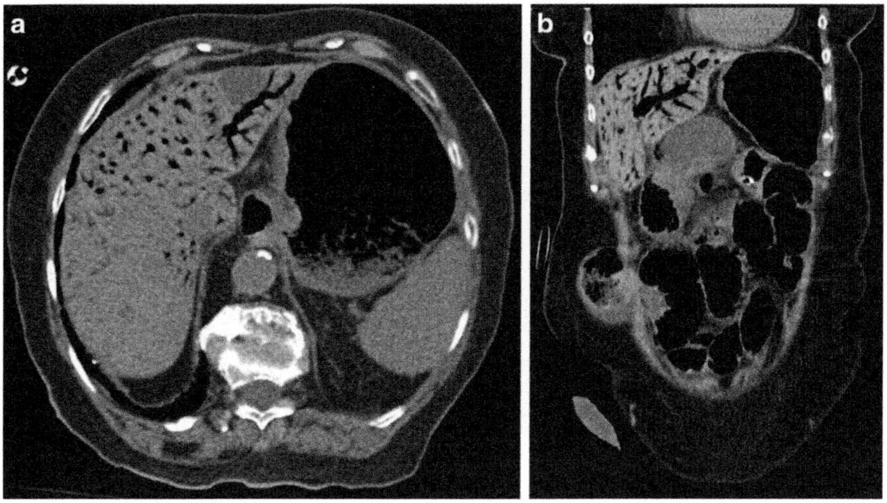

FIGURE 27.3 - PORTAL VENOUS GAS
Axial (**a**) and coronal (**b**) CT images demonstrating air within the portal veins in a more peripheral location than pneumobilia

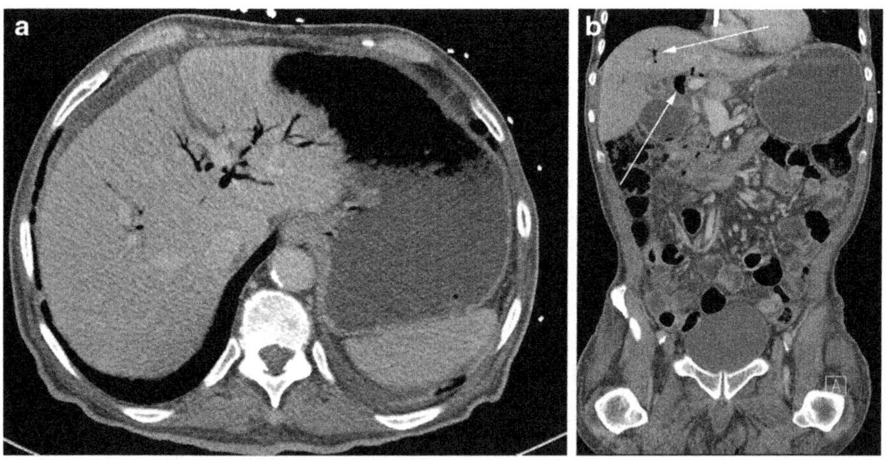

FIGURE 27.4 - PNEUMOBILIA
Axial (**a**) and coronal (**b**) CT images showing air more centrally located in the liver within the biliary tree (*arrows*)

28 Bowel Obstruction

Objectives:
1. Describe the radiologic findings of large and small bowel obstruction.
2. List criteria used to distinguish bowel obstruction from ileus.
3. Define the term "air-fluid" level.

Gas is normally present in the stomach and colon. Small accumulations of gas may be found in the duodenum and upper portion of the jejunum. Scattered collections of gas may be present throughout much of the small intestine in bedridden patients, patients on narcotics for pain relief, and those who swallow large amounts of air habitually. Air can be seen as individual accumulations of rounded or ovoid shaped air. If a single loop of normal intestine can be recognized because of gas filling, the shadow is seldom more than 5–8 cm in length. More often, the gas does not form any specific loop pattern.

Small Bowel Obstruction

When individual segments of small intestine are dilated 3–4 cm in transverse diameter, one should consider the possibility that the gas pattern is abnormal. Radiographic findings in small bowel obstruction develop over time as fluid and gas build up proximal to the obstructing process.

The gas is visualized readily in supine radiographs, but the presence of fluid can only be confirmed on upright or decubitus views. In the upright view, the gas rises above the fluid and the interface between gas and fluid forms a straight horizontal margin: an air-fluid level. Fig. 28.1 demonstrates an air-fluid level in the small bowel.

H. Singh et al. (eds.), *Radiology Fundamentals: Introduction to Imaging & Technology*, DOI 10.1007/978-3-319-10362-4_28

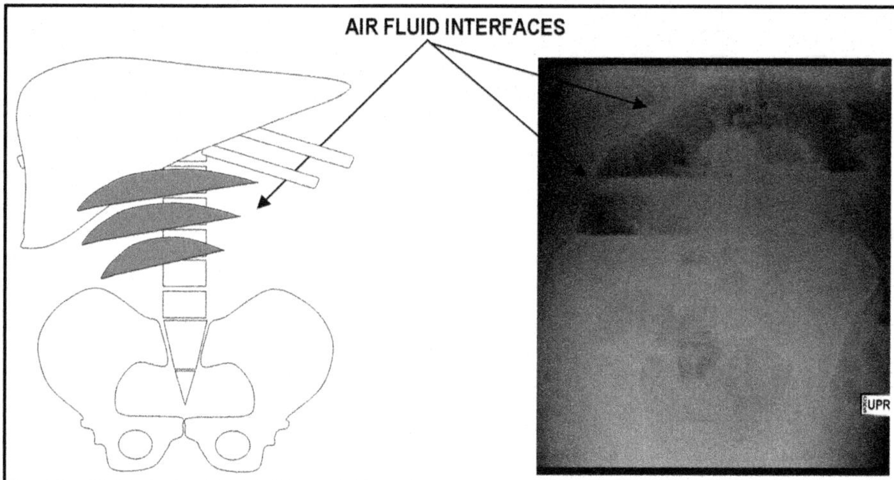

FIGURE 28.1 - AIR FLUID LEVELS
The gas rises above the fluid in the bowel lumen creating a gas-fluid interface. This can be seen normally in the stomach, but not in the small bowel

Air-fluid levels are generally considered to be abnormal in the small intestine. (Note that an air-fluid level is normally observed in the stomach because swallowed air is almost invariably present.) Air-fluid levels may be seen in the first portion of the duodenum where air may be trapped temporarily when the patient assumes the upright position. In the early stage of obstruction, only one or two such gas distended segments are visualized. With increasing time, more distended loops may become visible. For this reason, serial examinations may be necessary for the diagnosis of small bowel obstruction. As distension increases, more loops become visible and they tend to lie transversely, at different levels, so-called fighting loops. Gas-filled loops may be recognized as small intestine rather than colon when they occupy the central portion of the abdomen rather than the periphery. Also, the pattern of mucosal folds in the small bowel, the valvulae conniventes, is finer and closer together than the colonic haustra. Unlike the haustral markings of the colon, these folds traverse the entire width of the bowel loop (Fig. 28.2). This is referred to as the "stack of coins" appearance.

When two gas-filled loops of bowel lie adjacent to one another, the soft tissue density between them represents a double thickness of intestinal wall. Thus, information concerning wall thickness is available. In a simple obstruction, a double thickness of intestine wall seldom amounts to more than a few millimeters in width, since the walls are thinned considerably by the distension. Inflammatory changes in the wall or fluid in the peritoneal cavity interposed between the bowel loops results in a thickening of this soft tissue shadow. Abnormal thickening of the bowel wall is an important sign that the bowel obstruction you are dealing with is not a simple one.

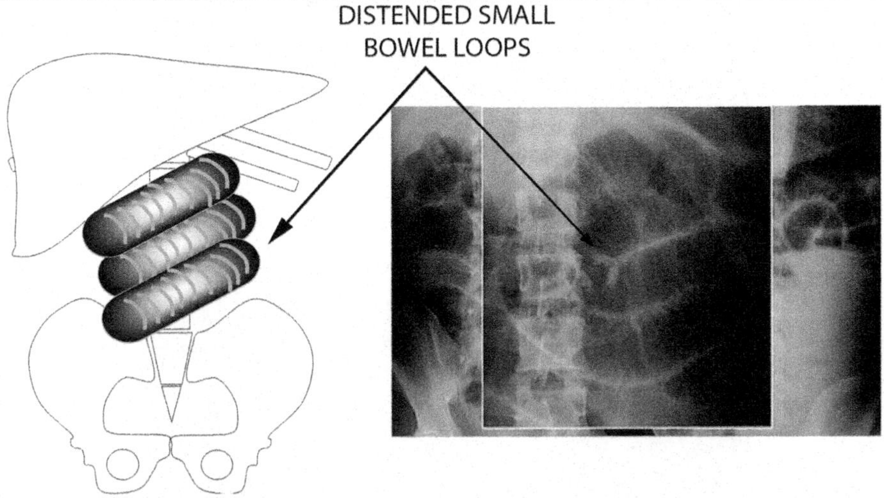

FIGURE 28.2 - DISTENDED BOWEL LOOPS
As the loops of the small bowel distend, they begin to lie on top of each other resembling a stack of coins. The mucosal markings, called valvulae conniventes, cross the small bowel in their entirety

If obstruction of the small intestine is complete, little or no gas will be found in the colon, a valuable differential point between mechanical obstruction and ileus.

If the obstruction is very proximal in the small intestine or if the patient has been decompressing the obstruction by vomiting, or if a nasogastric tube is used, the gas and fluid which would normally accumulate above an obstruction may not be present and the typical findings may not be seen on the radiograph.

Large Bowel Obstruction

As has been said previously, gas is normally present in the colon. Because of this, the diagnosis of colonic obstruction (large bowel obstruction) may be made only when the colon is thought to be dilated from the cecum to the level of the lesion. Usually the abnormally distended colon ends abruptly at the level of the lesion with the colon distal to the lesion being free of gas. This is similar to what was previously discussed for the small bowel, and the principle is the same. Namely, distended bowel is found proximal to the obstruction. There is a paucity of gas distal to the obstruction with time. The large bowel is considered pathologically dilated when the diameter is greater than 7 cm in the left colon or greater than 9 cm in the cecum.

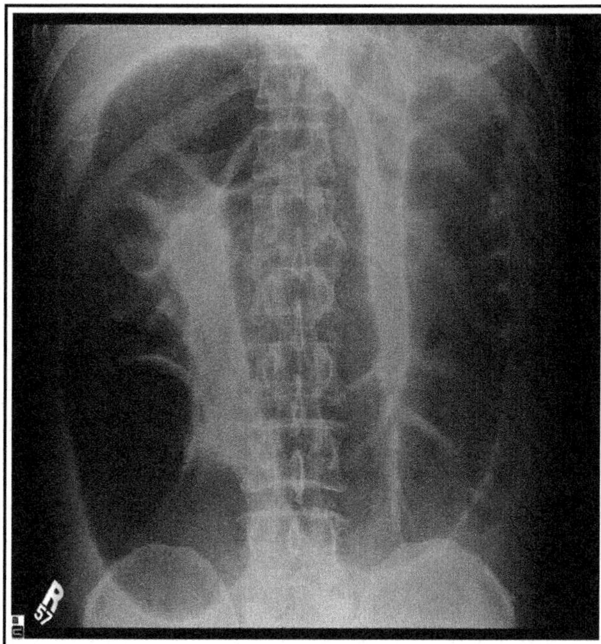

FIGURE 28.3 - TOTAL COLONIC OBSTRUCTION
Note the dilated, air-filled colon from the cecum to the proximal sigmoid. The cecum measures roughly 10 cm transversely

Fig. 28.3 shows the plain abdominal radiograph of a patient with a total colonic obstruction. Can you estimate the point within the large bowel at which the colon is obstructed?

The most likely site for obstruction of the large bowel, as might be expected, is in the rectosigmoid region since this is the most common site for colon carcinoma. The cecum undergoes the greatest distension in colonic obstruction and is the most likely site for perforation even when the obstruction is in the more distal colon. When the ileocecal valve is incompetent and the colon can decompress into the ileum and jejunum, there is less likelihood of perforation. When the cecum distends to ten or more centimeters, perforation becomes a very likely possibility. Fluid levels are of less significance in the diagnosis of colonic obstruction than they are in the small bowel.

Another common cause of large bowel obstruction is volvulus. Occurring typically in either the sigmoid colon or the cecum, volvulus is a twisting of the bowel around its mesentery causing a closed loop obstruction and proximal bowel dilation. Sigmoid volvulus is most common in elderly patients and on x-ray characteristically demonstrates a large air-filled bowel loop above the transverse colon known as the "northern exposure" sign. Cecal volvulus occurs in younger adults and often demonstrates an air-filled loop of large bowel located in the left upper quadrant.

Evaluation for Obstruction

Computed tomography (CT) is generally considered the study of choice for the evaluation of obstruction. CT may show the extent of obstruction, the cause of obstruction, transition points, free air, free fluid, and other pathology such as ischemic bowel and abnormal lymph nodes.

Contrast fluoroscopic evaluation is tailored to the area of concern. If the location of the obstruction is not known, the colon is studied first. Often, water-soluble contrast is used so that if there is a perforation, barium does not leak into the abdomen mixed with uncontained stool and bowel content. This combination could cause concretions in the abdomen.

If small bowel obstruction needs to be ruled out, and a fluoroscopic study is requested, barium can be given orally. Water-soluble contrast tastes bad and is not well tolerated by the patient. The dilated loop of bowel which is hard to see with water-soluble contrast due to dilution of the contrast at the site of obstruction may not be easy to identify. Barium will be diluted in the small bowel by small bowel fluid and will not cause concretions. If there is a concern of small bowel perforation, however, water-soluble contrast is the contrast of choice if a fluoroscopic study needs to be performed.

Ileus

There are many conditions which may reduce the motility of the large and small bowel. When this occurs, gas will accumulate within the bowel, giving a distended appearance both clinically and radiographically (Fig. 28.4). Note that the stomach and large and small bowel are all affected in equal proportion suggesting a diffuse rather than focal abnormality. These findings may be useful in distinguishing ileus from bowel obstruction, although certainly this differentiation can be difficult in some patients.

Occasionally ileus can present focally without diffuse bowel distention. Focal ileus is caused by local inflammation that impairs motility of a small segment of bowel. On plain radiography this has the appearance of a single dilated bowel loop which can be similar in appearance to bowel obstruction. CT can be used to differentiate from bowel obstruction and to find the etiology for the ileus (e.g., appendicitis, diverticulitis, cholecystitis, etc.). A focal loop of ileus, known as a "sentinel loop," can have the same appearance as an early small bowel obstruction. Serial clinical exams and follow-up radiography can help differentiate between them.

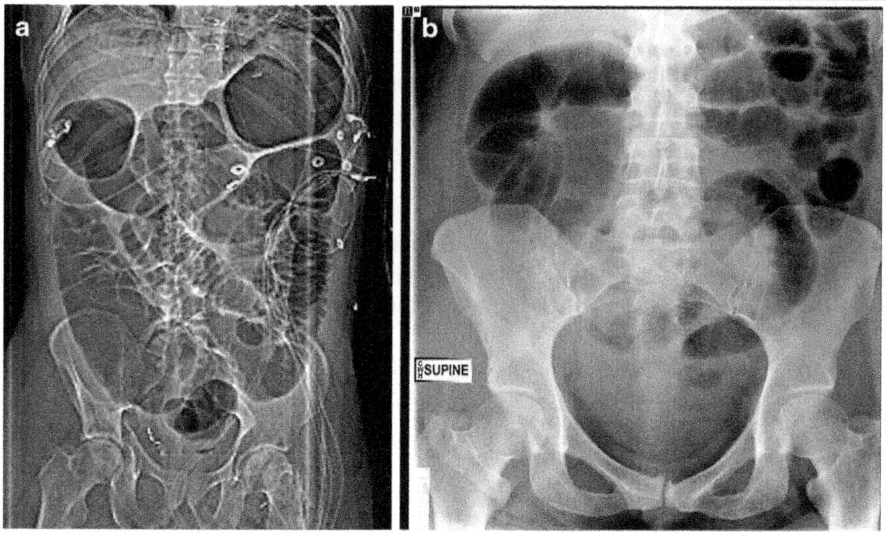

FIGURE 28.4 - ILEUS
Supine scout CT image (**a**) and radiograph (**b**) of two separate patients with ileus. Noted are multiple dilated, gas-filled small and large bowel loops measuring up to 5.5 cm in diameter throughout the abdomen and the upper portion of the pelvis. Equally distended loops of large bowel are seen extending down to the rectum

Mucosal Edema

Finally, the bowel wall may become edematous either in the presence of or the absence of obstruction. This is characterized by mucosal edema termed "thumbprinting." Bowel edema can be the result of infections, hemorrhage, or ischemia, among other causes.

Fig. 28.5 demonstrates a prominent transverse colon with thickened haustra. This usually indicates edema of the bowel wall. The acute development of these findings is concerning, and further diagnostic evaluation with CT is warranted. Conditions which chronically inflame the colon may give a similar appearance. Hence, as in all radiographic interpretations, the clinical history is essential.

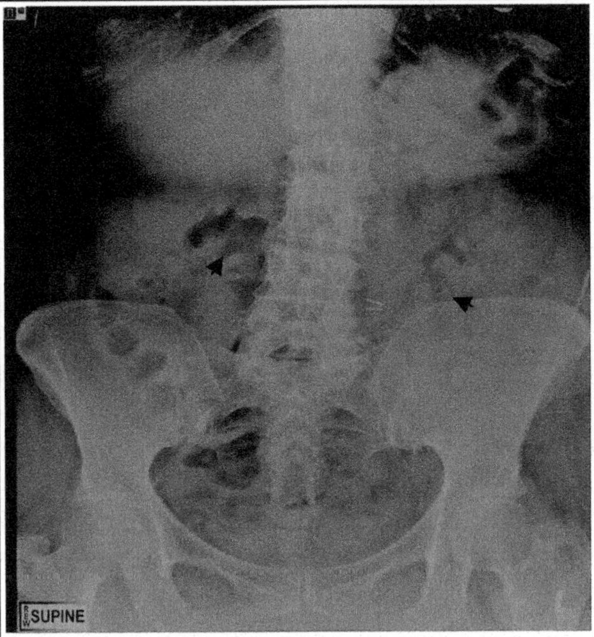

FIGURE 28.5 - LARGE BOWEL THUMBPRINTING
There is the suggestion of bowel wall thickening with thumb-printing of the transverse and descending colon (*arrows*)

29 CONCERNING ABDOMINAL MASSES

Objective:

1. Learn to recognize important masses in the abdomen including abscess, abdominal aortic aneurysm, renal cell cancer, pancreatic mass, and hepatocellular carcinoma.

Abscess

An abscess is a collection of infected fluid and inflammatory debris that has been walled off by the body's immune system. Any inflammatory process in the abdomen or pelvis such as appendicitis, diverticulitis, and Crohn's disease can lead to an abscess. Traumatic puncture wounds and foreign bodies can also result in abscess formation. Common locations for an abdominal abscess are the subphrenic and subhepatic spaces. Abscesses can also develop in organs, such as the liver (intrahepatic abscess) or kidney (renal abscess). An abscess must be promptly treated with antibiotics and either percutaneous or surgical drainage to prevent systemic infection or sepsis.

Patients with an abscess present with an increased white cell count and fever. Radiographically, an abscess appears as a loculated fluid collection with a thick, enhancing wall (Fig. 29.1). Free fluid tends to layer dependently, while fluid in an abscess remains loculated. Characteristic features of an abscess include fluid-fluid levels, septations, and, most notably, air.

Sometimes you will hear the term "phlegmon" used in similar clinical scenarios. A phlegmon is also a viscid collection of inflammatory debris that will resolve with antibiotics and generally does not require drainage or surgery. Disease processes such as appendicitis or pancreatitis can cause a phlegmon to develop. On CT, an

H. Singh et al. (eds.), *Radiology Fundamentals: Introduction to Imaging & Technology*, DOI 10.1007/978-3-319-10362-4_29

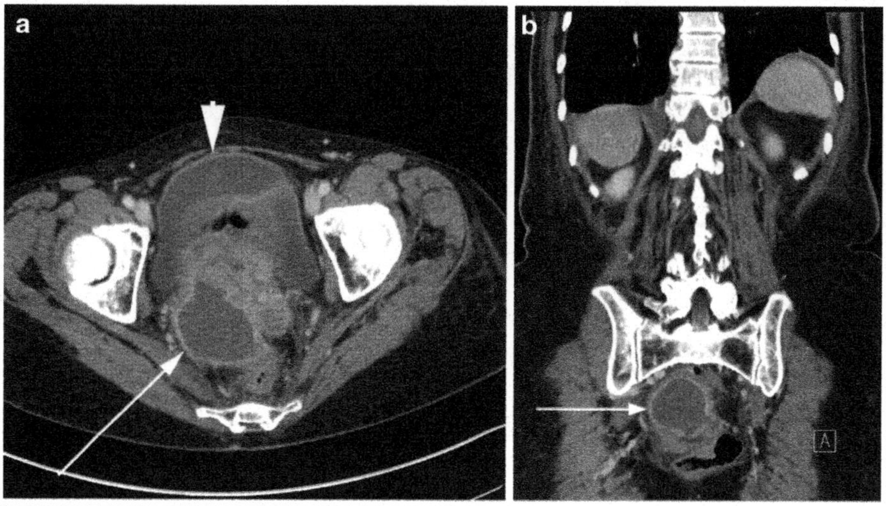

FIGURE 29.1 - ABSCESS
Axial (**a**) and coronal (**b**) CT images showing a peripherally enhancing encapsulated fluid-filled abscess (*arrow*). Note the normal appearance of the bladder (*arrowhead*) anteriorly

abscess will demonstrate fluid density (Hounsfield units < 20), while a phlegmon often demonstrates soft tissue density (Hounsfield units 20–40). A phlegmon and an abscess can be thought of as different points along the spectrum of inflammation.

Abdominal Aortic Aneurysm

Nearly 10 % of the population over age 65 has an abdominal aortic aneurysm (AAA). Smoking is a well-known risk factor. Guidelines state that ultrasound screening is indicated in any male over 65 years old with a smoking history. Once the abdominal aorta measures greater than 3 cm, it is considered to be an aneurysm. Ninety percent of AAAs are infrarenal (located below the renal arteries). Location is important for surgical or endovascular planning as repair of an aneurysm above the renal arteries is more complex.

With dissection of an aneurysm, the radiologist may see an intimal flap and the subsequent development of a false lumen. Dissection involving the origin of branch vessels (e.g., the celiac artery) can lead to ischemia of organs supplied by those branches. Worrisome radiographic findings include the hyperattenuating crescent sign which is a sign of impending aortic rupture and represents acute bleeding into the wall of the aneurysm and acute intramural hematoma (Fig. 29.2). Signs of rupture include evidence of hemorrhage in the surrounding retroperitoneal tissues or active extravasation of intravenous contrast.

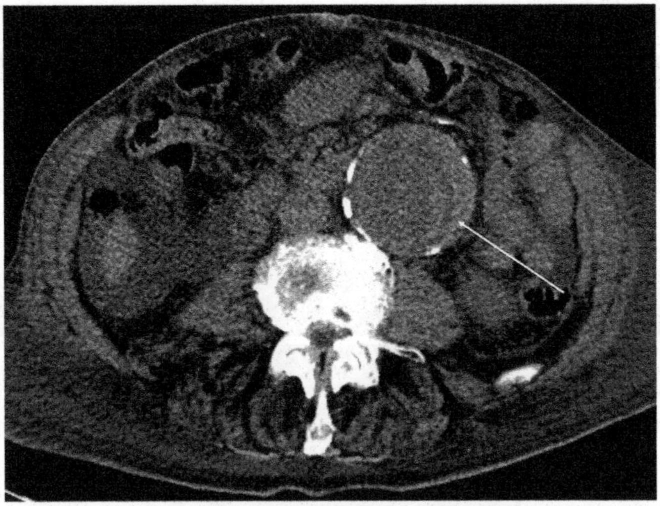

FIGURE 29.2 - ABDOMINAL AORTIC ANEURYSM
Rim calcified abdominal aortic aneurysm. *Arrow* points out the hyper-attenuating crescent sign, a sign of impending rupture

Renal Cell Cancer

Renal cell cancer (RCC) is by far the most common solid renal tumor. Smoking is a known risk factor. Other risk factors include Von Hippel–Lindau syndrome and acquired renal cystic disease from chronic hemodialysis. Renal cell cancer arises from the convoluted tubules in the renal cortex. The uncommon, yet classic, clinical triad associated with RCC is a palpable flank mass, flank pain, and hematuria. Other presenting features include fever and weight loss.

Radiographically, the tumors are heterogeneous in appearance on CT, and they appear as solid lesions or mixed cystic and solid lesions on ultrasound. The tumors show brisk enhancement after the administration of intravenous contrast (Fig. 29.3a, b). With every new diagnosis of RCC, the ipsilateral renal vein and the IVC must be examined carefully to look for tumor thrombus involvement, a relatively common occurrence with RCC (Fig. 29.3c). The surrounding renal hilar and pericaval and periaortic lymph nodes should also be examined for evidence of tumor involvement. Common sites of RCC metastasis include the lungs, bones, liver, brain, and adrenal glands. Renal cell cancer responds poorly to chemotherapy and radiation therapy. However, it is often curable with surgical resection when found early. Certain patients are candidates for less invasive techniques such as partial nephrectomy or ablation.

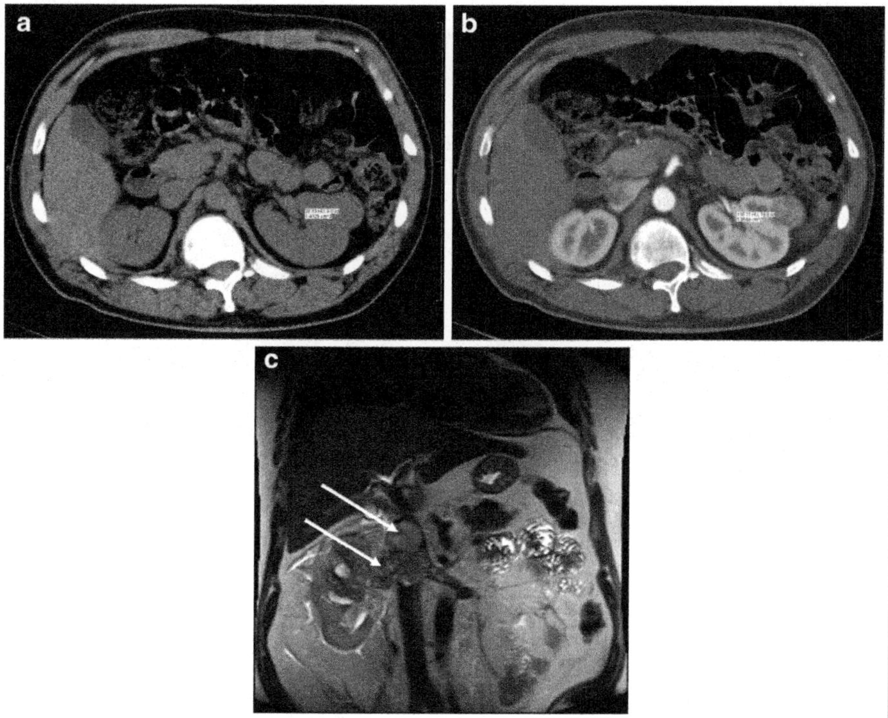

FIGURE 29.3 - LEFT RENAL MASS
(**a**) Noncontrast axial CT image shows a large isodense solid mass arising from the left kidney. Hounsfield units show a value of 30. (**b**) Enhanced CT during the arterial phase shows the same renal lesion as (**a**) which demonstrates rapid arterial enhancement. Hounsfield units measure 115, reflecting vascular enhancement in this case. (**c**) Coronal MRI image demonstrating extensive tumor thrombus in the right renal vein extending into the IVC

Hepatocellular Carcinoma

Hepatocellular carcinoma (HCC) is the most common primary hepatic malignancy in patients with chronic hepatic disease; it is very uncommon in patients without chronic liver disease. Common etiologies of chronic liver disease include chronic alcohol abuse, hepatitis B, and hepatitis C. Increasingly, hepatic steatosis and subsequent development of steatohepatitis are increasingly another cause of liver cirrhosis. Any solid hepatic mass in a cirrhotic patient is HCC until proven otherwise. HCCs develop along a pathologic continuum from a regenerative nodule to dysplastic nodule to HCC.

Patients often have clinical features of portal hypertension such as ascites, splenomegaly, variceal bleeding, and sometimes encephalopathy. The laboratory test,

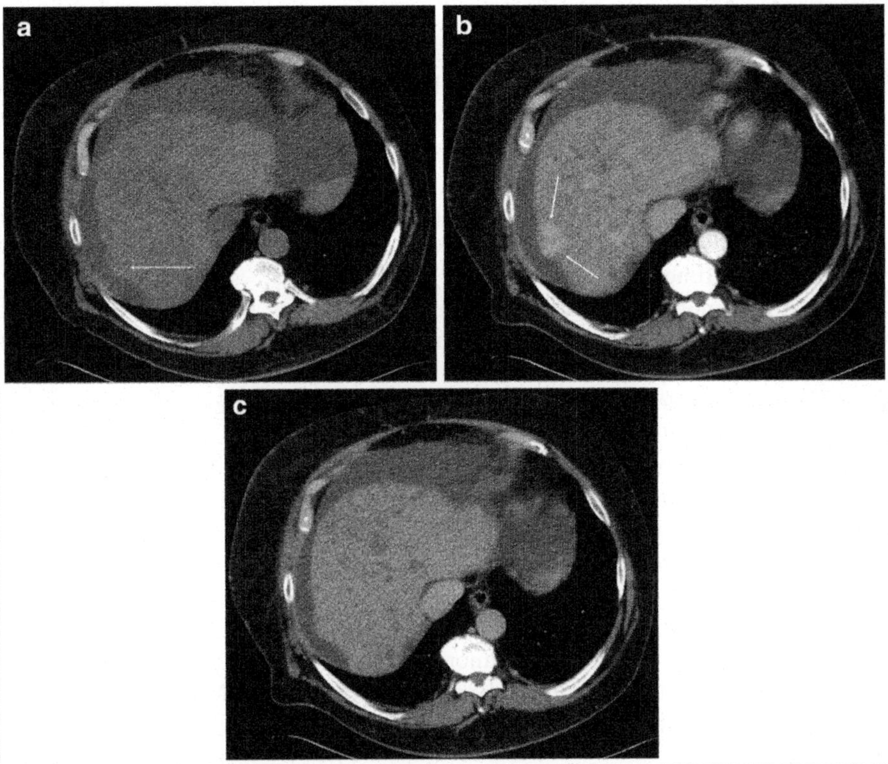

FIGURE 29.4 - HEPATOCELLULAR CARCINOMA
(**a**) Noncontrast CT shows a subtle isodense contour irregularity suggestive of a mass in the periphery of the right lobe of the liver. (**b**) Enhanced CT during the arterial phase shows avid enhancement of the mass seen in (**a**). (**c**) Enhanced CT during the venous phase shows that the mass in the periphery of the right liver has become isodense again consistent with rapid wash-out of contrast which is characteristic of a hepatocellular carcinoma

serum alpha-fetoprotein, can be used to monitor for HCC development or recurrence, in the appropriate clinical population. Radiographically, HCCs may be discrete masses but are often inconspicuous and infiltrating. The classic characteristic that assists in their identification is the fact that HCCs vigorously enhance following intravenous contrast administration (Fig. 29.4). Like renal cell carcinoma, vascular invasion by tumor thrombus is relatively common. The hepatic and portal veins must be assessed for involvement of tumor thrombus on pretreatment imaging. The definitive treatment is liver transplant. Temporizing treatments include partial hepatectomy, cryoablation, radiofrequency ablation, chemoembolization, and systemic chemotherapy. A newer treatment known as Yttrium-90 therapy is a radiation treatment delivered by radioactive spheres deposited in a similar manner as chemoembolization.

Pancreatic Mass

Solid masses in the pancreas are commonly neoplastic tumors which may be either benign or malignant. Pancreatic adenocarcinoma is a malignancy which has a very low five years survival rate despite aggressive surgical and medical treatment. The poor prognosis is due to the fact that the tumor does not manifest symptoms until late in the course of the disease. When symptoms present they often include vague abdominal pain, weight loss, and/or jaundice. Unfortunately, most tumors are not resectable at the time of diagnosis.

Pancreatic tumors are difficult to detect on imaging. Often they appear as a hypodense to isodense mass with minimal contrast enhancement on CT. They are difficult to diagnose with transabdominal ultrasound as the gland is often obscured by overlying bowel loops and bowel gas; however, lesions are often identified and biopsied with the use of endoscopic ultrasound. Sixty percent of pancreatic adenocarcinomas are located in the pancreatic head. Due to the inconspicuous nature of these tumors, indirect clues are important for determining the presence of a pancreatic tumor. The best known finding of these clues is the double duct sign (Fig. 29.5). This refers to dilation of both the common bile duct and the main pancreatic duct caused by tumor in the pancreatic head compressing the distal ends of both of the common bile duct and the pancreatic duct. When evaluating a pancreatic mass, the surgeon needs to know whether the tumor is resectable. Radiographic signs of unresectable tumor include vascular involvement (celiac artery, SMA, and portal vein) and extension beyond the pancreas into other organs.

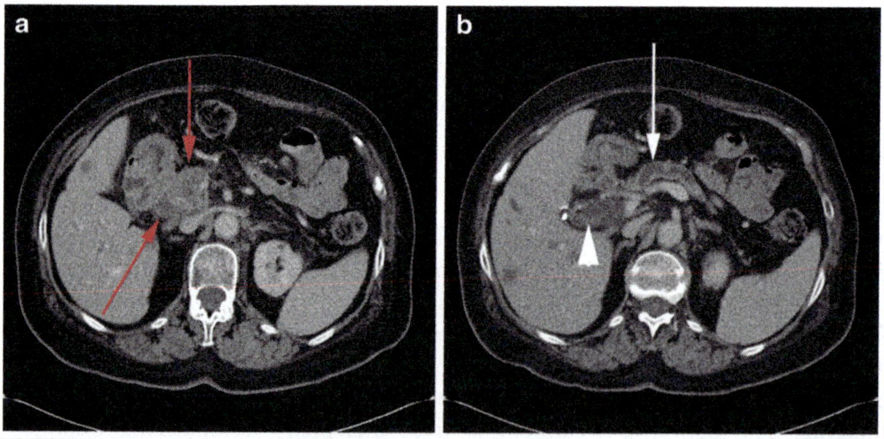

FIGURE 29.5 - PANCREATIC HEAD MASS
(**a**) Axial CT of the upper abdomen shows a heterogeneous enhancing mass in the pancreatic head (*red arrow*). (**b**) Axial slice superior to (**a**) demonstrating dilated pancreatic (*white arrow*) and common bile duct (*arrowhead*) known as the "double duct sign"

30 Fluoroscopic Evaluation of the Upper GI Tract and Small Bowel

Objectives:

1. Identify normal anatomy on a "barium swallow" and "upper GI" series.
2. Be able to differentiate mucosal versus extramucosal lesions based on radiographic findings.
3. Describe the radiographic features of malignant esophageal lesions.
4. Know the common locations for esophageal diverticuli and their radiographic appearance.
5. Name two separate methodologies for imaging the small bowel.

Radiopaque enteric contrast material is commonly employed for radiographic visualization of the gastrointestinal (GI) tract. Traditionally for the upper GI tract, a barium sulfate mixture is ingested and traced radiographically as it passes through the oropharynx, hypopharynx, esophagus, and more distal GI tract. When there is a concern of perforation or obstruction, water-soluble contrast may be used.

Fluoroscopy

GI studies are observed fluoroscopically (real-time imaging) so that peristalsis and the rate of flow of contrast can be ascertained. Close-up images of small anatomic areas are obtained at the time of fluoroscopy for the purpose of recording any specific abnormalities. Finally, static images (called overhead images), which are large images covering a large region of the GI tract, are acquired at the end of the study for the purpose of giving a geographic perspective of the contrast distribution within the GI tract.

H. Singh et al. (eds.), *Radiology Fundamentals: Introduction to Imaging & Technology*, DOI 10.1007/978-3-319-10362-4_30

Normal Esophageal Motility

Swallowed contrast is propelled by peristaltic waves, which are visible as smooth, segmental, and progressive narrowing of the esophagus. The normal peristaltic wave with swallowing is called the primary peristaltic wave. A secondary wave may occur if the patient swallows quickly after the primary swallow. These should not be confused with fixed abnormalities which may represent pathologic lesions (Fig. 30.1).

Figure 30.2 demonstrates a single image from a normal fluoroscopic exam of the esophagus. Sometimes abnormalities of esophageal motility may be manifest as so-called tertiary contractions. These appear as multiple disorganized small transient indentations of the contrast column within the esophagus and generally are related to abnormalities of the neurologic plexus, which propagate the peristaltic wave. They are commonly seen in older individuals.

When the neurologic plexus in the distal esophagus degenerates, spasm without relaxation of the lower esophageal sphincter may occur, producing a condition

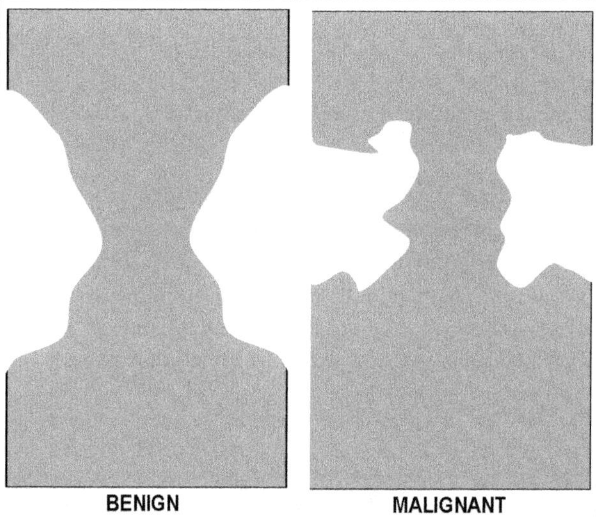

FIGURE 30.1 - CONTRAST ESOPHAGRAM
On contrast swallow studies, benign (*left*) and malignant (*right*) lesions have a different appearance. Note the gradual narrowing with smooth margins of the benign lesion versus the overhanging edges and abrupt appearance of the malignant lesion

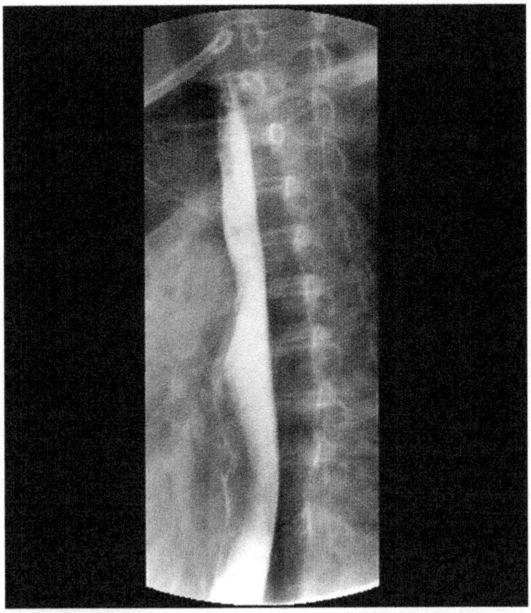

FIGURE 30.2 - NORMAL CONTRAST ESOPHAGRAM
Contrast UGI study, in this case barium, demonstrating a normal esophageal appearance

termed achalasia (Fig. 30.3). This results in distension of the proximal esophagus with collections of ingested food and secretions. A complication of achalasia is aspiration pneumonia.

Esophageal Carcinoma

Esophageal carcinomas are fixed narrowings, often with mucosal ulceration and overhanging edges or "shouldering" of the barium column.

Esophageal carcinomas occur most commonly in the mid to lower esophagus (Fig. 30.4). It may be difficult to distinguish an esophageal stricture caused by gastric acid reflux from one caused by a carcinoma. Endoscopic biopsy is often required.

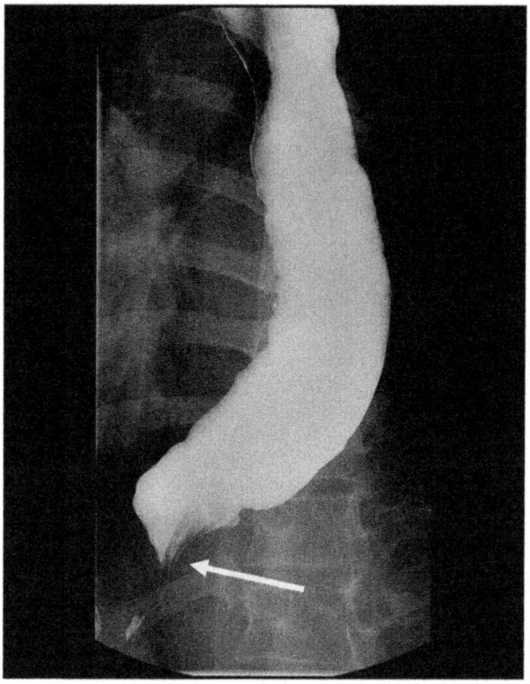

FIGURE 30.3 - ACHALASIA
Malfunction of the neurologic plexus leads to spasm of the lower esophageal sphincter resulting in a markedly distended esophagus and the classic "birds beak" (*arrow*) narrowing at the level of the lower esophageal sphincter

Esophageal Diverticuli

Diverticuli of the esophagus take two forms, traction diverticuli and pulsion diverticuli. Traction diverticuli most commonly arise in the region of the carina. They result from retraction of the inflamed subcarinal lymph nodes as they pull on the esophageal mucosa via fibrous adhesions. Pulsion diverticuli occur when the peristaltic waves exert a positive pressure within the esophageal lumen. Any weakness in the esophageal wall may lead to a "ballooning out" of the mucosa. A common location for an esophageal wall weakness is in the upper esophagus posteriorly where the constrictor muscles do not quite overlap to completely cover the esophageal wall. This is known as Killian's dehiscence. The pulsion diverticulum formed in this area is termed a Zenker's diverticulum and may be present as a mass in the upper neck. Another common location for pulsion diverticula is just above the lower esophageal sphincter. These diverticula are called epiphrenic diverticula.

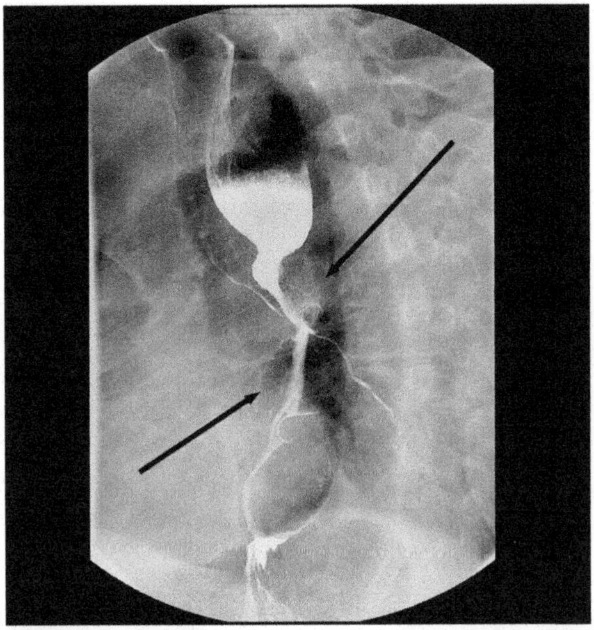

FIGURE 30.4 - ESOPHAGEAL CARCINOMA
Note the irregularity and overhanging edges (*arrows*)

Double and Single Contrast GI Studies

Standard upper GI studies include tailored evaluations of the esophagus, stomach, and duodenal bulb.

In a double contrast study, barium and air are the two contrast agents. Within the stomach, the barium is made to coat the gastric mucosa, and the air distension allows the mucosal folds of the stomach to be clearly evident (Fig. 30.5).

In a single contrast upper GI series, barium is the only contrast agent. The stomach is nearly filled with contrast material and the mucosal detail is not as evident. Single contrast studies are faster to perform and result in less radiation exposure. But, less diagnostic information is obtained.

Generally, static images of the duodenal bulb and proximal loop ("C" loop) of the duodenum as it curves around the head of the pancreas are then obtained. The duodenal bulb and post-bulbar portion of the duodenum are common places for ulceration and diverticuli formation. The duodenum ends anatomically at the ligament of Treitz which should be at the same craniocaudal level as the duodenal bulb and lies to the left of the midline.

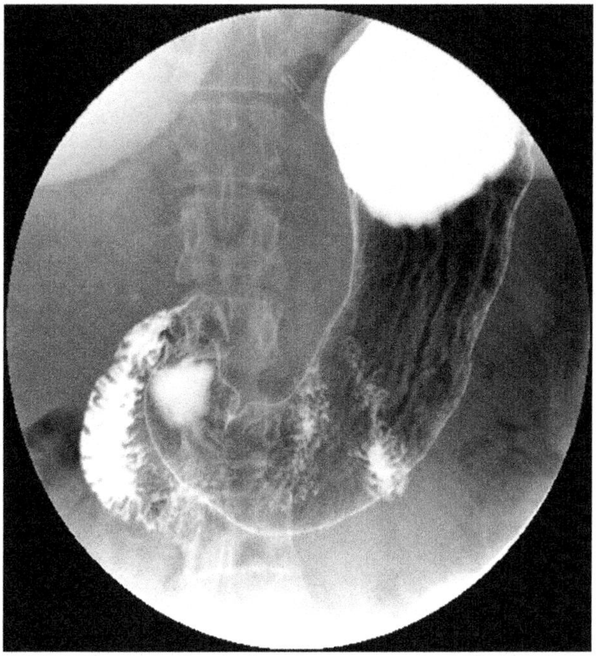

FIGURE 30.5 - DOUBLE CONTRAST GASTRIC STUDY
Note the detail of the gastric and duodenal mucosa

Filling of ulcer craters with barium produces small collections of contrast within the gastric wall. Gastric folds may radiate toward the ulcer as a result of inflammation. Ulcers may be malignant or benign and endoscopic biopsy is often required for evaluation.

Adenocarcinoma is the most common gastric malignancy and can present as an irregular solitary filling defect or as a diffuse infiltrative lesion that narrows the gastric body and antrum and makes it rigid, termed “linitis plastica.”

Small Bowel Follow-Through

A single contrast study of the contrast column may be followed through the small bowel as it passes distally through the GI tract, termed “a small bowel follow-through” (Fig. 30.6). This will reveal gross abnormalities such as mucosal masses, strictures, and mass effect displacing the small bowel loops. The small bowel follow-through terminates when contrast is seen within the cecum of the colon, having passed through the terminal ileum and the ileocecal valve.

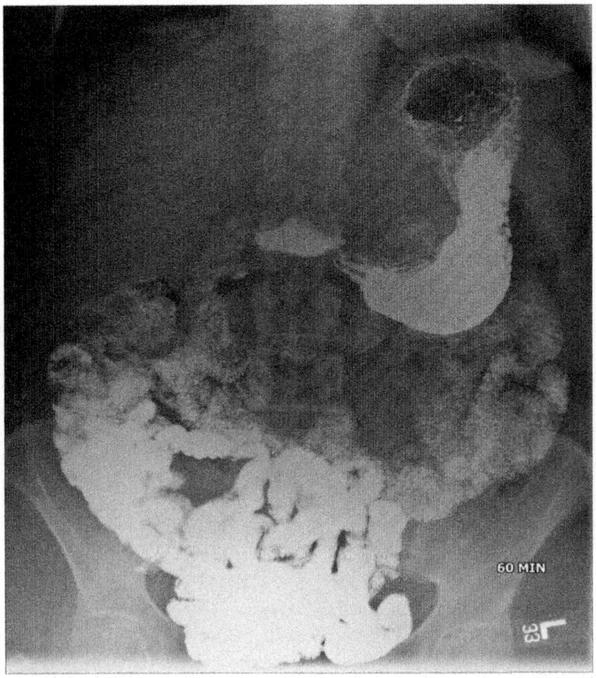

FIGURE 30.6 - SMALL BOWEL FOLLOW-THROUGH
Detail of the mucosal lining is visible as barium passes through the small bowel

Conventional Enteroclysis

A double contrast study of the small bowel, termed an "entcroclysis," may be performed for the purpose of further elucidating small bowel anatomy. By placing an enteric tube distal to the ligament of Treitz, occluding the jejunal lumen with a balloon and injecting soluble barium and methylcellulose as a "solid column," the double contrast effect is achieved. Multiple single exposure images of the small bowel are obtained with the fluoroscopy machine. The study is concluded once contrast reaches the cecum.

Small bowel malignancies may be either primary or metastatic and usually will appear as focal narrowing or strictures of the small bowel and/or nodular filling defects. This study is also useful for detecting low-grade small bowel obstruction secondary to Crohn's disease and postoperative adhesions (Fig. 30.7). Active Crohn's disease can also be detected with this type of examination.

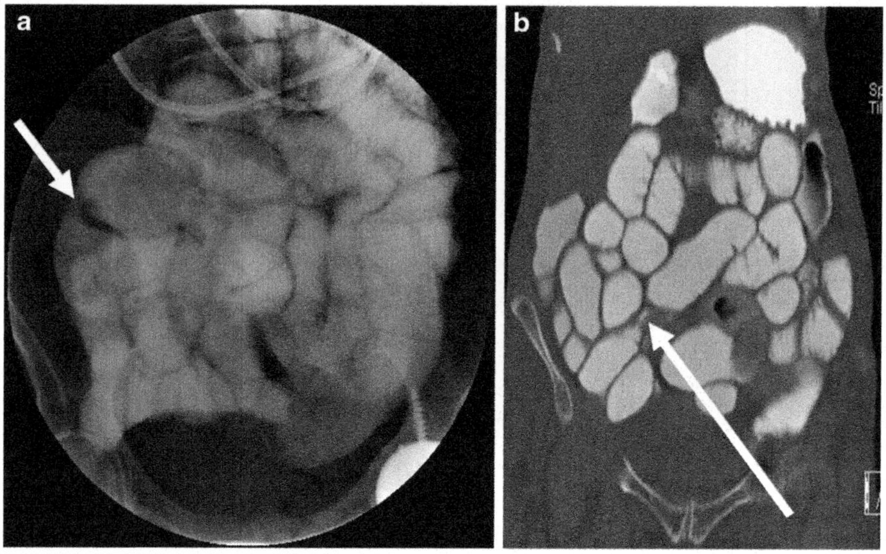

FIGURE 30.7 - CONVENTIONAL VERSUS CT ENTEROCLYSIS
(**a**) Conventional enteroclysis demonstrates a focal area of narrowing in the distal ileum (*arrow*). (**b**) Coronal image from a CT enteroclysis of the same patient demonstrates the focal area of narrowing in the distal ileum in the same location as the narrowing seen on conventional enteroclysis (*arrow*). CT enteroclysis had the added advantage of being able to demonstrate multiple different areas of narrowing in this patient (not shown) as well as evaluating bowel wall thickness and extraluminal pathology

This study is more difficult for the radiologist to perform and for the patient to tolerate. Therefore, it is used only in selected situations.

CT Enteroclysis

This type of study evaluates the small bowel in a similar manner to conventional enteroclysis. However, barium and methylcellulose are not used as contrast agents. The patient will receive either positive (radiopaque) contrast, such as barium or diluted water-soluble contrast, or negative (radiolucent) contrast, such as water, prior to being taken to the CT scanner. Typically the scan is performed once contrast has reached the cecum. CT enteroclysis is more sensitive for the detection of small strictures and mucosal inflammation such as in Crohn's disease.

Postoperative Imaging

Fluoroscopy is also useful in the postoperative evaluation of patients that have undergone partial GI resection. In the upper GI tract, fluoroscopy with a water-soluble nonionic contrast agent is commonly performed to identify anastomotic leakage or stenosis. Barium is contraindicated when leak is suspected because it can stimulate an inflammatory response and peritonitis.

31 Imaging of the Colon

Objectives:

1. Explain the difference between a single and double contrast barium enema.
2. List the typical findings seen in colonic malignancies.
3. Describe the radiographic appearance of colonic diverticuli and polyps.
4. Develop a basic understanding of the principles of CT colonography (virtual colonoscopy).

As with the upper GI series, fluoroscopic colonography can be performed in either a single or double contrast fashion. In single contrast studies, the colon is filled only with opaque contrast such as barium or water-soluble contrast. This demonstrates an extrinsic displacement of the colon, such as might be seen in a pelvic mass in a patient with a gynecological malignancy, to the greatest advantage. Strictures and large intraluminal filling defects may also be identified (Fig. 31.1). Double contrast studies involve partially filling the colon with barium followed by insufflation with air (or carbon dioxide) via a rectal tube placed in the rectum for the purpose of elucidating polyps, early carcinomas, or inflammatory bowel disease. If there is a concern of obstruction or perforation, single contrast water-soluble enema may be used (Fig. 31.2a).

An important part of the barium enema study is thorough bowel preparation for the examination. Barium studies cannot be performed without adequate preparation and this is often quite difficult for the patients. Patients who undergo barium enemas ingest a clear liquid diet and take laxatives a day or two before the examination for the purpose of clearing the GI tract of stool.

Figure 31.2b is a single image from normal double contrast barium enema study. On the normal barium enema study, you should be able to identify the rectal ampulla, the sigmoid colon, descending colon, transverse colon, ascending colon, and cecum. Filling of the appendix is variable, even when normal and present.

H. Singh et al. (eds.), *Radiology Fundamentals: Introduction to Imaging & Technology*, DOI 10.1007/978-3-319-10362-4_31

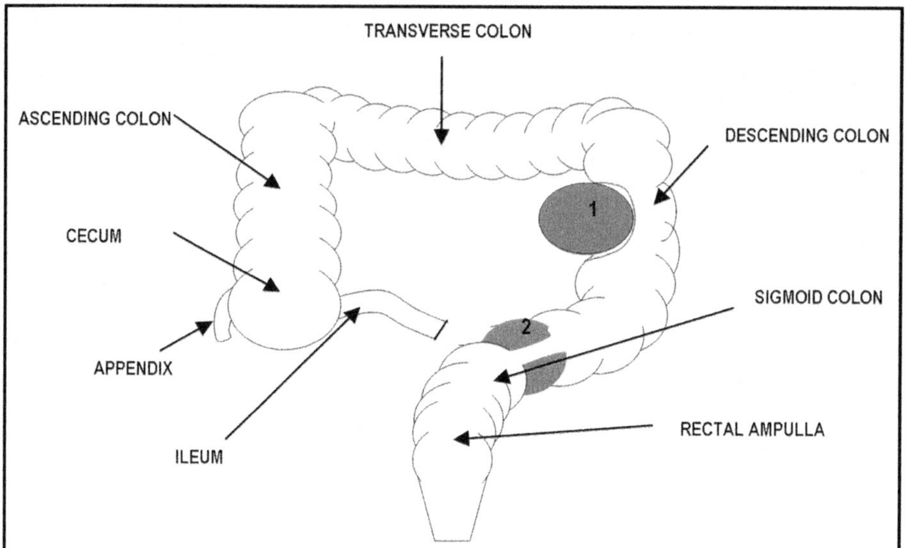

FIGURE 31.1 - SEGMENTS OF THE COLON
Note the different segments of the colon. Also note the different effects an extrinsic or mural mass (*1*) will have on the colon versus an intrinsic/mucosal lesion (*2*)

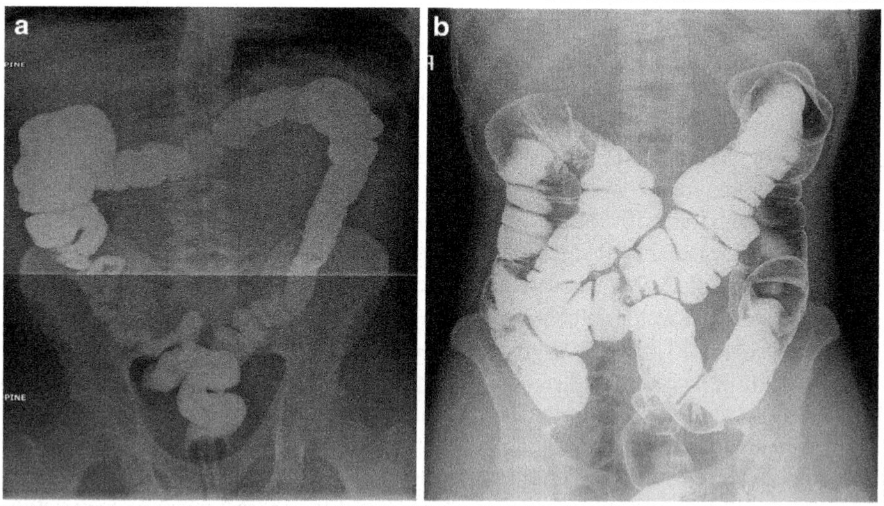

FIGURE 31.2 - (A) SINGLE CONTRAST AND (B) DOUBLE CONTRAST ENEMA
Although a single contrast study may be easier to perform, mucosal detail is better seen on the double contrast study

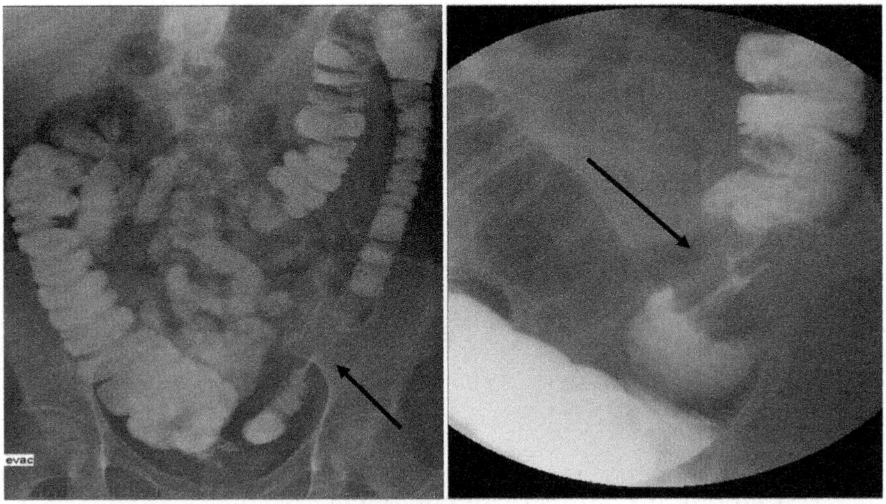

FIGURE 31.3 - APPLE CORE LESION OF THE SIGMOID COLON
Again note the abrupt caliber change and the irregular margins (*arrows*)

Note that the barium column is impinged upon by regularly occurring mucosal folds called haustra. These haustra are somewhat less prominent in the rectosigmoid region. Loss of normal haustral markings may indicate pathology.

Abnormalities of the colon may be intrinsic (mucosal) or extrinsic. Figure 31.3 demonstrates a typical "apple core" lesion of the sigmoid colon, in this case a colonic adenocarcinoma. This extrinsic abnormality on fluoroscopy did not represent normal colonic peristalsis. There are overhanging edges and there is disruption of the normal mucosal pattern within the narrowed segment. The rectosigmoid region is the most common site of colonic carcinoma.

Colonic Diverticula and Polyps

Figure 31.4 demonstrates numerous colonic diverticula in the region of the sigmoid colon. Diverticula are outpouchings of colonic mucosa between weak taenia coli muscles. They are more common with age.

Polyps can be either benign or premalignant. Adenomatous polyps are on the spectrum of premalignant lesions that with time progress to adenocarcinoma. Barium enema, especially a double contrast barium enema, is a relatively low-cost, low-risk procedure for the detection of these polyps. Please note that double contrast barium enema is less sensitive than colonoscopy at detecting small polyps. Colonoscopy has largely replaced barium enemas; however, it is more expensive and carries a higher risk of complications including perforation.

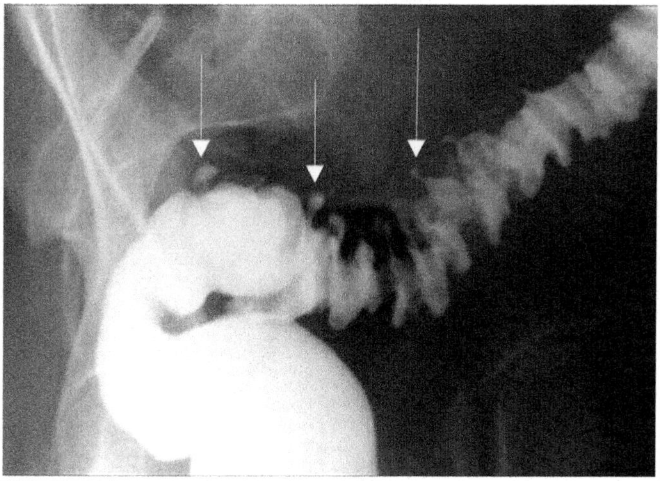

FIGURE 31.4 - SIGMOID DIVERTICULI
Multiple diverticular outpouchings within the sigmoid colon consistent with diverticulosis

CT Colonography (Virtual Colonoscopy)

Double contrast barium enemas (DCBEs) are becoming increasingly obsolete studies in the evaluation of the colon, because of the relatively lower sensitivity in detecting colonic polyps compared to optical colonoscopy.

There is a relatively new screening tool that is almost as sensitive as optical colonoscopy in the detection of small polyps > 5 mm in diameter. This tool is called computed tomography colonography (CTC) or "virtual colonoscopy." Several multicenter studies have shown that CTC is almost as sensitive (98–99 % sensitivity) in the detection of polyps greater than 5 mm as optical colonoscopy.

For this type of study, the large bowel is prepped in the same way as for an optical colonoscopy. The patient is placed in the CT scanner and a rectal tube is inserted in the rectum, and the colon is distended with carbon dioxide via a special insufflation pump. The CT scanner is used to obtain very thin slices through the abdomen and pelvis, and images are reconstructed in axial, coronal, and sagittal planes. The patient is then rescanned in the prone position (Figs. 31.5, 31.6, and 31.7).

The CT images are then reviewed using special software in either 2-D mode (axial, coronal, or sagittal) or 3-D mode (virtual colonoscopy) or both. Colonic polyps are considered significant if they measure > 5 mm from the base of the stalk to the top of the polyp. In general, polyps < 5 mm on CTC are not reported, or if they are reported, a recommendation of follow-up colonoscopy (optical or CT) in 5–7 years can be made.

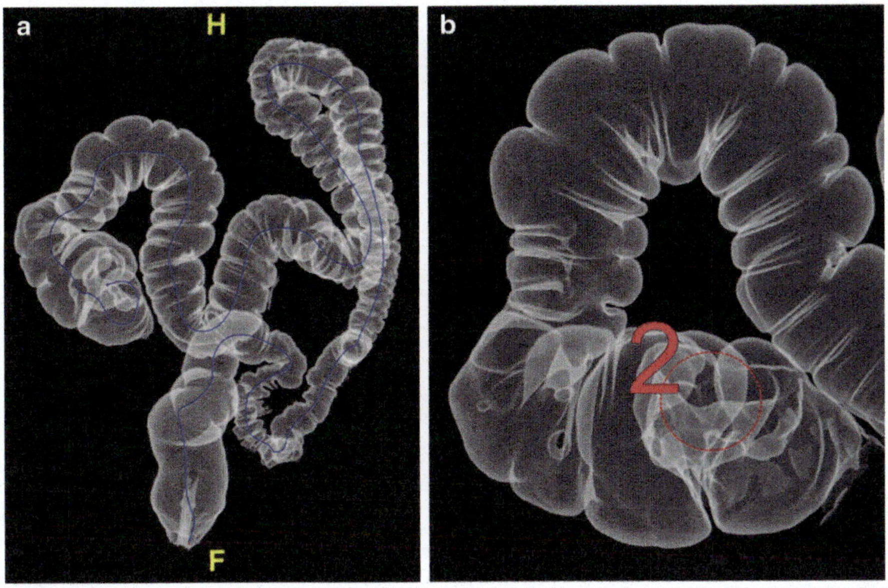

FIGURE 31.5 - CT COLONOGRAPHY
(**a**) This demonstrates a "double contrast" image obtained by the CT scanner and is used as a "road map" during the virtual colonoscopy portion of the study. (**b**) This is a magnified "double contrast" view of the cecum. There is a large filling defect in the cecum

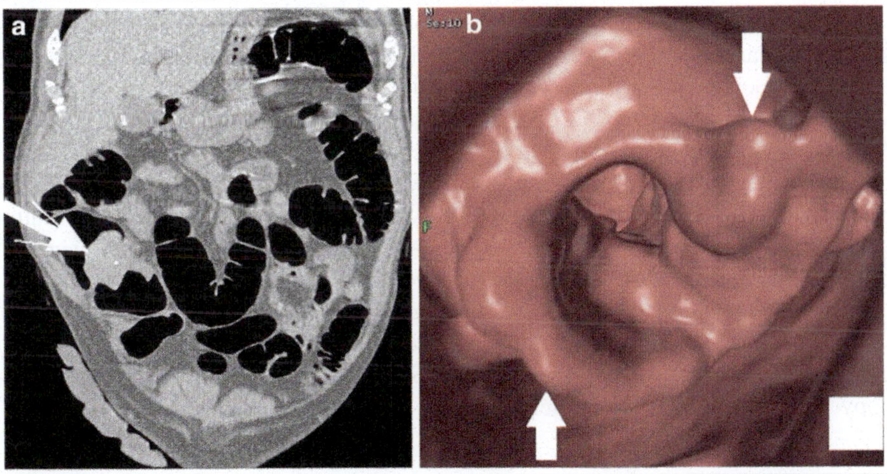

FIGURE 31.6 - CT COLONOGRAPHY
(**a**) Coronal 2-D CT image of the colon demonstrates a large irregular filling defect in the cecum (*arrow*). (**b**) This is a 3-D CT image of a "virtual colonoscopy" study demonstrating the same large mass in the cecum (*arrow*) as seen in (**a**). Biopsy specimen of this large mass came back as invasive adenocarcinoma, T4

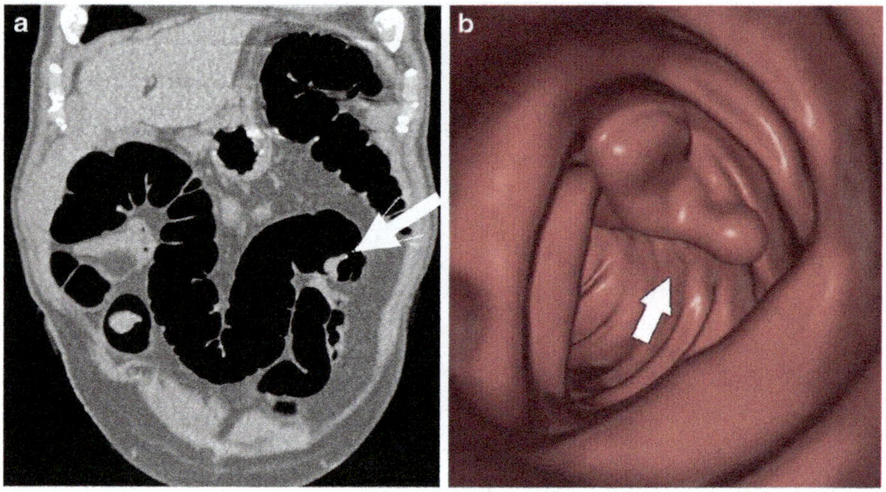

FIGURE 31.7 - CT COLONOGRAPHY
(**a**) Coronal 2-D CT image of the colon also shows a polyp in the transverse colon in the same patient (*arrow*). (**b**) This is a 3-D CT image of a "virtual colonoscopy" study in the same patient, demonstrating the polyp in the transverse colon (*arrow*). Biopsy specimen of this polyp came back as benign adenoma

There is some controversy over how polyps measuring between 6 and 9 mm should be managed. Ultimately it is the patient and treating physician preferences and any associated comorbid conditions that dictate how these polyps will be dealt with. In general, if there are 1–2 polyps measuring 8–9 mm and the patient is young, optical colonoscopy with polypectomy is recommended. In a young patient with < 3 polyps between 6 and 7 mm, follow-up in 3 years by colonoscopy (optical or CT) is recommended. If there are > 3 polyps, polypectomy is recommended, no matter what the age of the patient. Polyps > 10 mm at any age should be removed by optical colonoscopy and sent for pathology evaluation.

If the patient is 50 years and CTC is negative for significant polyps or masses, optical colonoscopy is recommended in 5 years. If the patient is 55 years and optical colonoscopy is negative for polyps or masses, follow-up every 10 years by colonoscopy (optical or CT) is recommended.

32 Imaging of the Gallbladder

Objectives:

1. State the strengths and weaknesses of each of the following radiographic tests used for evaluation of the gallbladder and related structures: ultrasound, IDA scan, percutaneous transhepatic cholangiogram, ERCP, and CT scan.
2. Understand the typical imaging findings of acute cholecystitis on ultrasound.

Right upper quadrant pain is one of the most common clinical presentations, and the gallbladder is one of the most frequently imaged organs in this setting. There are numerous radiographic tests for evaluation of the gallbladder. This section discusses each of these briefly, but is certainly not complete in its coverage of the various limitations and sequencing of these tests. Of note, radiology is not the only specialty to image the gallbladder as emergency department physicians and surgeons commonly image this organ at the bedside using ultrasound.

The Gallbladder on Plain Radiograph

Figure 32.1 shows discreet radiopacities in the right upper quadrant of the abdomen, each measuring approximately 1 cm in size. Based on the radiographic density compared to the ribs, one can easily surmise that these are densely calcified. They represent calcified gallstones within the gallbladder. Gallstones are composed primarily of cholesterol and therefore most are lucent on abdominal radiographs. Only 10–15 % of gallstones calcify sufficiently for visualization on a plain radiograph.

H. Singh et al. (eds.), *Radiology Fundamentals: Introduction to Imaging & Technology*, DOI 10.1007/978-3-319-10362-4_32

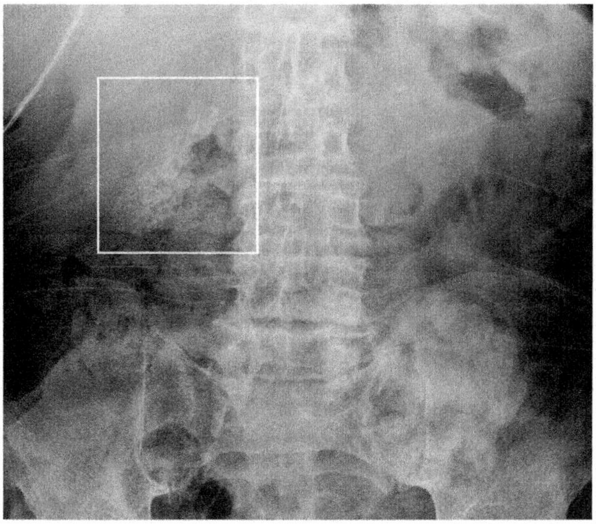

FIGURE 32.1 - GALLBLADDER STONES
The appearance and location of these calcifications are typical of gallstones

Visible gallstones are seen as lamellated calcific densities in the right upper quadrant of the abdomen, which are usually clustered in groups. They range in size from several millimeters to several centimeters.

A uniformly dense calcification of the entire gallbladder wall, termed "porcelain gallbladder," is associated with chronic gallbladder inflammation. Porcelain gallbladder is considered a premalignant condition that degenerates to gallbladder carcinoma in approximately 10 % of cases.

Gallbladder on Ultrasound

Ultrasound is the preferred method for detecting the presence of gallstones. Its advantages include the fact that no ionizing radiation is employed and that the test may be performed in a single appointment.

Gallstones within the gallbladder are seen as bright echoes within the anechoic, bile-filled gallbladder (Fig. 32.2). Distal to the bright echoes representing the gallstones, there is "shadowing" because of non-transmission of sound through the stones. This is seen as dark bands without any echoes similar in configuration to the beams of a car's headlights and is sometimes called the "headlight sign." Ultrasound is made more difficult in patients with copious bowel gas since sound is poorly

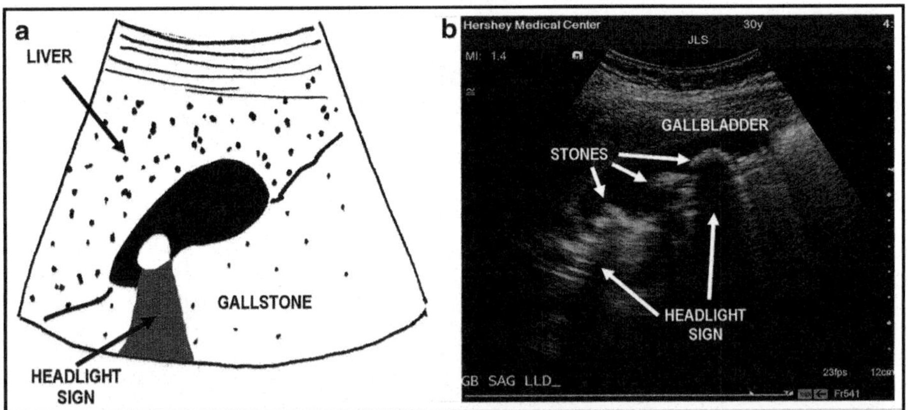

FIGURE 32.2 - GALLSTONES ON ULTRASOUND
In the above diagram (**a**) representing an ultrasound image (**b**), the gallstone in the gallbladder has an acoustic shadow behind it called the "headlight sign"

transmitted through air. Ultrasound is also difficult in very obese patients since the sound is greatly attenuated by the thick body wall.

Characteristic findings on ultrasound in acute cholecystitis include gallbladder distention, wall thickening (>3 mm), pericholecystic fluid, nonmobile stone in the gallbladder neck or common bile duct (CBD), and sonographic Murphy's sign. In the case of choledocolithiasis (stones in the CBD), the CBD may be dilated to 7 mm diameter or greater. Note that the CBD may be prominent if there is history of cholecystectomy.

Hepatobiliary Scintigraphy

Nuclear medicine studies may also be used in evaluating possible gallbladder dysfunction (see Chap. 37, "Gastrointestinal Nuclear Medicine"). These studies are often performed when other imaging is equivocal and additional evaluation is needed. A group of compounds in the iminodiacetic acid (IDA) group are employed. Each of these is labeled to a radioactive compound and injected intravenously. The compound is then selectively extracted from the blood pool by the hepatocytes and excreted through the bile ducts with subsequent filling of the gallbladder and spillage into the duodenum. This occurs according to a predictable time course.

Failure to visualize the gallbladder at the appropriate time may indicate a cystic duct obstruction (e.g., from gallstones) or some degree of dysfunction (such as seen in chronic cholecystitis). An example of a biliary leak on hepatobiliary scintigraphy is given (Fig. 32.3).

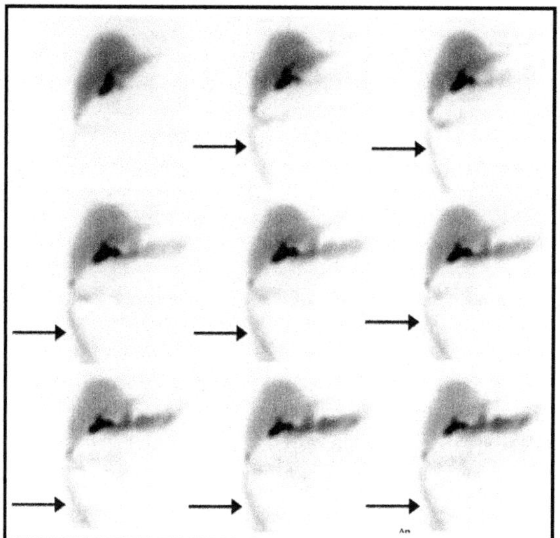

FIGURE 32.3 - BILIARY LEAK ON HIDA SCAN There is a normal hepatic extraction of radiotracer and excretion/clearance into the biliary system (*black* structures). Note the increased tracer activity within the abdominal cavity. The radiotracer tracks along the inferior edge of the right lobe of the liver. Findings are consistent with bile leak

Visualizing the Biliary Tree

Contrast may be used to directly opacify the biliary tree (Fig. 32.4). This can be done from one of two approaches (Fig. 32.5). A percutaneous transhepatic cholangiogram (PTC) is performed by placing a needle through the abdominal wall directly into one of the intrahepatic bile ducts. Contrast is then injected through the biliary tree and flows distally toward the point of obstruction. This is performed by interventional radiologists. Alternatively, gastroenterologists can cannulate the ampulla of Vater and inject contrast into the biliary tree in a retrograde manner through the endoscope in a procedure called endoscopic retrograde cholangiopancreatography (ERCP). This will likewise opacify the biliary tree and point out any filling defects or focal narrowing. An additional advantage of ERCP is that the pancreatic duct can also be visualized.

Often, following gallbladder removal, a "T-tube" is left in place to serve as a stent and prevent bile duct obstruction immediately following surgery. When the question of a retained gallstone within the biliary tree or obstruction to biliary flow due to postsurgical stricture or edema is raised, contrast may be infused through the T-tube, opacifying the biliary tree and demonstrating whether or not an abnormality is present (Fig. 32.6).

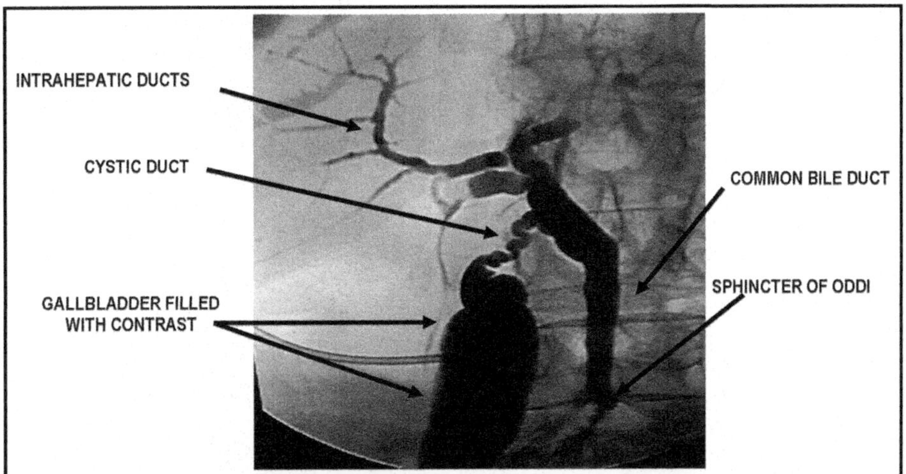

FIGURE 32.4 - GALLBLADDER AND ADJACENT STRUCTURES
On this cholecystostomy study, contrast is injected via the indwelling gallbladder drain. Note the contrast-opacified gallbladder and the cystic duct as well as the adjacent biliary structures

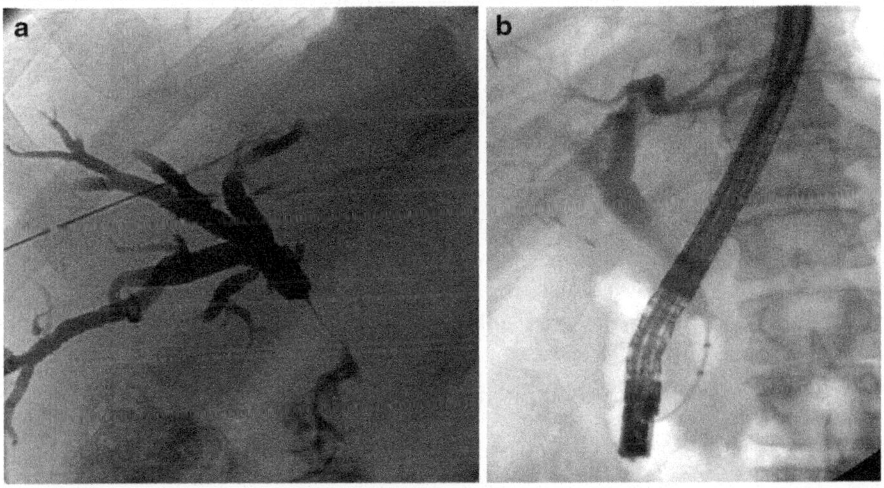

FIGURE 32.5 - PTC (A) AND ERCP (B)
In the PTC, contrast is introduced transhepatically. In the ERCP, contrast is introduced in a retrograde fashion

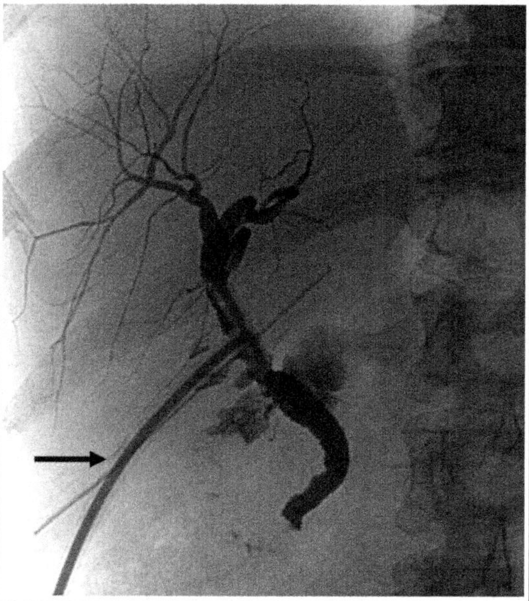

FIGURE 32.6 - CHOLANGIOGRAM
Contrast is injected through the T-tube (*arrow*) to opacify the biliary tree

Gallstones on CT

Finally, in the course of performing an abdominal CT for other reasons, gallstones may often be demonstrated as radiographically dense foci within the fluid-filled gallbladder (Fig. 32.7). Gallstones may not be seen on CT scan if they are composed mostly of cholesterol and not calcium.

Remember that the diagnosis of gallbladder disease and its complications remain complex and challenging. The use of a radiologist as a consultant to recommend and perform one or more of the appropriate studies described above will help to find the accurate diagnosis.

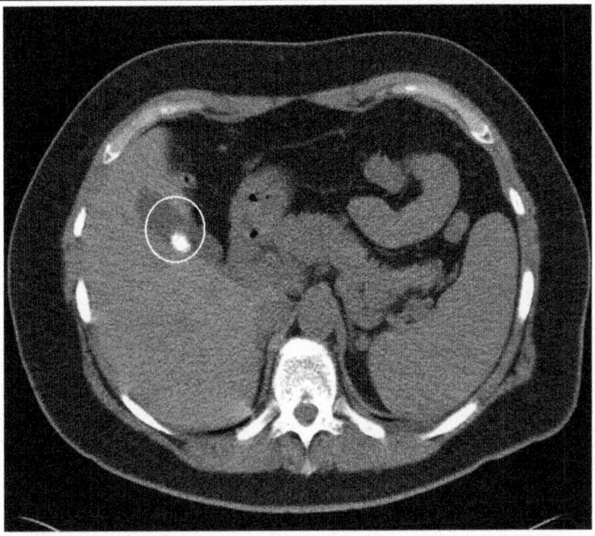

FIGURE 32.7 - GALLSTONE ON CT
Appearance of a gallstone with significant amounts of calcium, on CT

33 Incidental Abdominal Lesions

Objective:
Learn to recognize several lesions found incidentally on CT scans and understand a management algorithm.

Introduction

The advent of high-quality cross-sectional imaging has revolutionized medical and surgical diagnosis and treatment. However, it has also led to the discovery of numerous incidental findings that may require evaluation to determine whether they may be safely dismissed or if further workup is required.

This chapter discusses several of the most common incidental findings and offers evidence-based management recommendations based upon the *Journal of the American College of Radiology* article on this subject (Berland et al. 2010). The guidelines listed below assume a relatively healthy population with reasonable life expectancy. In patients with multiple or severe comorbidities or with limited life expectancy, these guidelines may not be appropriate and decisions should be tailored on an individual basis.

Incidental Cystic Renal Lesion

Renal cysts are some of the most commonly encountered incidental findings. The Bosniak criteria are a well-studied evidence-based approach to the management of renal cysts. The Bosniak criteria describe five (I, II, IIF, III, IV) categories of renal

H. Singh et al. (eds.), *Radiology Fundamentals: Introduction to Imaging & Technology*, DOI 10.1007/978-3-319-10362-4_33

cystic lesions based upon distinct imaging characteristics. The concept is that more purely cystic a lesion, the more likely it is benign. The more calcification, solid components, enhancement, or thickened walls a lesion has, the more likely it is to be malignant.

Categories I and II do not require follow-up and include simple cysts, cysts with fine calcifications and/or thin internal septa, and non-enhancing hyperdense cysts. Category IIF (F stands for "follow-up") has indeterminate features and should be followed up at 6 and 12 months and then yearly for 5 years to assure stability. Categories III and IV should be referred for surgical consideration at the time of diagnosis (Fig. 33.1).

Size is not a determinant in renal cystic lesions. Interval growth or stability of a lesion may delineate benign from malignant renal cystic lesions.

Incidental Solid Renal Lesion

Renal lesions which are greater than water density may be solid, proteinaceous, or hemorrhagic. Lesions less than 1 cm are too small to characterize with any imaging modality. Also it is important to thoroughly search for fat within a solid renal lesion. If fat is identified in the lesion, then the lesion can almost always be diagnosed as an angiomyolipoma, a benign lesion composed of vascular, muscular, and fatty elements. Of course there are always exceptions. Rarely, a renal cell carcinoma can incorporate fat. This would be the most compelling reason to follow "benign" lesions such as angiomyolipomas over time for evidence of change.

Solid renal lesions that are greater than 1 cm in size and lacking fatty elements have the potential to be malignant and need to be evaluated with an enhanced dynamic imaging study such as renal protocol CT or MRI (Fig. 33.2). Lesions that demonstrate any area of significant post-contrast enhancement are worrisome and should be referred for surgical evaluation.

Historically, biopsy of a renal lesion prior to surgical resection has not been routinely performed. Oncocytomas are benign solid renal tumors which, if correctly identified, do not need to be excised. In the few cases where an oncocytoma is suspected or the patient is a poor surgical candidate, image-guided renal biopsy can be performed for definitive diagnosis and planning.

Incidental Hepatic Lesion

Incidental hepatic lesions are very common. In fact, nearly half of patients without malignancy have benign hepatic lesions at autopsy. Any hepatic lesion in an oncology patient is extremely concerning for tumor. The recommended approach for evaluating incidental hepatic lesions involves assessing lesion size and patient risk.

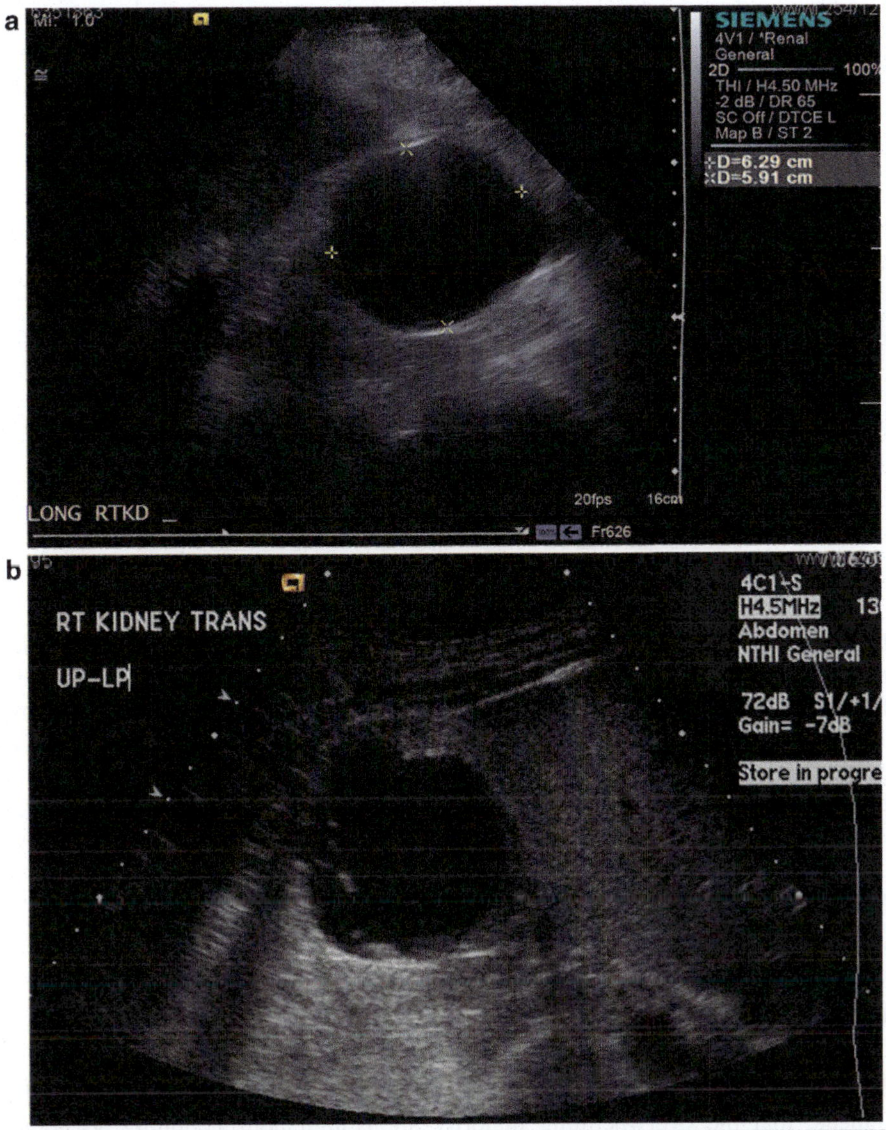

FIGURE 33.1 - (A) ULTRASOUND IMAGE OF A SIMPLE RENAL CYST
Features include well-circumscribed lesion; anechoic (*black*), well-defined wall; and posterior acoustic enhancement (whiter area behind the cyst) (**b**) Ultrasound image of a more complicated renal cyst. In comparison to image (**a**), this cyst has a nodular septation with portions of soft tissue nodularity along the wall

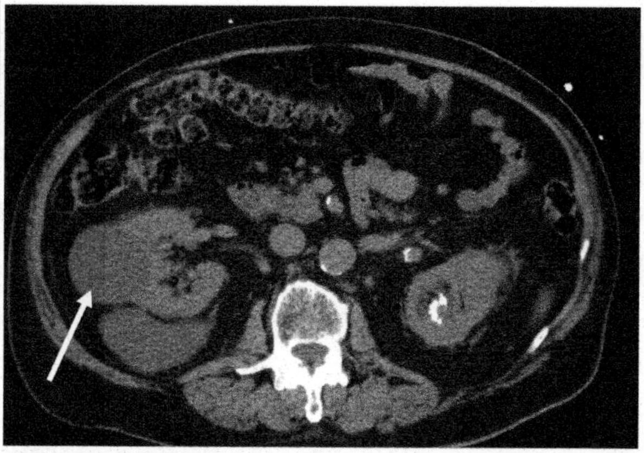

FIGURE 33.2 - LARGE SOLID RENAL LESION ARISING IN THE RIGHT KIDNEY
Given the intermediate density of the lesion, it is indeterminate and needs to be evaluated with further imaging

Despite a complex algorithm based upon these factors and imaging characteristics, the crux of the approach is that any size of a lesion in a high-risk patient needs further evaluation with advanced imaging (CT or MRI) and potential biopsy. The majority of benign lesions are hepatic cysts or hamartomas (which show no evidence of enhancement) and hemangiomas (which have a characteristic enhancement pattern) (Fig. 33.3). High-risk patients are those with known malignancy or cirrhosis or patients with risk factors predisposing to the development of cirrhosis (hepatitis, sclerosing cholangitis, etc.). In all other patients, the decision to dismiss or follow up is based upon size and specific imaging characteristics.

Incidental Adrenal Lesion

It is estimated that 3–7 % of the population has an incidental adrenal lesion. Studies indicate that the overwhelming majority are benign nonfunctioning adenomas. Therefore, it is important to definitively characterize these lesions on imaging.

The assessment of incidental adrenal lesions is primarily based upon imaging features. If an incidental adrenal lesion has Hounsfield units (HU) of less than 10 on a non-contrast CT exam, it can be definitively diagnosed as a benign adrenal adenoma (Fig. 33.4). For lesions 1–4 cm in size that are greater than 10 HU, it is recommended that the patient be rescanned using a specific CT adrenal protocol. This protocol scans the patient at different time points after intravenous contrast administration to calculate a value termed "adrenal washout." The concept is that a benign

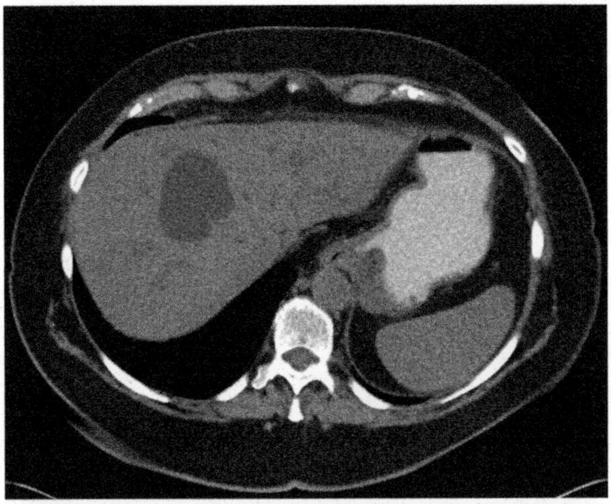

FIGURE 33.3 - LARGE HYPODENSITY IN THE CENTER OF THE LIVER
In a patient with a known malignancy, this would be concerning for metastasis. However, without that history, it most likely represents a large hepatic cyst

adrenal adenoma will enhance and then quickly wash out the contrast, whereas an adrenal metastasis (and presumably adrenal carcinoma) will enhance and retain the contrast (showing delayed washout). Biopsy should be recommended for a lesion with delayed washout. Of note, lesion size and patient history of malignancy are also important factors. Lesions larger than 4 cm are likely malignant and are referred for possible surgical excision. Of note functioning adrenal cortical tumors and pheochromocytomas are almost always associated with symptoms and elevated biochemical markers in blood or urine.

Incidental Pancreatic Lesion

Incidental pancreatic cysts in patients without clinical or laboratory findings of pancreatic disease are relatively common findings. The most common cystic lesion found in the pancreas is a pseudocyst, which is a low-density collection typically developing as a consequence of pancreatitis 4–6 weeks after onset. Cystic pancreatic neoplasms are generally benign or low-grade malignancies. There are three main categories of cystic pancreatic neoplasms: mucinous neoplasm, serous neoplasm, and intraductal papillary mucinous neoplasm (IPMN) (Fig. 33.5). Serous tumors are benign but can enlarge. Mucinous tumors and IPMNs have a malignant potential.

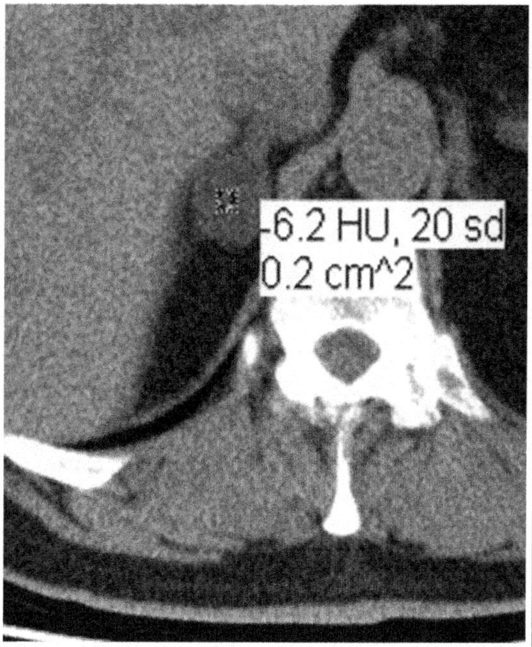

FIGURE 33.4 - NOTE THE ROUND LESION ARISING FROM THE RIGHT ADRENAL GLAND
The Hounsfield units measured –6.2 which is diagnostic of a benign lipid-rich adrenal adenoma

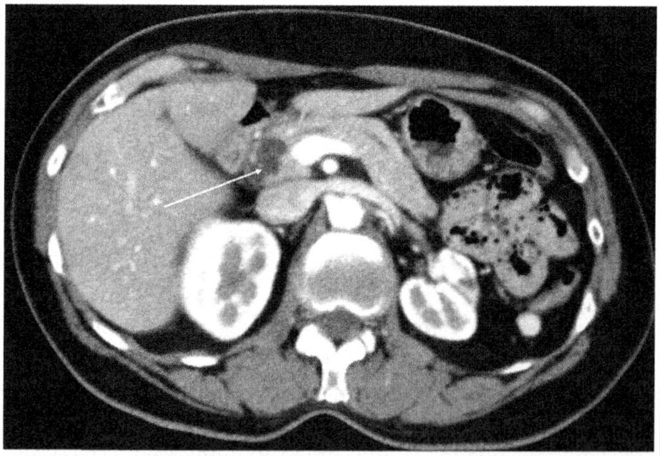

FIGURE 33.5 - AXIAL CT IMAGE AT THE LEVEL OF THE PANCREAS SHOWING A MULTICYSTIC LESION OF THE PANCREATIC HEAD

Table 33-1 Pancreatic cystic lesion follow-up

Lesion type	Follow up
Cystic lesions, 2 cm or less	F/U MRI or CT at 1 year
Cystic lesions, 2–3 cm	MRI with MRCP
Serous lesions	Follow q 2 years
Lesion without classic radiology findings	Follow q 6 months for at least 2 years
IPMN	Follow q 6 months for at least 2 years

Size is the predominant variable used in the evaluation of incidental pancreatic lesions. In the absence of a recent pancreatitis, pancreatic cystic lesions less than 2 cm should be followed up with CT or MRI in 1 year. If the lesion is unchanged in size and appearance, no further follow-up is needed. If the lesion grows or changes on follow-up or if the initial lesion is 2–3 cm in size, MRI with MRCP (MR cholangiopancreatography) is generally recommended. If a serous lesion is diagnosed, then it should be followed up every 2 years. If an IPMN is diagnosed, follow-up is recommended every 6 months for at least 2 years. If the lesion does not have classic radiology characteristics, then annual follow-up is recommended. If the initial lesion is greater than 3 cm and serous neoplasm cannot be definitively diagnosed, then cyst aspiration using endoscopic ultrasound guidance should be attempted. See Table 33.1.

Reference

Berland L, Silverman S, Gore R, et al. Managing incidental findings on abdominal CT: white paper of the ACR Incidental Findings Committee. J Am Coll Radiol. 2010;7(10):754–73.

34 Inflammatory and Infectious Bowel Disease

Objectives:

1. Know the radiographic manifestations of bowel inflammation and the three general etiologies.
2. Know the radiographic manifestations of Crohn's disease and ulcerative colitis on both plain radiographs and contrast studies.
3. Realize that there is considerable overlap in the radiographic findings found in these processes and that biopsy may be necessary for definitive diagnosis.
4. Understand the significance of toxic megacolon with respect to acute complication of these two processes.

Colitis

Colitis is defined radiographically as colonic wall thickening of 3 mm or more when the bowel is distended (Fig. 34.1). Often the bowel wall in colitis will enhance after intravenous contrast administration. There are three chief etiologies in the differential diagnosis of colitis: infection, inflammation, and ischemia.

Numerous types of infections can cause colitis. Two of the most severe forms are pseudomembranous colitis and typhlitis. Pseudomembranous colitis is often a pancolitis. The toxin of the *Clostridium difficile* bacteria causes colonic mucosal ulceration which leads to the formation of pseudomembranes composed of mucin, fibrin, and inflammatory cells. Typhlitis is a neutropenic colitis that is classically seen in leukemic patients. It involves the cecum and/or ascending colon. Both of these forms of colitis are very severe and cause marked wall thickening and pericolonic inflammation and can lead to colonic perforation.

H. Singh et al. (eds.), *Radiology Fundamentals: Introduction to Imaging & Technology*, DOI 10.1007/978-3-319-10362-4_34

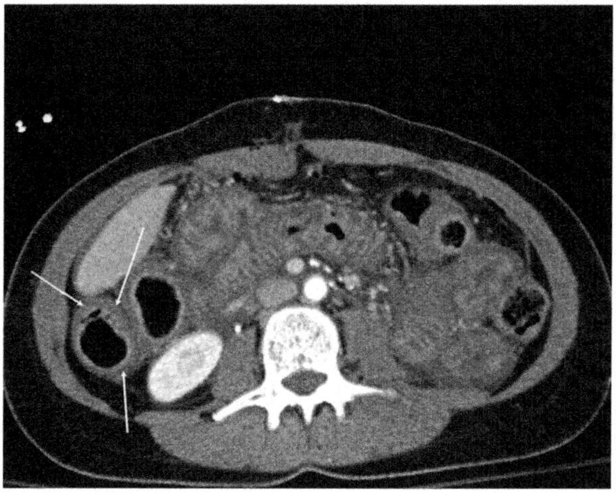

FIGURE 34.1 - COLITIS
Wall thickening of the ascending colon (*arrows*) related to a nonspecific colitis

Ischemia causes a segmental colitis. Segmental refers to the fact that only portions of the colon supplied by the vessel in question are affected. Ischemic colitis tends to occur at the watershed areas of vascular distribution: the splenic flexure and recto-sigmoid regions. Fig. 34.2 demonstrates ischemic colitis involving the cecum and ascending colon in a patient with atherosclerotic disease. When ischemic colitis occurs, it can progress to bowel necrosis with air in the bowel wall (pneumatosis).

There are two common types of inflammatory colitis: ulcerative colitis and Crohn's disease (Fig. 34.3).

Crohn's Disease (CD)

In Crohn's disease, also termed regional enteritis, bowel inflammation is transmural (involving the entire thickness of the bowel wall), may be discontinuous (with intervening skip areas of normal bowel between affected segments), and involves the entire GI system, anywhere from the mouth to the anus. The distal ileum and colon are most commonly involved. The earliest radiographic findings on double contrast examinations of the colon are tiny aphthous ulcers which appear as white "pin-pricks" in the mucosa as barium fills the tiny ulcers. These are very difficult to visualize with single contrast technique. A double contrast barium enema can detect the more subtle surface changes and thus detect early Crohn's disease with a high degree of accuracy. CT scan does not show the mucosal abnormalities as well as fluoroscopy studies but can show distribution and extent of disease.

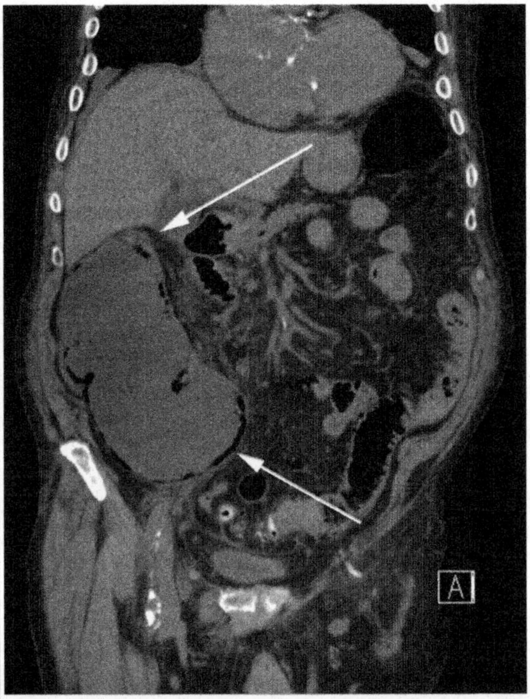

FIGURE 34.2 - ISCHEMIC COLITIS
Coronal CT image demonstrating ischemic changes in the cecum and ascending colon. Note the pneumatosis in the bowel wall (*arrows*) and inflammatory stranding in the pericolonic fat. Vascular calcifications are present in the right common femoral artery indicative of long-standing atherosclerotic disease

Crohn's Cobblestoning

Deep linear ulcers may form in Crohn's disease creating an intersecting network of ulceration which results in a characteristic appearance called cobblestoning (Fig. 34.4). Note how the ulcers are larger and deeper, not aphthous any longer. Cobblestoning may also occur in advanced ulcerative colitis, an example of the radiographic overlap in appearance between ulcerative colitis and Crohn's disease. Notice that patches of ulceration are often separated by completely normal mucosa commonly referred to as "skip" areas. With advanced disease, the bowel wall thickens and becomes fibrotic, sometimes with stricture formation. Again, strictures may form in either ulcerative colitis or Crohn's disease, another example of the radiographic similarity which may be present in these two processes.

CROHN'S DISEASE	ULCERATIVE COLITIS
Skip Lesions, Entire GI Tract	Confined to Colon
Eccentric	Concentric
Fistulae Common	Fistulae Rare
Pseudopolyps Seen	Pseudopolyps, 20 %
Toxic Dilatation Very Uncommon	Toxic Dilatation, Uncommon
Rectal Involvement 50%	Rectal Involvement 95%
Perianal Fistulae and Fissures	Anus Normal
Terminal Ileum Strictured and Irregular	Terminal Ileum Dilated and Wide Open

FIGURE 34.3 - CROHN'S DISEASE VERSUS ULCERATIVE COLITIS
There are several distinguishing characteristics separating the two entities, helping to distinguish them radiographically

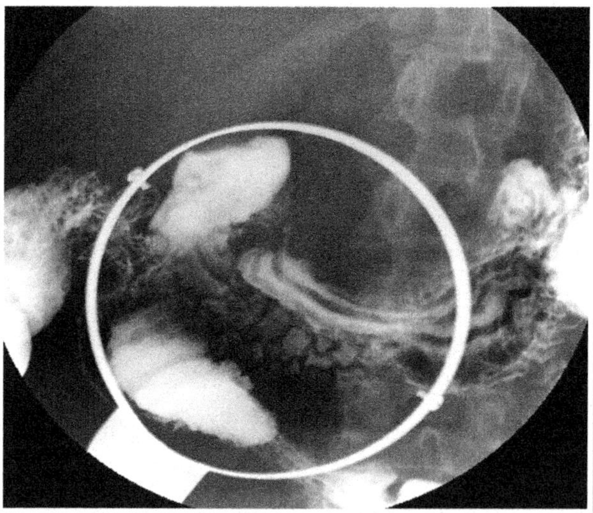

FIGURE 34.4 - CROHN'S COBBLESTONING
Cobblestone appearance of the 2nd and 3rd portion of the duodenum in a patient with known Crohn's disease. The ulcers fill with white barium and show up as white cobblestones

The "String Sign" and "Lead Pipe" Appearance

Narrowing of the terminal ileum, often referred to as the "string sign," also occurs in Crohn's disease and is related to both spasm as well as stricture formation. Fistulas are a frequent complication of Crohn's disease and may extend from the cecum and ascending colon to the terminal ileum or the sigmoid colon. There is also a significant increase in the frequency of ileoileal fistula. Fistulas are best shown by single contrast examination. Other complications of Crohn's disease are perforation, hemorrhage, and colonic malignancy.

At a more chronic stage, CD may cause diffuse fibrosis and spasm of the longitudinal muscles of the wall of the affected colon, giving a characteristic "lead pipe" appearance (Fig. 34.5) due to obliteration of the normal colonic haustral folds and typically involving the descending colon. Complications of CD include not only small and large bowel fistulas but also enterocutaneous fistulas, abdominal abscess formation, small bowel strictures, bowel obstruction, and even perforation.

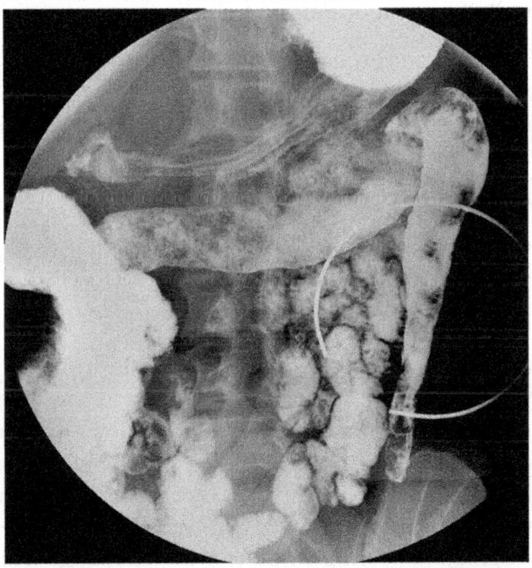

FIGURE 34.5 - LEAD PIPE APPEARANCE
Single contrast enema in a patient with a long history of Crohn's disease shows the "lead pipe" appearance of the transverse and descending colon

Ulcerative Colitis

Ulcerative colitis begins in the rectum and progresses proximally. The rectum is spared in about 5 % of patients. The colonic involvement is relatively uniform and symmetric. During the early stages of ulcerative colitis, the mucosa loses its normal even texture and demonstrates a finely stippled appearance through the barium coating of the mucosa. This is related to multiple shallow ulcerations with surrounding edema, which provide a granular appearance. In ulcerative colitis, inflammation involves the mucosa only and does not extend throughout the bowel wall. For this reason, fistula formation is much less common in ulcerative colitis than in Crohn's disease.

Polypoid Changes in Inflammatory Bowel Disease

Three types of polypoid changes may be seen in both ulcerative colitis and Crohn's disease:

1. Pseudopolyps are islands of inflamed edematous mucosa seen between denuded and ulcerated areas of the bowel wall.
2. Inflammatory polyps are areas of inflamed mucosa resulting in polypoid elevation.
3. Postinflammatory polyps are seen in the quiescent phase of ulcerative colitis and may be composed of normal or inflamed mucosa.

These "polyps" are thought to have originated from ulcerations of the mucosa with severe undermining. Long fingerlike outgrowths, called filiform polyps, are thought to be related to a reparative process. With healing, the colon may regain a normal appearance or may lose its haustra and shorten, resulting in the "lead pipe" colon, a sign of "burnt-out colitis."

Ulcerative Colitis and Colon Cancer

Patients with extensive, long-standing ulcerative colitis are at an increased risk of developing colorectal carcinoma. The incidence begins to rise steeply after 10 years of active disease. The risk is greatest when total colitis is present. Carcinoma in patients with ulcerative colitis is more likely to occur in multiple sites.

Rather than producing an intraluminal mass, colon carcinoma associated with inflammatory bowel disease may infiltrate and spread along the bowel wall giving rise to deceptively benign appearing strictures. Colon cancer is also more difficult to diagnose in patients with chronic ulcerative colitis because it is associated with symptoms related to or mimicked by the underlying disease. Colonoscopy and biopsy are used for long-term follow-up in patients with chronic pancolitis. In some patients, prophylactic colectomy may be performed.

Toxic Megacolon

Fig. 34.6 shows a patient with toxic megacolon. Toxic megacolon is an acute non-obstructive dilation of the colon which is seen in different kinds of inflammatory bowel disease. This patient, with a diagnosis of ulcerative colitis, presented with fever, bloody diarrhea, and abdominal distension.

The diagnosis of toxic megacolon is manifested here by a dilated transverse colon, paucity of haustral markings, and some thickening of the bowel wall. Attempts should be made to identify this condition on plain radiograph because of the high risk of perforation if a subsequent barium enema is attempted. One of the most dramatic and ominous signs that may develop in the course of ulcerative colitis is this rapid development of extensive colonic dilatation and edema.

Note that since the underlying colon is diseased, the chance of perforation is extremely high. Therefore, *barium enema is contraindicated in the presence of toxic megacolon.*

Enterography and Advanced Imaging

Small bowel enterography can be used to evaluate for active Crohn's disease. When traditionally performed with CT, the patient is instructed to drink dilute oral contrast and also receives intravenous contrast in an effort to demonstrate mucosal

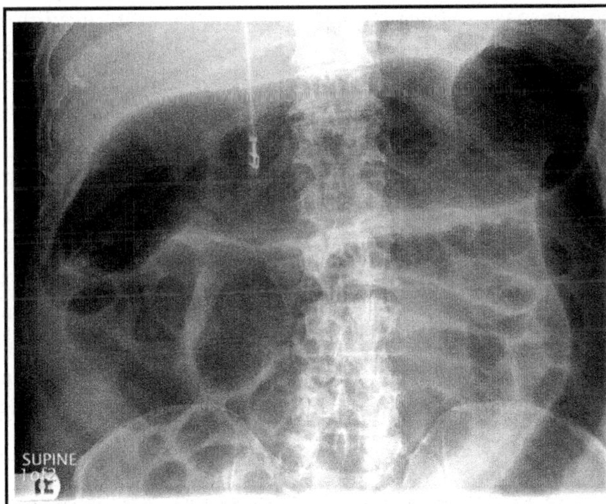

FIGURE 34.6 - TOXIC MEGACOLON
Megacolon appearance with a dilated transverse colon

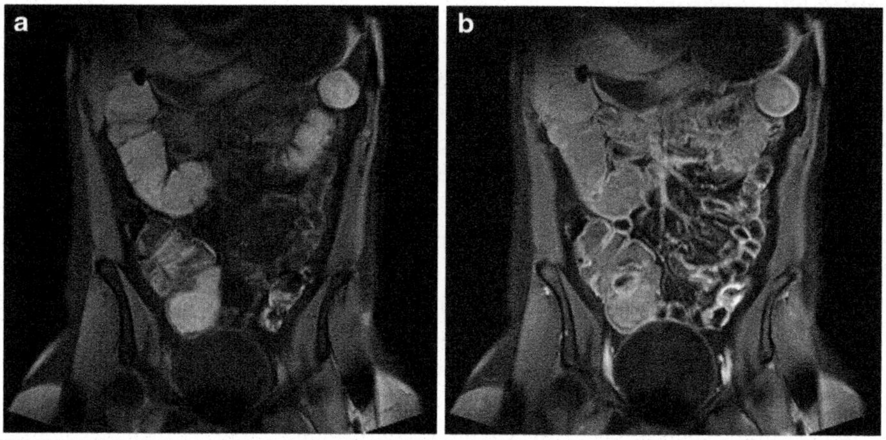

FIGURE 34.7 - MRI ENTEROGRAPHY
(**a**) T1 weighted image with fat saturation showing a normal image from MRI enterography. Note the PO contrast within the loops of large and small bowel. (**b**) T1 weighted post contrast image with fat saturation demonstrating typical bowel wall enhancement and no focal inflammatory change

enhancement often seen with inflammation from Crohn's disease. In addition to mucosal enhancement, bowel wall thickening will be appreciated due to the inflammatory change and distention with oral contrast.

MRI is increasingly being utilized in the setting of inflammatory bowel disease, particularly Crohn's disease. Although CT is currently widely used in this setting, MRI has certain advantages including comparable diagnostic information while avoiding ionizing radiation. Decreasing radiation is of particular concern for these children, adolescents, and young adults given the chronic nature of their disease and frequent imaging. MRI is also superior to CT when evaluating perianal disease. Recent advances in MR technology allow faster acquisition times which decrease the effects of bowel motion which had previously degraded image quality. Before the exam the patient will drink oral contrast to provide bowel distention as they would with CT enterography. Bowel wall enhancement is assessed with intravenous gadolinium administration (Fig. 34.7). MRI findings in the setting of inflammatory bowel disease again will include bowel wall thickening, luminal narrowing, and avid enhancement in the setting of active disease. MR enterography has the added advantage of differentiating a fibrotic lesion from an inflammatory stricture and therefore helps determine surgical versus medical management.

35 Intra-abdominal Lymphadenopathy

Objectives:

1. List the various radiographic modalities which may be employed for the purpose of detecting abdominal and pelvic lymphadenopathy.
2. List two limitations of computerized tomography in the evaluation of abdominal lymphadenopathy.
3. Identify the following structures on a normal abdominal CT scan: aorta, inferior vena cava, kidneys, liver, pancreas, and spleen.
4. State the indications for intravenous and/or gastrointestinal contrast prior to an abdominal CT scan.

Lymphadenopathy

Lymph node enlargement (lymphadenopathy) may be found in many conditions, both benign and malignant. Benign lymph node enlargement can occur in response to different infections such as tuberculosis and fungal disease. Malignant lymphadenopathy can occur in primary lymphatic diseases such as Hodgkin's disease and non-Hodgkin's lymphoma as well as other malignancies that metastasize to regional lymph nodes.

In the past, the presence of intra-abdominal lymph node enlargement could only be surmised by the extrinsic mass effect of the enlarged lymph nodes and various contiguous structures as seen on radiograph or barium studies of the abdomen. Now, CT scanning is used to identify locations and size of abdominal lymph nodes.

H. Singh et al. (eds.), *Radiology Fundamentals: Introduction to Imaging & Technology*, DOI 10.1007/978-3-319-10362-4_35

Lymphangiogram (Historical Perspective)

The lymphangiogram was performed by cannulating the lymphatics located in the web spaces between the toes of the feet and injecting an oily contrast material directly into the lymphatic vessels. It is a 2-day examination. On the first day of the examination, contrast could be seen within the lymphatic vessels themselves. By day 2, the uptake of contrast by the lymph nodes made them directly visible. The problem with the lymphangiogram is that it is extremely uncomfortable and time consuming for the patient. We have imaging modalities that allow us to detect lymphadenopathy noninvasively and with minimal discomfort to the patient.

Computerized Tomography (CT) Scanning

CT scanning is an extremely useful method for detecting intra-abdominal lymph node enlargement. Lymph nodes appear as round or ovoid soft tissue structures many times surrounded by fat (Fig. 35.1).

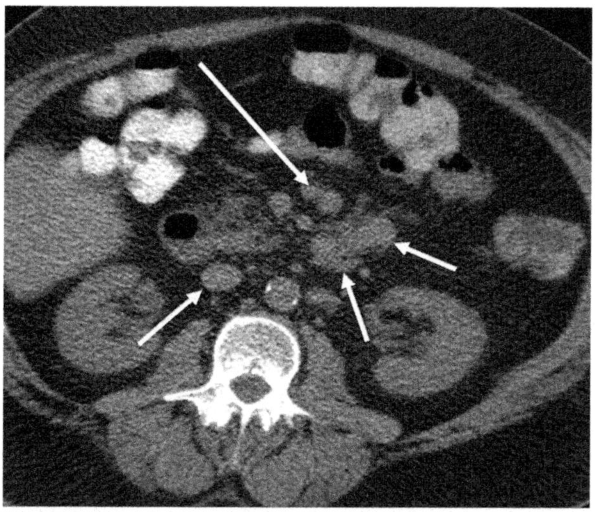

FIGURE 35.1 - ABDOMINAL LYMPH NODES
Mesenteric lymph nodes and para-aortic lymph nodes can be seen if they calcify on plain film or abnormal soft tissue densities on CT scan

Lymph nodes are considered abnormal on CT when they are enlarged. Normal size criteria for a lymph node depend on its location within the body. One of the limitations of CT is that some lymph nodes may be replaced with tumor but not enlarged. Hence, there will be some false negatives where disease has replaced nodal tissue but has not enlarged the nodes. Similarly, not all enlarged nodes herald a malignancy; thus, false-positive cases may be encountered. Another limitation of CT scanning relates to the presence or absence of intra-abdominal fat. Since fat has a very low density on CT scan, it serves to separate and define the normal abdominal structures. In patients who are very thin or have paucity of intra-abdominal fat, it may be difficult to distinguish the borders of normal anatomic structures from enlarged lymph nodes, thus limiting the study. The injection of intravenous contrast or the placement of contrast within the GI tract either orally or by rectum may help to define bowel loops and normal anatomic structures from abnormal masses. For this reason, patients may be asked to drink a low-density barium mixture; normal barium as used in an upper GI series would be too dense and create artifacts on the scan prior to a scan for the detection of abnormal lymph nodes. Other water-soluble contrast agents may also be used.

Intrinsic to the detection of abnormal lymph nodes in the abdomen is the ability to define normal anatomic structures. You should be able to detect abnormal lymph nodes as extra densities by knowing which structures in the abdomen represent normal anatomy (Fig. 35.2). Small blood vessels in the abdomen and pelvis can be confused with lymph nodes on single axial images. However, with the ability to electronically scroll through the examination, ovoid/round lymph nodes can easily be differentiated from linear vessels. Because of its capacity to distinguish different tissue densities such as soft tissue, air, fat, and bone, CT is the primary modality of choice in patients in whom an abdominal mass lesion or lymphadenopathy is suspected.

In the case of malignant neoplasm spread, tumors can have typical nodal groups that will be involved in the earlier stages of the disease prior to diffuse metastasis. Organs often have a regional nodal chain that is responsible for lymph drainage and subsequently can be seeded with tumor causing enlargement. Malignancy of the esophagus and stomach characteristically involves the celiac, perisplenic, and gastrohepatic nodes. Hepatic and biliary cancer will spread to the portal and pancreaticoduodenal nodes. Lymphadenopathy of mesenteric nodes is associated with small bowel cancer. Right-sided colon carcinoma involves the superior mesenteric nodes, while left-sided cancers spread to the inferior mesenteric nodes. Classically testicular cancers will spread to the periaortic retroperitoneal lymph nodes due to their embryologic origin. Findings of periaortic lymphadenopathy in an otherwise young healthy male should prompt testicular ultrasound.

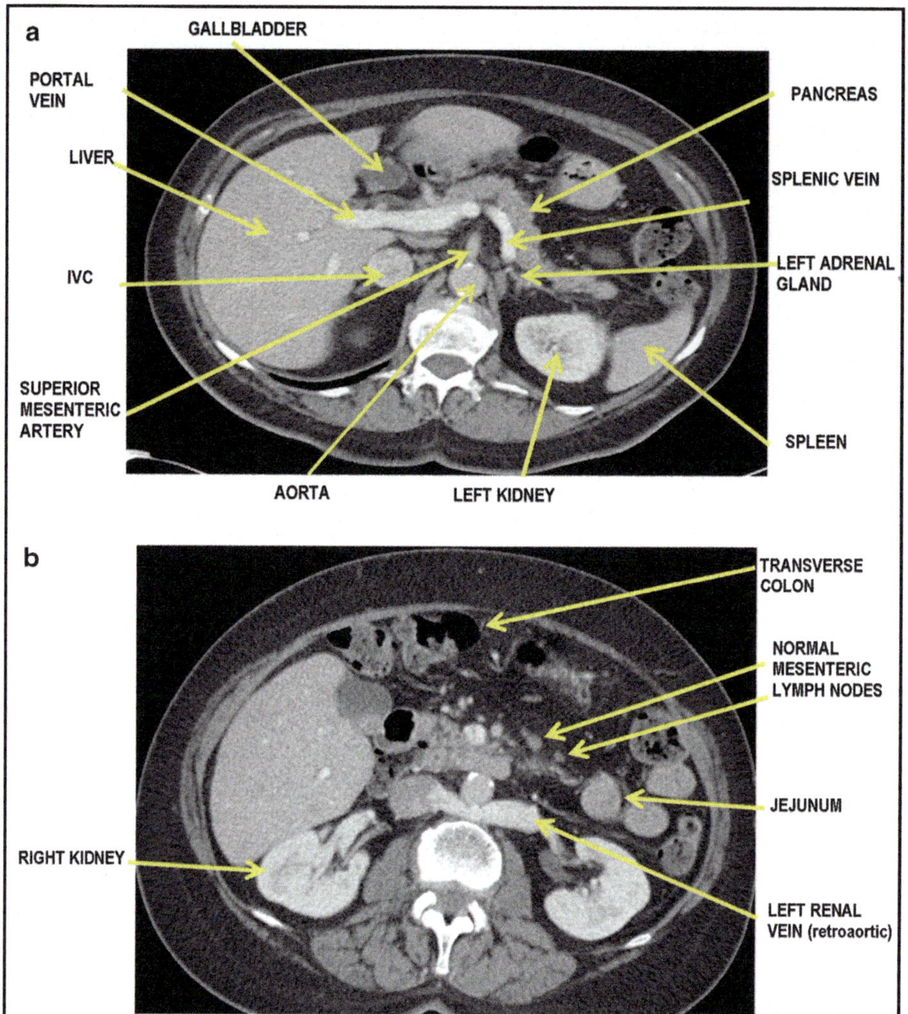

FIGURE 35.2 - NORMAL ANATOMY ON CT
You should be familiar with normal cross-sectional anatomy in order to help identify abnormalities such as lymphadenopathy

Part V
Nuclear Medicine Section

36 Nuclear Medicine Cardiac Imaging

Objectives:

1. List advantages of radionuclide imaging for calculation of the left ventricular ejection fraction over cardiac catheterization and echocardiography.
2. Describe principles of "electrocardiogram-gated" (ECG-gated) imaging.
3. Describe the physiologic rationale for myocardial perfusion imaging (MPI) of the myocardium.
4. Identify which type of stress is better for MPI.
5. List common radiopharmaceuticals used in MPI.
6. Define redistribution and which MPI radiotracer has this property.
7. Define normal, ischemic, and infarction patterns on MPI.
8. Define myocardial viability and list imaging approaches.

Nuclear medicine cardiac imaging includes modalities that are capable of evaluating the ventricular wall motion, global and regional left and right ventricular ejection fraction, myocardial perfusion, and myocardial metabolic activity that includes viability.

The *radionuclide ventriculography*, which is also called *multigated acquisition (MUGA) scan*, *gated blood pool imaging*, and *radionuclide angiography*, is based on labeling a patient's red blood cells with ^{99m}Tc pertechnetate and imaging the blood pool within the cardiac chambers, synchronized to the beating heart. The camera starts imaging each beat when triggered by the Q-wave on the electrocardiogram (ECG) – this type of acquisition is called *ECG-gated.* It takes 10–15 min to obtain one planar projection. During this acquisition each beat is split into 16–32 (depending on the desired temporal resolution) frames or intervals. Activity in every interval (1, 2, 3, etc. up to 16–32) of each beat is summed up in their corresponding composite interval, and together they form a composite beat. It takes about 500 individual beats to obtain a satisfactory composite multi-interval image of an average beat,

H. Singh et al. (eds.), *Radiology Fundamentals: Introduction to Imaging & Technology*, DOI 10.1007/978-3-319-10362-4_36

which can then be displayed as a blind-loop movie, called *cine*. The clinical imaging is usually obtained using planar MUGA, while SPECT MugA can be used for research or advanced clinical purposes.

Usually, three planar views are obtained (Fig. 36.1) – anterior, left anterior oblique (LAO), and left lateral views. The projection that provides the optimal angle for differentiating the activity of the left ventricle and right ventricle is the LAO view, because the LV and RV are clearly separated by the septum; hence, the other name for this projection is the *best septal view*. The processing computer is able to detect and follow the edge of the left ventricle in LAO view, determining the counts in it at each interval of the cycle and graphing the information as the time-activity curve (defined in Chapter 7). Because those counts are linearly related to the corresponding LV volume, this curve is also called the "volume curve."

Therefore, MUGA calculation of left ventricular ejection fraction (LVEF) is volume based (LV activity at end diastole minus that at end systole over end diastole and multiplied by 100 %). LVEF can also be calculated using cardiac catheterization and echocardiography, where the volume is estimated by a geometrical formula that assumes an elliptical LV shape – an assumption that varies in accuracy depending on the actual shape of the LV. The other volume-based method used for calculation of LVEF are SPECT MUGA and MRI, where voxels render actual LV volumes, but the higher cost limits feasibility of their broader applications. Currently, the main indication for MUGA is the determination and monitoring of systolic function (LVEF) in patients with cardiac disease or at risk for developing drug cardiotoxicity, particularly from chemotherapy (e.g., doxorubicin, trade name Adriamycin). Normal LVEF is equal to or greater than 50 %. The images can also provide information on chamber size and volume, qualitative regional wall motion, chambers' contractile synchrony, and diastolic function.

Myocardial perfusion imaging (MPI) is a technique that primarily depicts coronary blood flow at the level of myocardial tissue perfusion. It was initially imaged using planar scintigraphy, but currently SPECT is most commonly used because it improves accuracy. This imaging can be obtained ECG-gated, which allows for assessment of wall motion and an estimated volume-based LVEF in addition to depicting tomographic perfusion. While there is evidence that SPECT/CT may provide the best accuracy, it is rarely used because of the additional radiation exposure required from CT. The gamma-emitting RFs used are Thallium-201 Chloride (^{201}Tl) and ^{99m}Tc labeled agents, such as sestamibi and tetrofosmin (Baggish and Boucher 2008). ^{82}Rubidium chloride (^{82}Rb) is a positron emitter used for MPI and imaged with PET or PET/CT.

^{201}Tl is a potassium cation analogue and thus is transported in and out of the myocardium by Na^+/K^+ cellular pumps. ^{201}Tl uptake therefore reflects perfusion and myocardial cell viability. It is extracted avidly (85 % on first pass through myocardium) and myocardial accumulation is proportional to coronary blood flow. However, even in cases of significant coronary stenoses, such as 75–85 % diameter narrowing, myocardial perfusion in the affected myocardial segment may be undistinguishable from a segment perfused by a totally normal coronary in the resting state. This is because the segment supplied by the diseased (*jeopardized*) artery

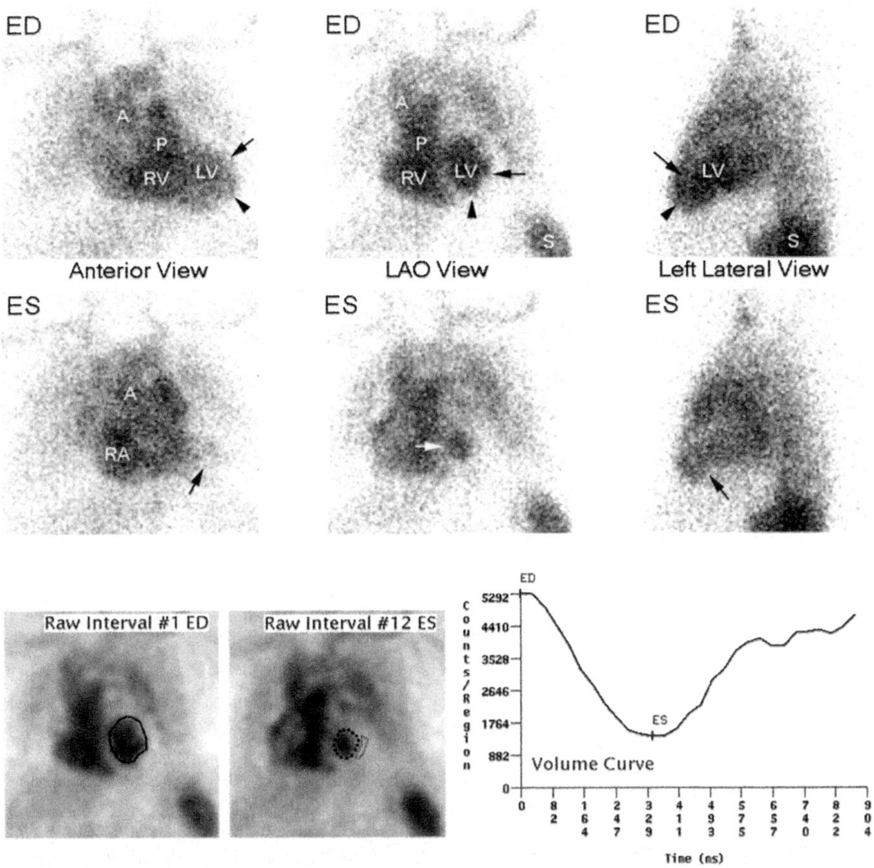

FIGURE 36.1 - MUGA SCAN
Representative images for MUGA scan. The acquisitions were obtained in anterior, left anterior oblique (*LAO*), and left lateral views for 29 intervals each. Only end diastolic (*ED*) and end systolic (*ES*) frames (intervals) are displayed. Seen on anterior ED frame is activity in the left ventricle (*LV*), right ventricle (*RV*), pulmonary outflow conus (*P*), anterolateral wall (*arrow*), and apex (*arrow head*), while ES frame shows filled right atrium (RA), more activity in the aorta, and inferior septal segment (*arrow*) that is better exposed by retracted RV. LAO view depicts normal activity in the spleen (*S*) and location of lateral (black *arrow*) and inferior apical (*arrow head*) segments on ED frame, while the septal segment is pointed out (*white arrow*) on ES frame. The anterior (*arrow*) and apical (*arrowhead*) segments are annotated on ED frame, while the inferior segment (*arrow*) is annotated on ES frame. Lower panel shows the ED and ES intervals with the LV regions of interest automatically identified by computer edge detection algorithm. In actuality the same is done on every frame of 29 intervals and those LV counts are plotted as the volume curve shown to the right.

compensates during resting state by vasodilation (mediated by intrinsic adenosine), which in turn can normalize perfusion to the affected segment. It is during maximum coronary vasodilation, produced by exercise or coronary vasodilator drugs (here forth referred as "stress"), that the difference in myocardial perfusion between normal and jeopardized segments may be unveiled. While a normal artery can triple or quadruple its blood flow (normal *coronary blood flow reserve*) via compensatory dilation during stress, the diseased artery has already reached its maximal compensatory dilation at rest and therefore would not be able to increase the flow any further at stress (abnormal reserve). Therefore, post-stress imaging of the myocardium associated with the jeopardized artery would show less activity (a *perfusion defect*) than the myocardium perfused by the normal segment. Thallium washout can also help distinguish between jeopardized myocardium and normal myocardium. ^{201}Tl normally washes out of myocardial cells over time with the rate of about 10 % per hour. The washout is much slower from an ischemic jeopardized myocardial segment. By 4 h, which is when delayed images are obtained, the activity in the normal and ischemic segments can come close to one another (becomes *homogeneous*) – a phenomenon called *redistribution*. ^{201}Tl washes out from a myocardial scar (infarcted) tissue as rapidly or faster than from normal myocardium; therefore, no redistribution occurs in areas of prior infarct.

The best form of stress is physical exercise, usually done on a treadmill. The exercise increases coronary blood flow and is also helpful in assessing exercise tolerance, relationship of symptoms to exercise level and ECG findings, as well as hemodynamic response (blood pressure and heart rate increase) during the test. All of these findings are important for diagnostic and prognostic purposes, as well as clinical management. ^{201}Tl is injected intravenously at peak stress, and images are obtained in 10–15 min. Areas of ischemia and infarction are displayed as decreased activity on the image. The patient is then allowed to rest, and *delayed* (*redistribution*) images are obtained 4 h later. Therefore, the study could be completed in about 5 h.

The ^{99m}Tc labeled agents are taken up in the myocardium by passive diffusion and not as avidly as ^{201}Tl (65–70 % first pass extraction). They bind to the intracellular structures and remain there without any significant washout (no redistribution). Therefore, the imaging approach is different from that of ^{201}Tl. Typically, a smaller amount of activity will be injected at rest and imaged first. Then at peak stress, a larger amount of activity is injected in order to override the residual activity injected at rest on post stress imaging. The study is usually completed in 2–3 h. The imaging is acquired using ECG-gated SPECT.

A normal study should show homogeneous tracer distribution (Fig. 36.2). A perfectly normal study is rare in SPECT imaging, as different artifacts (particularly attenuation) frequently cause areas of decreased activity even in patients with normal perfusion – considerable skill is required to distinguish those artifacts from real perfusion defects. Ischemic areas would show redistribution, i.e., normalization (Fig. 36.3). If no redistribution is seen, the defect is called *fixed* and implies an area of infarction (fibrosis). There is a spectrum of defect severity, from slight to severe and sometimes totally absent activity. The likelihood of coronary artery disease

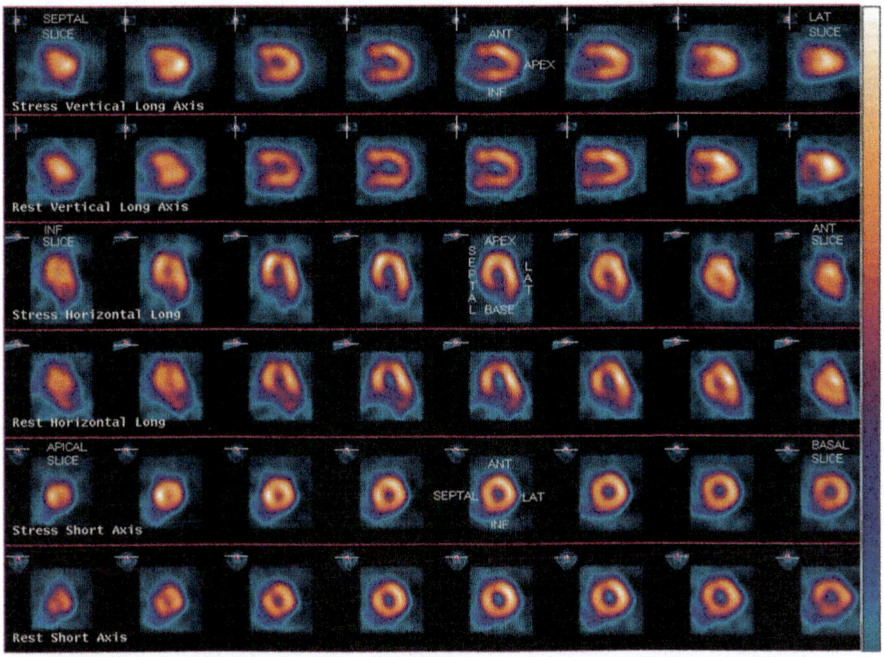

FIGURE 36.2 - NORMAL THALLIUM MIOCARDIAL PERFUSION SCAN
Normal thallium-201 SPECT slices are shown in three standard axes, post-stress on the top and resting (or redistribution) slices on the lower row at closely matched anatomical slice position. The ventricle is reoriented during computer processing such that the slices are generated in relationship to the long axis of the left ventricle rather than the standard body axes. The major left ventricular segments are anterior (*ANT*) wall, inferior (*INF*) wall, lateral (*LAT*) wall, septal wall, and the apex. The opposite end of the left ventricle from the apex is called the base. The beginning and the ending slices of each post-stress row are labeled according to their anatomical location. Notice the *color bar* at the right edge that shows relative color coding of activity (called a color lookup table), from lowest at the bottom to the highest at the top. Color coded images of myocardial perfusion are preferred to the grayscale images because the defects are easier to appreciate on visual inspection and grade them in relation to the most intense (presumably normal) region.

and risk of cardiac events and cardiac death increases with increasing severity of ischemic perfusion defect.

Myocardial viability imaging (MVI) is indicated for characterization of myocardial cells in dysfunctional segments as either living (amenable to recovery of function) or irreversibly damaged and replaced by fibrosis. This information is critical in some patients with coronary disease prior to bypass surgery. Since ^{201}Tl can characterize both perfusion and cellular metabolism (Na^+/K^+ pump function), it is used for assessment of viability in clinical practice. ^{201}Tl can be injected at rest with images obtained at 30 min and 4 h later (some patients may need another

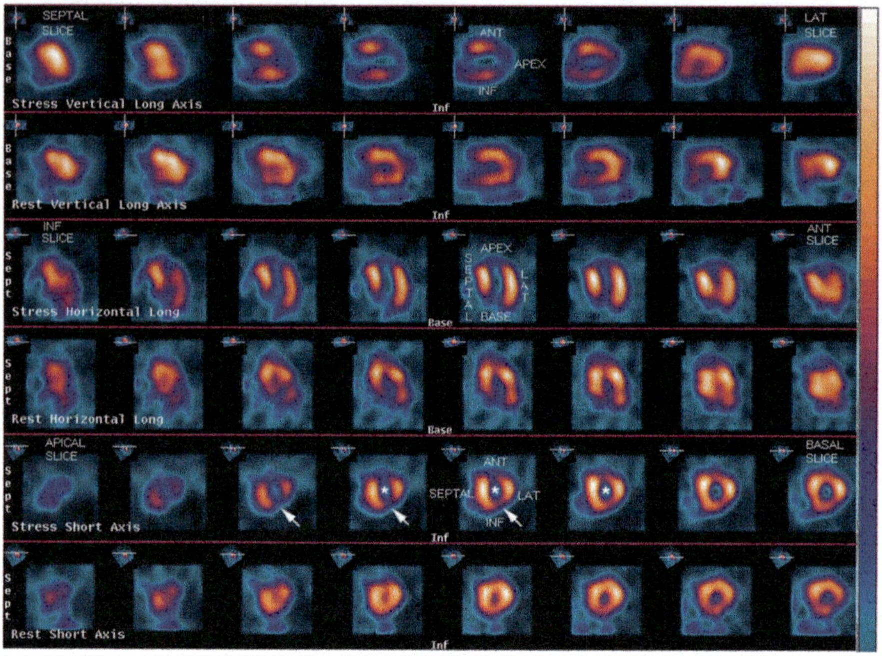

FIGURE 36.3 - ABNORMAL THALLIUM MIOCARDIAL PERFUSION SCAN
Thallium-201 chloride SPECT showing severe perfusion defect on post-stress images involving the distal anterior wall, extending to the apex and periapical region. The 4-h-delay images show complete redistribution, consistent with severe ischemia in the left anterior descending (*LAD*) coronary artery distribution. The lesion is likely in the mid to distal LAD, distal to the major septal branches takeoff, based on spared septal activity. Compare the inner cavity size on the post-stress, mid-ventricular short axis slices (annotated by asterisks) to the cavity size on the resting images. This is an example of transient ischemic dilation (*TID*), which speaks in support of significant stress-induced ischemia that usually involves more than one vessel. Indeed, there is also a moderate-to-severe inferolateral perfusion defect (*arrows*) that redistributes, consistent with ischemia in the left circumflex coronary artery

image at 24 h) for characterization of viability. Myocardial regions with greater than 50 % of normal segment uptake on any of the imaging sequences are considered viable.

References

Baggish AL, Boucher CA. Radiopharmaceutical agents for myocardial perfusion imaging. Circulation. 2008;118(16):1668–74.

Mylonas I, Beanlands RS. Radionuclide imaging of viable myocardium: is it underutilized? Curr Cardiovasc Imaging Rep. 2011;4(3):251–61.

37 Gastrointestinal Nuclear Medicine

Objectives:

1. Define hepatobiliary scintigraphy.
2. Understand common indications for HBS.
3. List essential diagnostic criteria for HBS indications.
4. Define the gastric emptying test (GET).
5. List the indications for GET.
6. Understand the essentials about gastrointestinal (GI) bleeding scan test.
7. List the appropriate indications for GI bleeding scan.
8. Understand the critical plans that should be optimally made prior to GI bleeding scan.
9. Define the Meckel's scan and its indication.

Hepatobiliary scintigraphy is an NM test that uses bilirubin-like radiotracer that offers dynamic visualization of the hepatocyte function (clearance of radiotracer from the blood by the liver), bile flow (radiotracer passage from the liver), and patency of the biliary tree (radiotracer tracking through), as well as its intestinal passage. The common RF used is ^{99m}Tc-mebrofenin. The most common indications for this test include *acute cholecystitis* (AC), chronic abdominal pain due to *functional gallbladder disorders* (goes by many other terms, e.g., "gallbladder dyskinesia", etc.), and *biliary leak*. The imaging is usually carried out in a dynamic planar mode (Fig 37.1a), but static planar imaging and occasionally SPECT or SPECT/CT may be helpful to clarify or resolve uncertain findings.

The essential part of AC pathophysiology is obstruction of the cystic duct; hence, demonstrating obstruction would be the most specific diagnostic finding. The nonvisualization of gallbladder (GB) activity on HBS functionally demonstrates obstruction, which cannot be directly imaged by any other noninvasive test. Hence, HBS has the advantage of the highest specificity over other modalities such as ultrasound, CT,

H. Singh et al. (eds.), *Radiology Fundamentals: Introduction to Imaging & Technology*, DOI 10.1007/978-3-319-10362-4_37

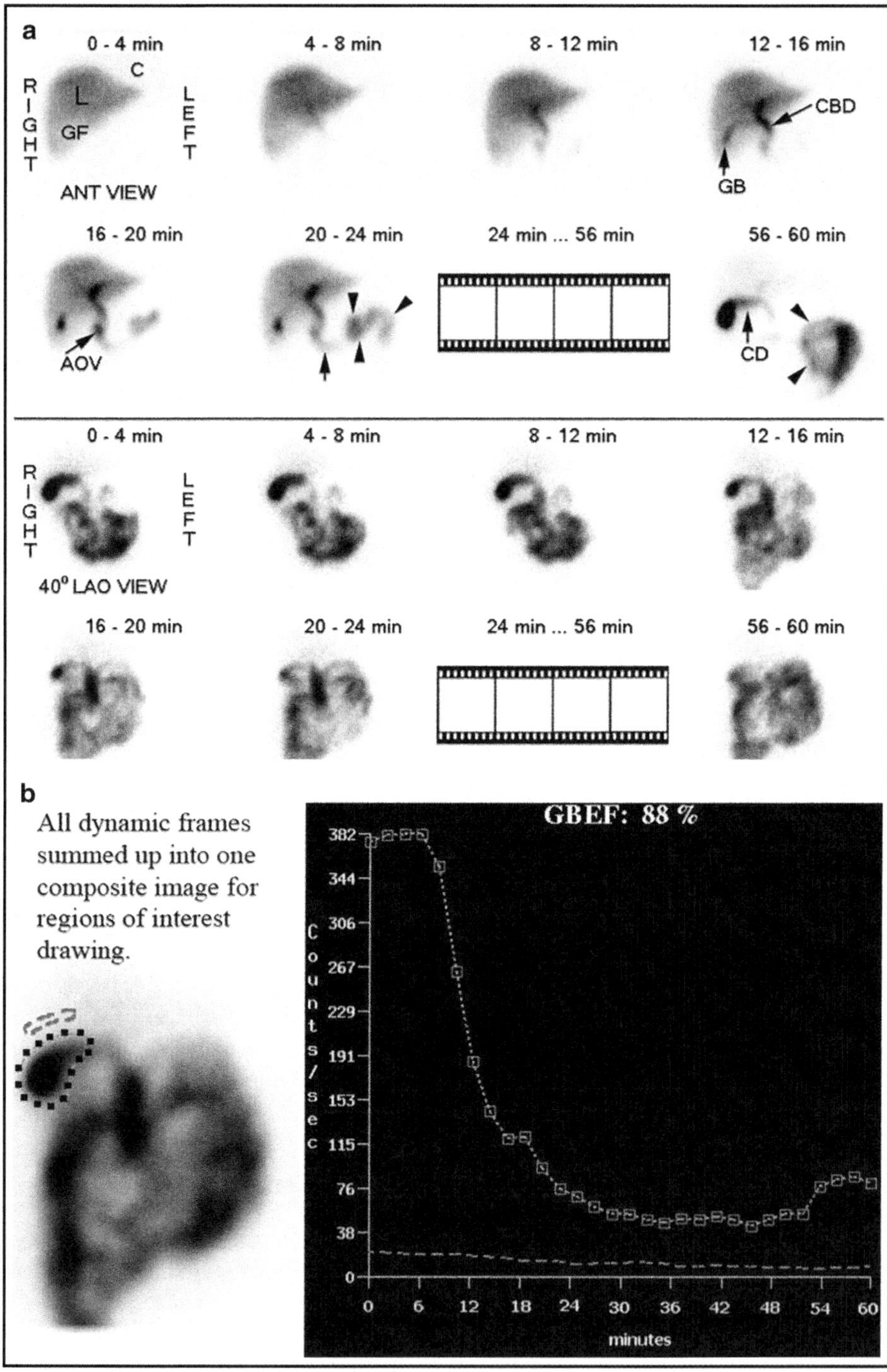
a
0 - 4 min
4 - 8 min
8 - 12 min
12 - 16 min
RIGHT
LEFT
C
L
GF
CBD
GB
ANT VIEW
16 - 20 min
20 - 24 min
24 min ... 56 min
56 - 60 min
AOV
CD
40° LAO VIEW
b
All dynamic frames summed up into one composite image for regions of interest drawing.
GBEF: 88 %
Counts/sec
minutes

and MRI, which show indirect signs of GB inflammation. Therefore, HBS is indicated when other tests render equivocal or clinically doubtful results. The key to obtaining reliable HBS results is in careful patient preparation. If the test is done shortly after meal which stimulates GB contraction, radioactive bile will not be able to enter the gallbladder during the test and could cause false-positive result. Treating a patient's pain for over 24 h with morphine before the test results in constriction of the sphincter of Oddi, which would in turn drive bile back into the GB due to the resulting back pressure, which can also result in a false-positive test, as radioactive bile cannot enter once the GB is filled to its maximum capacity. Avoiding morphine or other narcotic medications is essential prior to the test. Conversely, administering morphine during the HBS test would expedite GB filling by the same back pressure in the properly prepared patient, expediting the results and enhancing specificity of the test.

The essential finding in *functional gallbladder disorder* is abnormal gallbladder emptying, tested on HBS by calculating ejection fraction (EF) following sincalide (synthetic cholecystokinin) stimulation. The normal GB EF is 38 % or greater (Fig. 37.1b) when 0.02 mcg of sincalide is infused over 60 min (the infusion rate is critical). Patients with abnormal GB EF often undergo laparoscopic cholecystectomy, which sometimes may be complicated by a *bile leak* from incompletely closed

FIGURE 37.1 - (A) HEPATOBILIARY IMAGING

This is a patient with chronic abdominal pain who was referred for HBS with GB EF. The *top* two panels of baseline images represent a dynamic sequence obtained over 60 min, displayed in 4 min per frame formatting in the anterior (*ANT*) view. The first frame shows that all activity is concentrated in the liver (*L*), and no activity is seen in the area corresponding to the cardiac blood pool (*C*), which indicates normal hepatocellular function. The area of decreased activity at the inferior edge of the liver corresponds to the gallbladder fossa (*GF*). Subsequent frames show progressive drainage of the bile into the biliary tree. On the 12–16-min frame, the gallbladder (*GB*) and common bile duct (*CBD*) activities are visualized. On the next frame, a small collection of bile is seen at the point of the ampulla of Vater (*AOV*), as it drips into the descending (second) part of the duodenum. The third part of the duodenum is better seen on a 20–24-min frame (*arrow*). The activity is also seen to progress into the proximal jejunum (*arrowheads*). Frames from min 24 through 56 are not displayed. The last frame (56–60 min) shows the most intense activity in the GB connecting via cystic duct (*CD*) to faint activity in the CBD. Most of the activity has been cleared from the liver, and some activity is still seen in the loops of the small bowel (*arrowheads*). Below the black line of separation are post-sincalide frames that were acquired in the left anterior oblique (*LAO*) projection that were displayed in a similar format as on baseline images. The GB shows rapid and vigorous emptying.

(b) GALLBLADDER EJECTION FRACTION

The post-sincalide composite image shows the GB region of interest (*ROI*) delineated by the *black dotted* outline. The background ROI is drawn on the liver just above the GB as shown by the *gray broken* outline. The GB activity corrected by the background activity is plotted on the graph in *white squires* connected by the *dotted white line*. The GB EF is calculated from this curve by taking and subtracting the minimal count from the maximal count and dividing by the maximal count. The liver background counts are plotted for reference (*gray dashes*), showing the expected gradual decline.

cystic duct or from injury to other parts of the biliary tree. HBS can specifically diagnose it by showing radiolabeled bile as it escapes (leaks) outside the biliary system or bowel lumen, showing its spread and extraluminal collections.

Gastric emptying test (*GET*) quantifies and depicts the process of radioactively labeled meal emptying. The international standard solid meal consists of egg whites (equal to 2 eggs) fried with ^{99m}Tc-sulfur colloid, 2 slices of bread, strawberry jam, and 120 mL of water. Indications for GET include functional dyspepsia, diabetic gastroparesis, and assessment of emptying before surgery (i.e., fundoplication, etc.). Static images are obtained in anterior and posterior projections at times 0 h (immediately following food consumption), 1, 2, and 4 h. The normal ranges for percent of meal emptied from the stomach are ≥10, ≥40, and ≥90, respectively. Emptying of greater than 70 % at 1 h is considered accelerated (dumping syndrome). Of note, solid meals empty in a linear fashion. If a solid meal cannot be used, 300–500 mL of water labeled with ^{99m}Tc-labeled RF can be an alternative. Liquid meals empty exponentially, and T1/2 is used for quantification. Normal T1/2 is <18 min. Both tests are appropriate for adults only. Whole milk or feeding formula labeled with ^{99m}Tc-sulfur colloid can be used for gastric emptying in small children and the test is called "*milk scan.*" In addition to GET the study also evaluates gastroesophageal reflux, which is another common problem in small children or neonates who have failure to thrive.

Gastrointestinal (GI) bleeding scintigraphy or scan dynamically depicts the blood pool distribution and identifies active extravasation of blood into the intestinal lumen. The RF is ^{99m}Tc labeled autologous red blood cells (^{99m}Tc-RBCs). The labeling procedure can be performed in any NM facility using a commercial kit. It requires 1–3 mL of whole blood, and the entire labeling process is completed within 20 min. However, it may not be possible to achieve efficient labeling in a rare patient on interfering medications (e.g., propranolol). Once started, GI bleeding scan can continuously and/or intermittently monitor for bleeding during ensuing 24 h. It is the most sensitive modality for detection of occult GI bleeding, as it is able to detect as little as 0.04 mL/min of blood loss. GI bleeding is typically intermittent and active blood loss is difficult to evaluate clinically. Even bright red blood per rectum is often not due to active bleeding, but rather from retained blood being evacuated well after the active bleeding has stopped.

Figure 37.2 demonstrates a normal ^{99m}Tc-RBCs distribution first, followed by appearance of a small bowel bleeding. If the patient is taken at that point for angiography, the results from the study will demonstrate the location of active bleeding and thus help identify culprit vessel, which can subsequently be therapeutically occluded during the same procedure. The longer the time elapsed following visualization of active bleed on GI bleeding scan, the less likely it will still be present on angiography (as bleeding is typically intermittent). Therefore, it is critical to have a clear plan in place with the involved services (angiography and/or surgery) informed and ready before a patient arrives in NM for GI bleeding scan. If the next step in clinical management is not considered until after active bleeding has been found on the GI bleeding scan, the decision making often leads to a long enough delay that allows the bleeding to stop and render subsequent angiography futile.

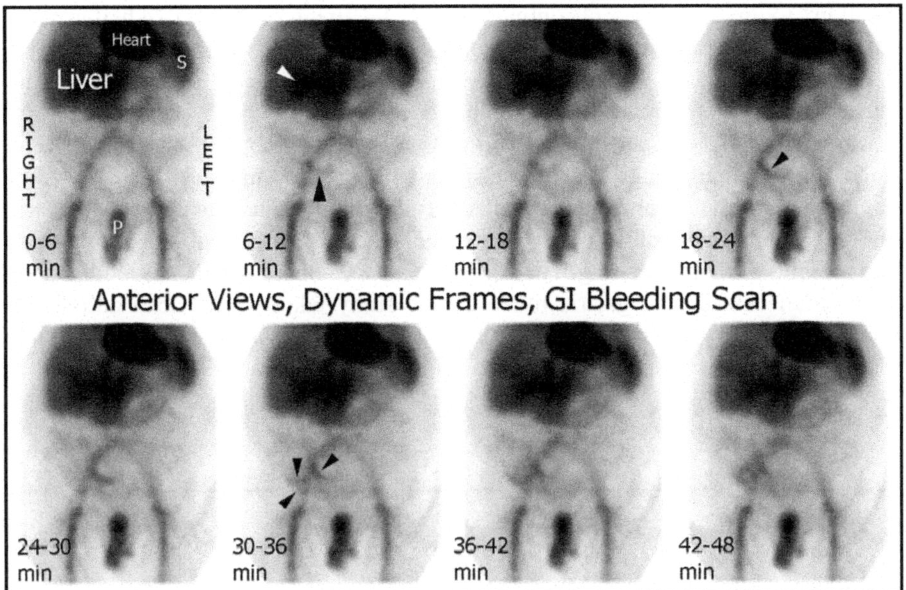

FIGURE 37.2 - GASTROINTESTINAL BLEEDING SCAN
Gastrointestinal bleeding scan showing small bowel bleeding at a relatively slow rate. The first frame obtained from injection (0 min) to 6 min shows normal distribution of blood pool in the heart, liver, spleen (*S*), and the cavernous body of the penis (*P*). One can clearly see blood pool in the large vessels, such as the aorta and vena cava, which show up as double-barrel channels along the midline of the body, eventually splitting into symmetrical iliac vasculature that continues down to the thighs. The curvilinear activity along the liver (*white arrowhead*) is blood pool in the porto-hepatic vasculature. The first sign of the bleeding is observed on the 6–12-min frame as a curvilinear subtle area of activity (*black arrowheads*) to the right of the abdominal midline. The central position suggests small bowel. However, diagnostic definition of active GI bleeding requires two additional criteria – change in intensity and movement. The intensity of this activity grows with time, as seen on the 18–34-min frame. Finally, on image 30–36 min, the activity moves in a loopy zigzag pattern, which is also typical for the small bowel. The activity in the penis can be confused with rectal bleeding. While this activity also becomes more intense, it doesn't move, therefore, not fulfilling the bleeding criteria.

Although a GI bleeding study can diagnose upper GI bleeding (above ligament of Treitz) with high sensitivity, it is not indicated as the initial workup. If gastric aspirates through nasogastric tube and/or endoscopy are negative, then it becomes reasonable to pursue the GI bleeding scan. However, GI bleeding scan is indicated in the initial workup of acute lower GI bleeding. Colonoscopy is of limited value because intraluminal blood makes visual identification of the bleeding source difficult. Angiography can be used to both diagnose and treat a lower GI bleed. However, to detect bleeding during angiography, the patient must be actively bleeding at approximately 1 mL/min during the few seconds it takes for the iodinated contrast to pass through the arteries. A tagged RBC study does not have this limitation, given the ability to image the patient continuously for 1–2-h intervals, over 24 h, if needed. Continuous imaging increases the likelihood of detecting an intermittent active bleed and allows for localization of the site of bleeding (small bowel, ascending colon, transverse colon, descending colon, or rectum).

Meckel's scan is aimed at identifying presence of ectopic gastric mucosa in Meckel's diverticulum in the small intestine, which is present at birth and is a vestigial remnant of the omphalomesenteric duct. It contains heterotopic rests of gastric mucosa, which may lead to peptic ulceration. The typical patient is a young child who presents with GI bleeding. The RF is ^{99m}Tc-pertechnetate, which is avidly taken up by chief cells in the gastric mucosa. The study takes about 1.5 h and shows uptake in the right lower abdominal quadrant that typically appears simultaneously with normal gastric uptake and increases in activity over time (Fig. 37.3).

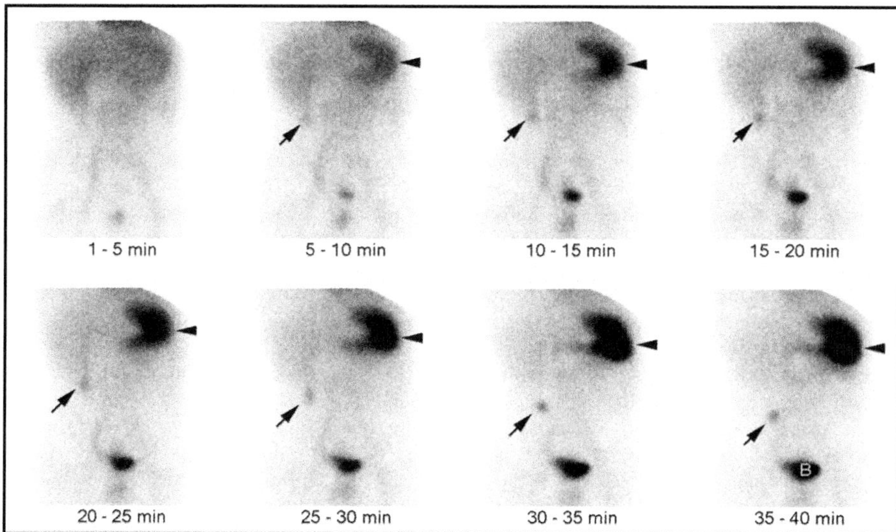

FIGURE 37.3 - MECKEL'S SCAN
Meckel's scan on a 3-year-old child with episode of blood per rectum 24 h ago. The images were obtained in anterior view using dynamic mode and displayed in 5 min per frame format. There is a clear tracer uptake in the stomach (*arrowhead*) and an extra-gastric focus of activity (*arrow*) in the right upper abdominal quadrant. Over time, both areas show progressively increasing activity that occurs simultaneously, which is consistent with Meckel's diverticulum. The extra-gastric focus moves during the acquisition, which is captured on some frames as linear smearing of activity. This can be best appreciated on image 25–30 min. Such movement is appropriate for the diverticulum on the small bowel, which is rather mobile on a relatively long mesentery. Accumulation of the tracer in the urinary bladder (*B*) is physiological.

38 Oncologic Nuclear Medicine

Objectives:
1. Explain the principle of positron emission tomography (PET).
2. Describe the patient preparation for F-18 FDG PET/CT.
3. List the most common indications for F-18 FDG PET/CT.
4. State the most common PET pitfalls.
5. List common indications for lymphoscintigraphy.
6. Explain the concept of sentinel lymph node.
7. State the principle of radioactive iodine whole body scan and treatment for thyroid cancer.

Nuclear medicine plays a multifaceted role in oncology, including diagnostic imaging and therapy. The few examples given in this chapter highlight some of the more common tests and applications, but there are many more that could not be included due to the limited space and scope. Metastatic skeletal disease is covered in the chapter on skeletal nuclear medicine.

Positron emission tomography (*PET*) is an imaging method that depicts the distribution of positron emitting RFs in the body. Oncological imaging is currently the main clinical application of PET, but numerous other applications, such as cardiac imaging (see Chapter 36, "Nuclear Medicine Cardiac Imaging"), as well as other clinical applications that continue to develop.

A positron is a positively charged counterpart of an electron emitted during a subtype of beta decay (see Chap. 7, "Introduction to Nuclear Medicine"). It is emitted from the nucleus and undergoes an annihilation reaction with an electron outside the molecule, transforming their combined mass into two 511 keV gamma photons traveling in 180° opposite directions. These photons strike the PET scanner's ring of detectors simultaneously, and computational algorithms reconstruct the tomographic image by localizing the annihilation events from the collected data (Fig. 38.1).

H. Singh et al. (eds.), *Radiology Fundamentals: Introduction to Imaging & Technology*, DOI 10.1007/978-3-319-10362-4_38

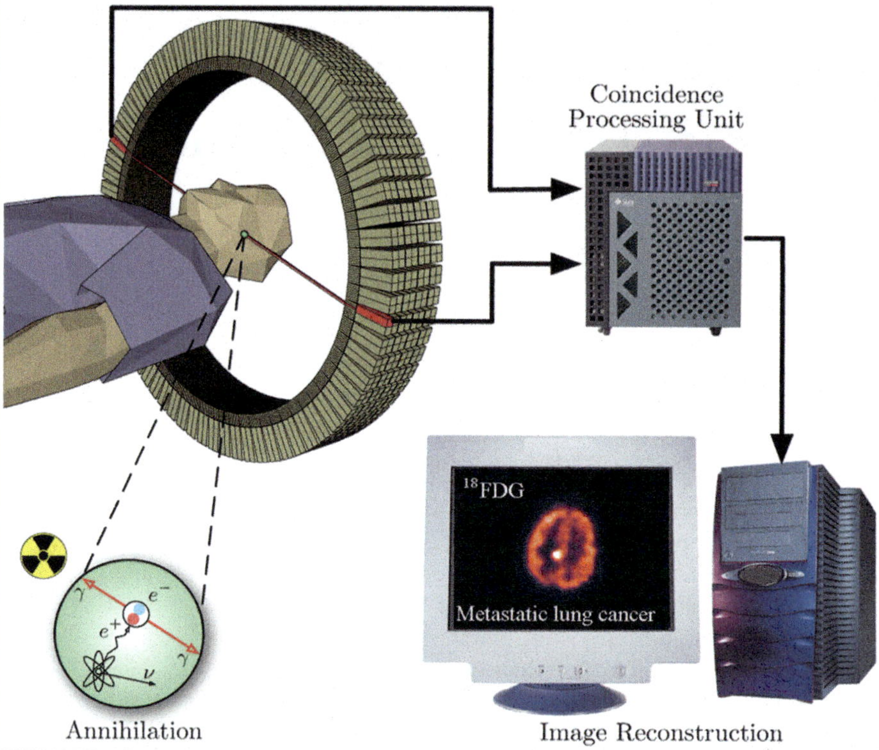

FIGURE 38.1 - PET PRINCIPLES
The image illustrates the processing principles of a positron emission tomography (*PET*). It shows how positron (e^+) is emitted from the nucleus of the isotope and collides with an electron (e^-), which results in the annihilation event that transforms their mass into two gamma photons emitted in diametrically opposite directions. These photons are registered by the scanner's detector (the green-colored ring). After the registration, the data is forwarded to a processing unit which determines if the two registered events are coincidence events (occurring at the same time) or not. All coincidences are forwarded to the image processing unit where the final image is produced via mathematical image reconstruction procedures. (This figure is modified from the image released into the public domain by the author, Jens Langner.)

The most commonly used positron-emitting isotope and RF in medicine today are fluorine-18 (^{18}F) and ^{18}F-fluorodeoxyglucose (^{18}FDG), respectively. ^{18}FDG is administered IV and most facilities today use hybrid PET/CT cameras to image it (Fig. 38.2). The ^{18}FDG is a glucose analogue that reflects its cellular uptake and hexokinase phosphorylation, i.e., glycolysis. Unlike glucose, a phosphorylated ^{18}FDG product is trapped in the cells and cannot progress further along the glycolytic pathway. An overwhelming majority of tumors display intense glycolysis and increased hexokinase activity that provides the energy for its growth. This process is elegantly portrayed on the ^{18}FDG PET/CT images (Fig. 38.3).

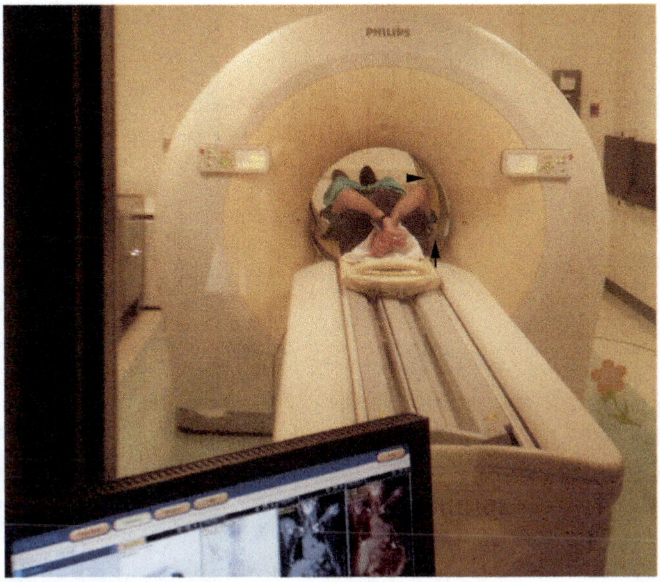

FIGURE 38.2 - A PET/CT SCANNER
This is a photograph of PET/CT camera taken from the control room that is separated from the camera room by a leaded glass and wall to shield the staff from the CT generated X-rays and patient emitted gamma rays. The camera contains two imaging rings, the CT gantry (*arrow*) and the PET detector (*arrowhead*). The images are reconstructed by a dedicated imaging computer and checked by the technologist before submitting the study for evaluation to physicians

Careful patient preparation is important for two reasons: (1) to decrease ^{18}FDG uptake in a normal myocardium, which improves sensitivity for tumor detection in a myocardium or pericardium, and (2) to create a favorable environment for ^{18}FDG uptake in a tumor. Myocardium favors glycolysis for its energy needs but can also use fatty acids during carbohydrate deprivation. Therefore, the patients are instructed to maintain a low-carbohydrate diet for a couple of days. They also fast for at least 6 h prior to ^{18}FDG injection. Fasting prevents the physiological movement of glucose and ^{18}FDG into skeletal muscles, which limits the available ^{18}FDG for tumor uptake. Special care is needed in preparing patients with diabetes mellitus as high glucose levels (usually above 200 mg/dL) can competitively inhibit ^{18}FDG uptake by tumors. Furthermore, administration of insulin to decrease glucose levels within a few hours of the test causes similar glucose and ^{18}FDG movement into the skeletal muscle and must be avoided. Increased glucose utilization in the brown adipose tissue can be stimulated by exposure to cold and is reflected by intense ^{18}FDG uptake. This can obscure findings in the same areas and degrade test accuracy. Therefore, patients are encouraged to wear warm, comfortable clothing and use warm blankets while in the imaging facility.

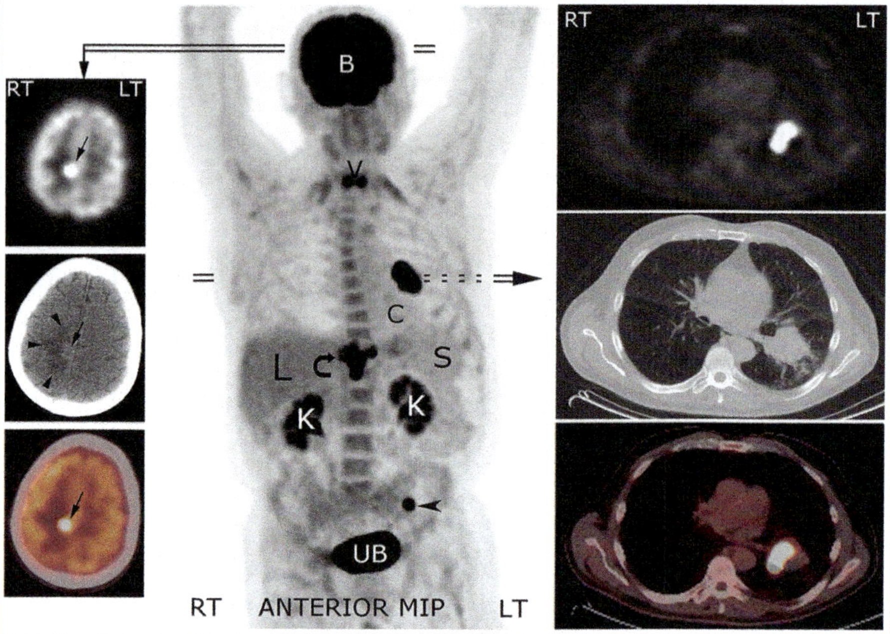

FIGURE 38.3 - PET/CT SCAN
^{18}FDG PET/CT images of a 72 year-old male with the recent diagnosis of non-small cell lung cancer, referred for staging. All images are labeled with the patient's left (*LT*) and right (*RT*) side. The anterior projection of the MIP image shows biodistribution of ^{18}FDG after carbohydrate depravation diet and 8 h of fasting, showing optimal pattern with no appreciable cardiac (*C*) activity. There is obligatory carbohydrate metabolism in the brain (*B*), shown here as intensely ^{18}FDG avid. Physiological, intense uptake is seen in the vocal cords (*V*), kidneys (*K*) that excrete ^{18}FDG into the urinary bladder (*UB*), moderate in the liver (*L*) and subtle activity in the spleen (*S*). There is a metastatic brain focus seen on properly intensity adjusted slices through the region marked with the double line leading to the left. The top slice is PET image that shows intense focal activity at the corticomedullary junction (*arrow*) – typical metastatic location. Corresponding CT slice shows surrounding edema (*arrowheads*). The fusion image overlays color-coded PET onto the CT for precise anatomical localization. The representative slice through the intensely ^{18}FDG-avid primary lung tumor is taken at the level shown by the *dashed double line*. The intense ^{18}FDG activity extends over part of the consolidation shown on CT with the spared part representing collapsed lung tissue from the obstruction by the tumor of proximal segmental bronchus. There are also skeletal metastases in the lower thoracic spine (*curved arrow*) and the left iliac bone (*concave base arrowhead*)

The first ^{18}FDG PET/CT indication approved by Medicare for payment was to evaluate solitary pulmonary nodules for the likelihood of malignancy. ^{18}FDG PET/CT is currently indicated to stage, restage, assess response to treatment, and conduct surveillance in a wide variety of malignancies (Fig. 38.3). Prostate and renal cell cancers have variable ^{18}FDG uptake and, therefore, are not among the approved indications. Because ^{18}FDG uptake is not specific for a malignant tumor, its uptake should not be used for the definitive diagnosis of malignancy. One of the most common benign causes of ^{18}FDG uptake is active inflammation. In fact, ^{18}FDG PET/CT has been used for the work-up of fever of unknown origin but currently is not approved for this indication by Medicare. Other benign causes of ^{18}FDG uptake include benign tumors, trauma, bone fracture, healing surgical site, and hematomas. False-negative studies do occur with greater frequency in tumors that commonly display poor ^{18}FDG uptake, such as bronchioloalveolar carcinoma (subtype of lung adenocarcinoma), marginal zone lymphoma, and mucinous colonic neoplasms.

Lymphoscintigraphy is a test that depicts lymphatic flow and nodal distribution. It is commonly used in oncology to identify the sentinel lymph node, which is the first node that receives lymph from the tumor-affected region. The most commonly used RF is ^{99m}Tc-labeled sulfur colloid injected intradermally in cases of skin cancer and subareolar in breast cancer. If tumor spreads along the lymphatics, the sentinel node should be the first to receive it. Lymphoscintigraphy has proven utility in the regional lymph node staging of breast cancer and skin cancer (e.g., melanoma). Because there is expected drainage to the axilla in breast cancer, the planar images are sufficient to provide guidance to surgeons who are well familiar with axillary anatomy (Fig. 38.4). Since melanoma can involve various skin regions with less predictable lymphatic drainage, SPECT/CT is used to localize the sentinel node anatomically, which helps to locate it at surgery. The test takes about 1–1.5 h and is usually done within 24 h of planned surgery.

Previously, radical lymphadenectomy was done in these cancers to determine the presence of tumor (staging) and to remove regional tumor spread, but it caused significant morbidity (e.g., lymphedema). Identifying and removing just the sentinel lymph node markedly decreases the extent of the surgery, particularly when no tumor is found in the sentinel node, and minimizes morbidity.

The whole body radioactive iodine (WB RAI) scan is a test that uses iodine isotopes to define RAI avidity in *differentiated thyroid cancer* (DTC). Iodine uptake makes DTC amenable to RAI imaging, treatment, and surveillance (Fig. 38.5). The most commonly used gamma-emitting isotopes for the imaging are ^{131}I and ^{123}I, which are given orally in the form of sodium iodide. Some DTC is incidentally found and sub-centimeter in size, which requires only a thyroidectomy. A larger DTC needs additional RAI therapy after the surgery. Because surgery cannot remove all thyroid tissues safely, the first RAI treatment completes the thyroidectomy by mainly targeting the benign remnant thyroid tissue, which is called RAI *ablation*. Ablation allows a subsequent effective use of thyroglobulin (Tg) for DTC surveillance. Since Tg is produced by either normal or cancerous thyroid cells, ablation is necessary for the detection of residual or recurrent DTC.

One of the critical prerequisites to using RAI for either diagnosis or treatment is depleting the body of iodine, which markedly improved RAI uptake by the tumor. The patient is placed on low-iodine diet for 2 weeks, which is a very challenging

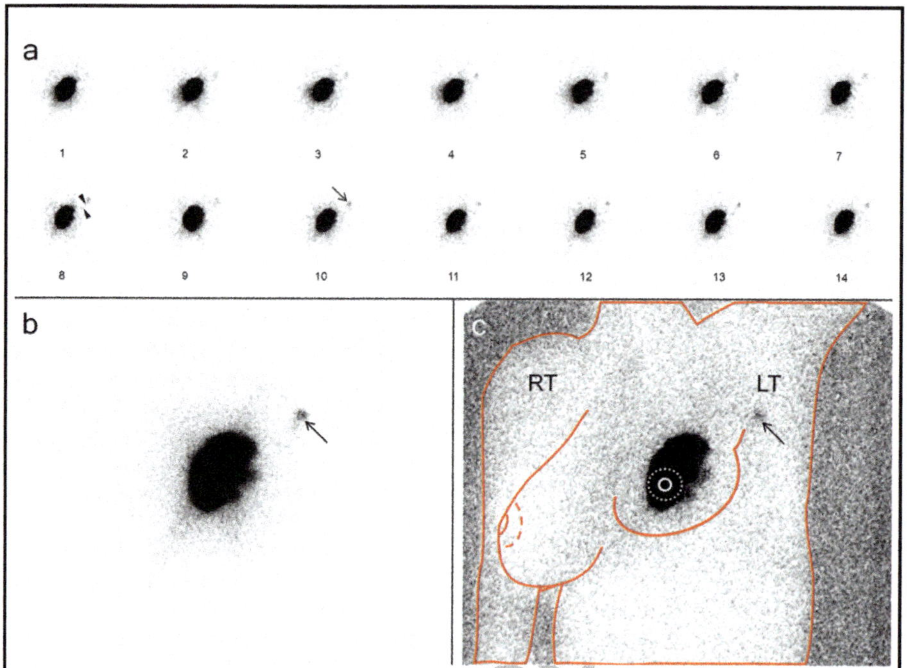

FIGURE 38.4 - LYMPHOSCINTIGRAPHY SCAN
(**a**) After the left breast subareolar injection (the intense focal activity on frame 1), dynamic images of the chest in 35° left anterior oblique (*LAO*) projection are obtained for 1 min per frame. The images show migration of the radiotracer into the left axillary lymph node (*arrow*) at the end of a channel that can be faintly visualized on frames 3–8 (*arrowheads*). The activity in the node becomes more distinct with time. (**b**) A static image in the same LAO view obtained at 30 min after injection shows clear focus of activity consistent with sentinel node. (**c**) To better appreciate its location, a transmission view is obtained in the same LAO projection. Transmission image is like a radiograph, but instead of the x-ray tube a flat and uniform source of radioactivity is placed behind the patient's back. The drawn-in outline of the patient's body is in light orange helps to appreciate that the left (*LT*) breast is pooled up and displaced medially, fixed in place by adhesive tape, so that it does not attenuate activity in the axilla. The right (*RT*) breast is naturally laying over the right axilla

diet to follow. The other critical prerequisite for iodine uptake is to have thyroid tissue stimulated with either intrinsic thyroid-stimulating hormone (by stopping hormone replacement, which caused iatrogenic hypothryoidism) or a human recombinant analogue administered by IM injection.

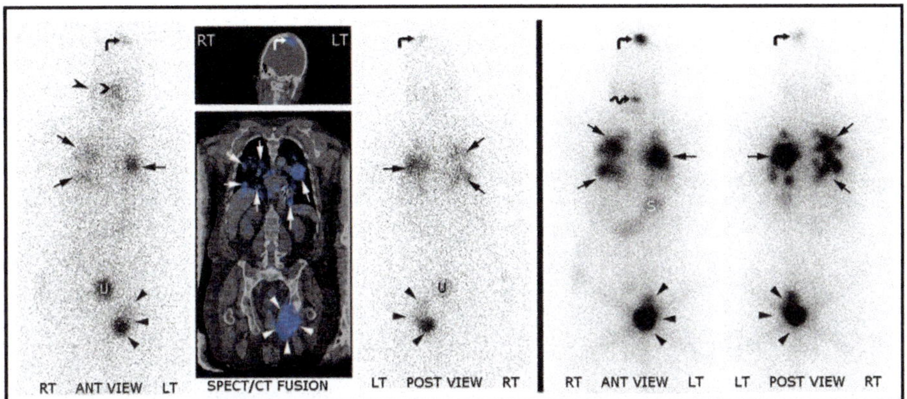

FIGURE 38.5 - I-131 SCAN
Diagnostic images obtained in whole body planar mode and SPECT/CT at 48 h after a 5 mCi I-131 dose are shown on the *left side* of the vertical divider line. Anterior (*ANT*) whole body view demonstrates abnormal activity in the lungs (*arrows*), left pelvis, and cranial vertex (*curved arrow*). There is physiological activity in the nasopharynx (*open arrowhead*), right salivary gland (*concave arrowhead*), left salivary gland (less obvious), and the urinary bladder (*U*). It is difficult to place those lesions anatomically due to inherent poor image clarity and lack of anatomical landmarks. The SPECT/CT fusion image overlays I-131 SPECT information color-coded in blue over the coronal CT slices. This technique gives clear anatomical localization to the findings. The left pelvic lesion (*white arrowheads*) is clearly seen to destroy the left iliac bone and the pulmonary lesions (*white arrows*) correlate with multiple nodular densities. The cranial lesion (*white curved arrow*) destroys the bony skull and is shown to extend into the brain tissue. The scan was repeated in whole body planar mode only, imaging the uptake of the 100 mCi treatment dose on day 7, showing the same sites, but much more clearly and with more foci of pulmonary metastases appreciable. There is physiological activity in the stomach (*S*) and most of the salivary activity had cleared with some remaining in the mouth (*squiggly arrow*). Urinary activity is not well seen because all of it had been excreted by the 7th day

39 Pulmonary Nuclear Medicine

Objectives:

1. Define ventilation-perfusion lung scintigraphy.
2. Define the radiopharmaceuticals used in lung perfusion and ventilation scans and the physiologic rationale for this examination.
3. Describe the differences in probability-based and trinary systems of interpretation of ventilation-perfusion lung scans.
4. Describe the principles of quantitative (differential) lung scintigraphy.
5. List the main indications of quantitative (differential) lung scintigraphy.

Ventilation-perfusion (or Quotient; hence, abbreviation V/Q) scan is an imaging technique aimed at interrogating the physiology and, to lesser degree, the anatomy of respective body functions. It is mostly indicated for *pulmonary embolism* (PE) or *thromboembolism*.

Assessment of ventilation is performed following inhalation of either a radioactive gas (e.g., Xenon-133) or aerosol (e.g., ^{99m}Tc-DTPA aerosol dispensed by a nebulizer) through a tightly fitted face mask. It allows for regional assessment of pulmonary airflow. The ventilation part of the V/Q scan is usually done first, as the radiotracer used during ventilation is either eliminated through expiration or given in a small enough activity that the radiotracer used during perfusion overrides the residual activity from the ventilation portion of the study. The perfusion imaging is done following intravenous injection of *^{99m}Tc-macroaggregated albumin* (MAA), which consists of small particles (average size of 15–30 μm). These particles are larger than the pulmonary capillary vasculature (about 7 μm); thus, nearly all radiolabeled particles are filtered out by the lungs during its first pass through in proportion with the regional pulmonary artery blood flow. The test can be performed using planar (the most common method in contemporary practice) or SPECT imaging (Reinartz et al. 2004).

H. Singh et al. (eds.), *Radiology Fundamentals: Introduction to Imaging & Technology*, DOI 10.1007/978-3-319-10362-4_39

Perfusion is imaged after an I.V. injection of about 300,000–500,000 ^{99m}Tc-MAA particles. There are 300–500 million alveoli in the lungs that are surrounded by a capillary network. A conservative estimate is that less than 1 in 1,000 capillaries would be occluded, which is generally very safe. Exception is a patient with severe pulmonary arterial hypertension that is associated with marked reduction in the alveoli and capillaries. Blocking additional capillaries with ^{99m}Tc-MAA can precipitate right heart failure in these patients; therefore, the study is contraindicated in severe pulmonary hypertension, and caution is advised in cases with signs of right heart strain. Another contraindication includes hypersensitivity to human albumin products (very rare).

The essential V/Q scan principle for detecting PE is based on detecting perfusion defect(s) with normal ventilation, called *V/Q mismatch*. The larger the perfusion defect and the greater their number, the higher is the probability of PE. At least two large segmental mismatches are needed to be reasonably convinced that the patient has a PE (called *high probability* or *positive scan for PE*). If a perfusion defect is matched by a ventilation abnormality, then the likelihood of PE is low. Such finding reflects airspace-based disease that often causes regional hypoxia-mediated vasoconstriction, which in turn can result in a *matched V/Q defect*. Different patterns on V/Q scan are comprised of variations in size, number, the anatomical distribution of perfusion defects, as well as corresponding chest X-ray (CXR) findings. Those patterns can be grouped in probabilistic interpretational categories that define the likelihood of PE, which include essentially normal or negative perfusion, *very low*, *low*, *intermediate* (or *indeterminate*), and *high probability*. This probabilistic reporting has to be combined with clinical pretest probability in order to estimate the post-test probability of PE, which is often confusing for managing physicians. More recently, a simplified approach was developed where the first three categories are reported as *negative study for PE*, the last category as *positive study for PE*, and the indeterminate as *inconclusive*. This system of interpreting is called *trinary*. Pregnancy is a specific concern as the whole body receives radiation exposure, albeit small, particularly from ^{99m}Tc-DTPA which is cleared into the urinary bladder, which is in close proximity to the uterus. Therefore, the ventilation portion of the examination should be initially omitted in pregnant patients and perfusion done with lowest possible activity. If perfusion images show suspicious defects, ventilation can be done later (Fig. 39.1).

Spiral CT pulmonary angiography (CTPA) supplanted V/Q scanning as the initial diagnostic imaging for PE (Wikipedia Contributors 2013). However, concern has been raised recently that it may be too sensitive, resulting in overdiagnosis and overtreatment. Its major strengths include: (a) readily available around the clock in most hospitals, (b) can be performed quickly, and (c) the interpretation is simple to understand-positive, negative, or indeterminate (usually for technical factors).

The indeterminate or inconclusive V/Q result is least helpful in clinical management and is most likely in the presence of CXR opacities, which is where CTPA should be favored. V/Q scanning may take several hours to obtain, or even longer if

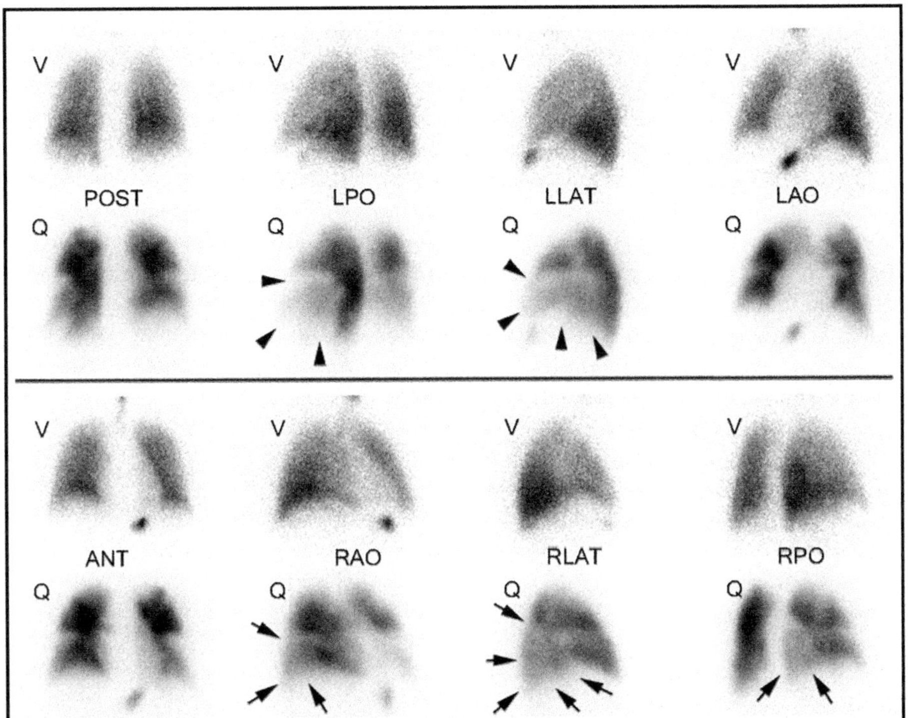

FIGURE 39.1 - HIGH PROBABILITY V/Q SCAN

V/Q scan with findings consistent with "High Probability" or "Positive for PE" interpretation. The chest X-ray was normal. The ventilation (*V*) obtained with ^{99m}Tc-DTPA aerosol are on top and perfusion (*Q*) obtained with ^{99m}Tc-MAA are on the bottom, paired according to the eight standard views: posterior (*POST*), left posterior oblique (*LPO*), left lateral (*LLAT*), left anterior oblique (*LAO*), anterior (*ANT*), right anterior oblique (*RAO*), right lateral (*RLAT*), and right posterior oblique (*RPO*). The ventilation images show normal physiological distribution of activity. The Q images show multiple, large, wedge-shaped perfusion defects. The largest one is severe in count deficit (photopenia) and involves most of the left lower lobe segments and both lingula (*arrowheads*) segments, sparing only the posterior basal segment of the lower lobe. The normal V in those segments defines "mismatch". There is an almost comparable in size mismatched defect that is milder in photopenia and involves all segments of the right lower lobe (*arrows*). There are multiple other smaller defects (not annotated).

ordered after regular work hours, as a technologist often needs to be called in from home and radiopharmaceuticals freshly prepared. Contraindications to CTPA include contrast allergy and renal insufficiency, which is when V/Q scan becomes the preferred modality. Pulmonary hypertension from chronic PE is another circumstance where V/Q may be more sensitive than CTPA (Tunariu et al. 2007). Pulmonary angiography still remains the gold standard for the diagnosis of PE and may be necessary if the diagnosis remains in doubt after V/Q or CTPA scans are performed.

Quantitative lung scintigraphy or differential pulmonary function scan is performed to (1) predict pulmonary function after lung surgery (pneumonectomy or lobectomy) and (2) to quantify asymmetry in patients with compromised pulmonary artery flow, which is usually part of congenital heart syndromes.

The common principle for both indications is based on the fact that perfusion images performed with ^{99m}Tc-MAA are the best correlates for both the lung blood flow and the lung respiratory gas exchange function. It has been shown that performing a ventilation study does not add significant information over perfusion alone in quantifying gas exchange function. This is because the blood flow and gas exchange functions are coupled.

The critical question in patients with lung cancer and abnormal baseline lung function is whether the remaining lung function after surgery would suffice for a

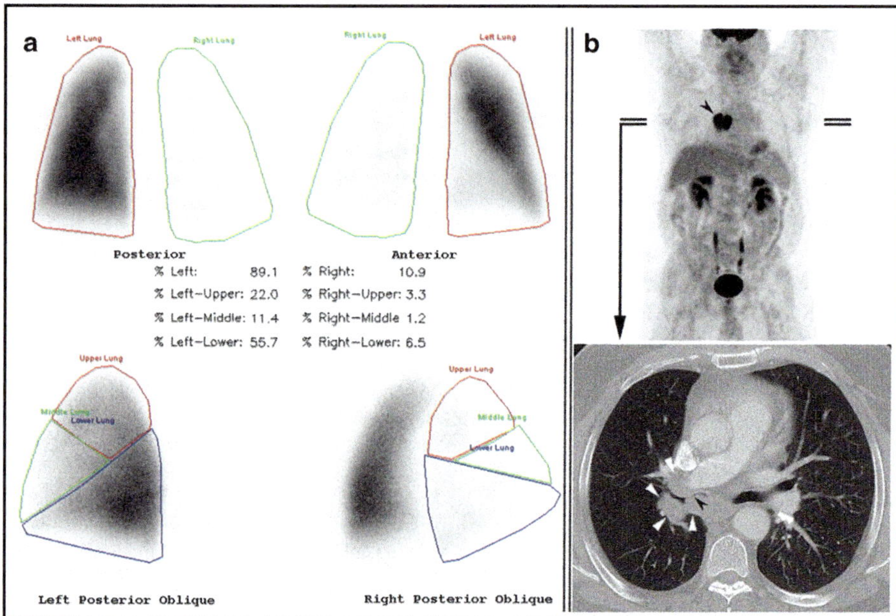

FIGURE 39.2 - APPLICATION OF QUANTITATIVE LUNG FUNCTION SCAN
This is a patient with right lung cancer who had FEV1 of 1.92 L/min, which would be concerning for pneumonectomy clearance and requires further evaluation. (**a**) The perfusion images in the anterior and posterior projections allow for count-based calculations of each lung contribution to lung function. Proportional calculations predict a post right pneumonectomy FEV1 of 1.71 L/min, which is adequate to maintain gas exchange after surgery. The lower panel shows posterior oblique images that allows calculation of individual lobe contributions to the overall pulmonary function and can be used for prediction of post lobectomy function. (**b**) The patient's non-small cell lung cancer was at the right hilum as seen on the top PET/CT MIP image (*arrowhead*) without metastases. The CT slice taken at the level of the mass is shown on the lower panel. The tumor (outlined by *white arrowheads*) compressed the right mainstem bronchus (*black arrowhead*), responsible for the lack of ventilation.

patient to live on, particularly during the perioperative period when the patient is first weaned off ventilator support. The essential lung function parameters in this context which predict complications are preoperative and predicted postoperative forced expiratory volume in one second (FEV_1). The example in Fig. 39.2 demonstrates how predicted postsurgical FEV_1 is calculated.

Pulmonary artery stenosis is often part of congenital heart disease and is typically unilateral. These patients have procedures, such as balloon angioplasty and stenting, which can correct or improve it. The asymmetry in pulmonary blood flow can be detected, quantified, and followed for the surveillance of restenosis using the same left versus right whole-lung quantification on the ^{99m}Tc-MAA images.

References

Reinartz P, Wildberger JE, Schaefer W, Nowak B, Mahnken AH, Buell U. Tomographic imaging in the diagnosis of pulmonary embolism: a comparison between V/Q lung scintigraphy in SPECT technique and multislice spiral CT. J Nuc Med. 2004;45(9):1501–8. Official publication, Society of Nuclear Medicine.

Tunariu N, Gibbs SJ, Win Z, et al. Ventilation-perfusion scintigraphy is more sensitive than multidetector CTPA in detecting chronic thromboembolic pulmonary disease as a treatable cause of pulmonary hypertension. J Nuc Med. 2007;48(5):680–4. Official publication, Society of Nuclear Medicine.

Wikipedia Contributors. CT pulmonary angiogram. 8 August 2013 10:35 UTC; http://en.wikipedia.org/w/index.php?title=CT_pulmonary_angiogram&oldid=567660359. Accessed 16 Dec 2013, 18:13 UTC, 2013.

40 Skeletal Nuclear Medicine

Objectives:

1. Describe the physiological rationale for tracer uptake on a bone scan.
2. Describe the sensitivity and specificity of the bone scan.
3. List the common causes of locally increased radiotracer uptake.
4. Describe the advantages of SPECT/CT over SPECT and planar bone scans.

Bone scan or bone scintigraphy (*BS*) is among the earliest diagnostic applications in NM imaging that remains useful today since its establishment in the early 1970s (Wikipedia Contributors 2013). Current bone-seeking radiotracers can be divided into those emitting gamma rays (imaged with gamma cameras) or positrons (imaged with PET/CT). The former group is collectively called ^{99m}Tc-polyphosphonates (^{99m}Tc-PPs), which include ^{99m}Tc-methylene diphosphonate and ^{99m}Tc-hydroxymethylene diphosphonate. The latter group includes ^{18}F-labeled sodium fluoride (Na^{18}F). They are all administered intravenously and taken up by the skeleton through a process called *chemabsorption* whereby the tracer is incorporated into the calcium hydroxyapatite crystal (CHAC) matrix of the bone, which is laid down by osteoblasts. Thus, bone-seeking radiotracers reflect skeletal osteoblastic activity (Wong and Piert 2013). Sometimes the radiotracers can localize to pathological or dystrophic calcium depositions in soft tissues such as calcified metastatic liver lesions from colorectal cancer or calcium deposits in the lungs or stomach in hyperparathyroidism.

^{111}In-labeled white blood cells (WBCs) can be used with ^{99m}Tc-PPs as an adjunct radiotracer to increase specificity for osteomyelitis indication (Fig. 40.1). Because of significant differences in emissions of the two isotopes, the images of both can be obtained simultaneously in their respective energy windows. Alternatively, ^{99m}Tc-WBCs can be used but must be performed on a different day from the bone scan owing to the same isotope label, which precludes differentiation of one from the other on

H. Singh et al. (eds.), *Radiology Fundamentals: Introduction to Imaging & Technology*, DOI 10.1007/978-3-319-10362-4_40

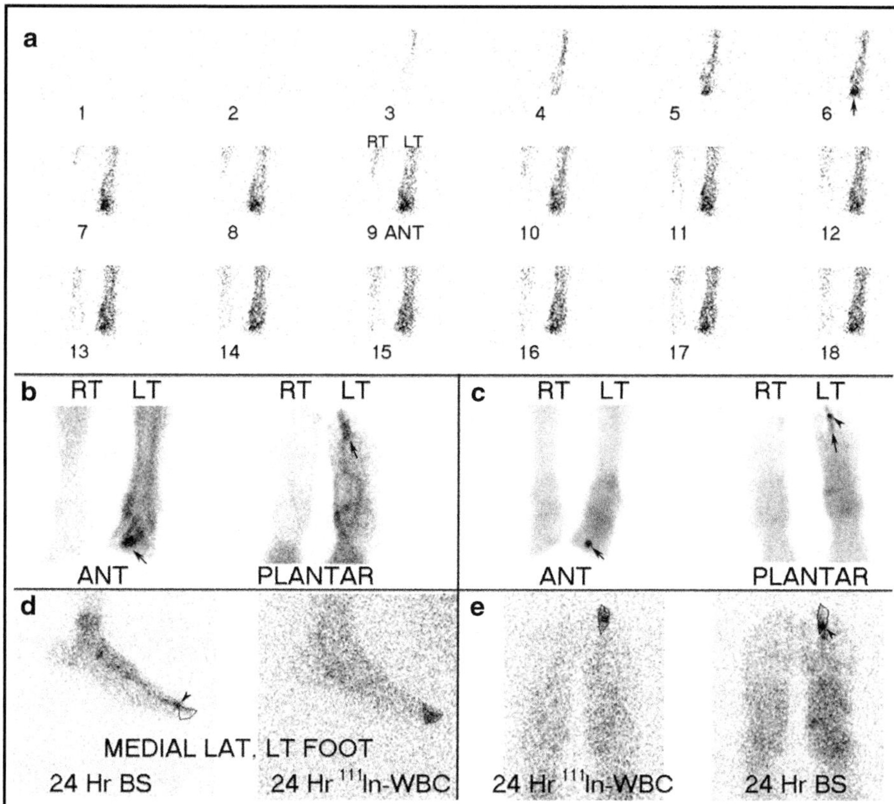

FIGURE 40.1 - 3-PHASE BONE SCAN

3-phase limited ^{99m}Tc-PPs bone scan (*BS*) in a patient with suspected osteomyelitis of the left second toe. The arterial (first phase) is 3 s per frame dynamic imaging (**a**) obtained in anterior view (*ANT*). The tracer appears on frame 3 in the left foot with intense focal activity (frame 6, *arrow*) corresponding to the affected toe. On frame 7 there is normal activity arriving on the unaffected side. The most intense focal activity is seen during the arterial phase (frames 4–9). The intensity decreases during the venous phase (frames 10 onwards). Frame 9 is annotated with left (*LT*) and right (*RT*) feet. The blood pool (second) phase (**b**) shows similar findings in ANT view (*arrow*). The plantar view is obtained with feet placed flat on the camera detector and best lays out the affected tow. The hyperemia is moderate over entire LT foot and intense focally in the toe (*arrow*). Delayed (3 h) spot images (**c**) show focal intense activity in the toe (*arrow*) on ANT view. The plantar view reveals the intense focus (*arrowhead*) in the distal third with milder activity proximally (*arrow*). There is less activity distally, which correlates with bone destruction on the radiograph and increased activity on the ^{111}In-labeled white blood cell (*WBC*) scan (**d** and **e**). It is the increased pressure of inflammatory focus (*irregular black outline*) on the ^{111}In- WBC scan that decreases osteoblastic activity. The lateral (*LAT*) (**d**) and plantar (**e**) views are orthogonal projections that best represent distribution of the findings imaging. The advantage of the former approach is that the BS and ^{111}In-WBC scans can be acquired concurrently and inherently co-registered to each other. Accordingly, drawing a region of interest on the ^{111}In-WBC focus makes it possible to place it on the identical location of the BS image. In osteomyelitis it would overlie the bone (Figs. 40.1d and e), whereas in cellulitis it would fall on the soft tissues away from bone.

^{99m}Tc-PPs are the most commonly used radiotracers for bone scintigraphy; thus, the term "bone scan" is typically synonymous with gamma-camera scanning. Although the bone's maximum uptake of ^{99m}Tc-PPs is reached within the first 20–30 min after injection, the high background activity created by interfering activity from soft tissues would preclude good skeletal visualization. As the radiotracer is cleared by the kidneys, skeletal visualization improves and reaches optimal quality by 2–3 h. Drinking fluids during this time improves tracer clearance and the sharpness, or contrast, of skeletal visualization.

The uptake of radiotracers depends on two variables: (1) blood flow and (2) amount of amorphous (newly formed) CHAC. Skeletal regions with increased blood flow (hyperemia) would simply receive greater delivery of the radiotracer, resulting in greater uptake. Osteoblasts lay down amorphous CHAC in actively growing, metabolizing, or repairing bone, which offers greater surface area for chemabsorption, i.e., greater uptake of the bone-seeking radiotracer.

Common indications for bone scanning include: primary skeletal tumors, benign neoplasms, metastatic skeletal disease (prostate cancer, non-small cell lung cancer, breast cancer, osteosarcoma, etc.), osteomyelitis, active facet arthropathy in patients with spinal (i.e., back) pain, stress fractures, occult fractures, and metabolic bone diseases (e.g., Paget's disease, fibrous dysplasia, etc.). An abnormality on the scan is not specific in and of itself. The combination of the pattern (location, distribution, intensity, etc.), correlation with other imaging modalities, and the patient's clinical presentation allow the interpreter to offer a list of likely specific diagnoses (a differential). A differential can be narrowed by applying other correlative imaging findings and/or by obtaining more detailed history and physical findings. One may repeat this deductive reasoning until the etiology is determined within a clinically acceptable degree of certainty.

Gamma imaging is most often performed using planar scintigraphy. But depending on clinical indication and a specific clinical dilemma, the imaging procedure (protocol) would vary. The 3-phase imaging includes: (1) dynamic blood flow sequence obtained immediately after injection (Fig. 40.1a), (2) static imaging of the blood pool that is obtained during the first 5–15 min after injection (Fig. 40.1b), and (3) static delays that are obtained 2–3 h later (Fig. 40.1c). This method is most useful in evaluating traumatic injuries (fractures, stress fractures, etc.) and osteomyelitis (Fig. 40.1). Because those indications typically involve small parts of the skeleton, the spot images would be sufficient. This type of scan is often referred to as "limited," meaning to the area of concern. For the detection of skeletal metastatic disease, only the static delay images are needed and they are usually obtained using the whole-body imaging mode (Fig. 40.2). See Introduction to NM for additional details.

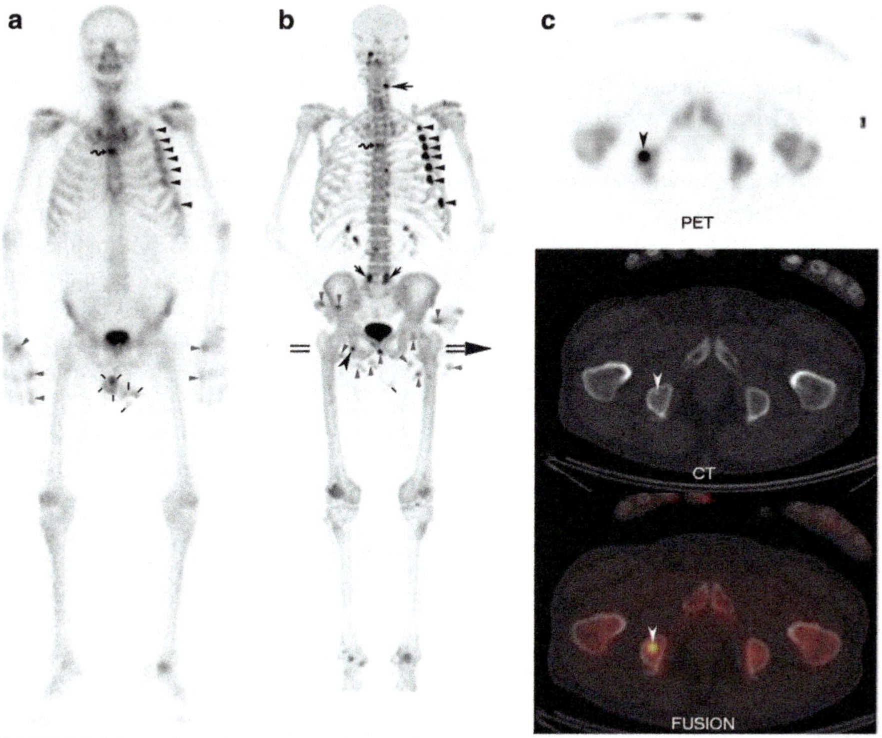

FIGURE 40.2 - METASTATIC DISEASE ON BONE SCAN
This is a 65-year-old male with a history of treated prostate cancer was found to have newly elevated prostate specific antigen on laboratory surveillance. The anterior projection of the ^{99m}Tc-PPs whole body bone scan (**a**) showed mild foci of uptake in the left chest (*black arrowheads*), which are distributed (lined up along consecutive ribs) in a typical pattern for rib fractures (corroborated by local pain and history of fall). There are joint-centered areas of mild uptake in the hands (*gray arrowheads*) and moderate uptake in the sternomanubrial joint (*squiggly arrow*), as well as in the knees, left ankle and elbow – typical of osteoarthritis. The splotchy activity in the groin is due to urinary contamination (*gray lines*). No metastatic disease was found. The anterior view of maximum intensity projection image of the Na^{18}F scan (**b**) few days later show the key finding in the right inferior ramus of the pelvis (*concave-base arrowhead*). There are multiple other spots scattered over the pelvis (*gray arrowheads*), which are all related to patient's arthritic foci in the hands placed over the pelvis. The axial section through the lesion was taken at the level shown by the *double line* with the *arrow* pointing to the column of tomographic slices (**c**). The intense lesion is seen on PET images in the inferior ischeal ramus where CT showed a small blastic lesion. The fusion image shows it as well. Notice the foci in the cervical and lumbar spine (*concave-base arrows*) that corresponds to benign active facet arthropathy (Images courtesy of Dr. Andrei H Iagaru)

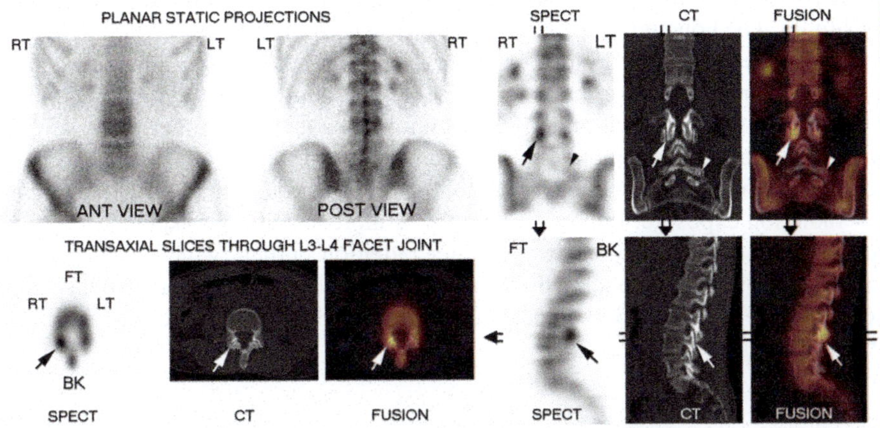

FIGURE 40.3 - DEGENERATIVE SPINE DISEASE ON BONE SCAN
A 56-year-old male with back pain who underwent 3-phase limited planar bone scan and SPECT/CT. The blood flow and pool images were normal (not shown). The spot images in anterior (*ANT*) and posterior (*POST*) views show no obvious abnormality. The sides relative to the patient are annotated for left (*LT*) and right (*RT*) on all image series. To the right of planar scans displayed are coronal slices through the lumbar spine at the level that reveals the key finding – intense focal uptake (*arrow*) in the right facet joint at L3/L4 level. There is mild uptake in the opposite side of the same level, which is less significant. For comparison, notice normal activity (*arrowheads*) at L5/S1 facets. Sagittal section through the intense focus is denoted on coronal slices by *double tick-lines* (on *top* and *bottom* edges of images) with the *arrow pointing down* to the corresponding sagittal slices. The same findings are depicted on the axial slice through the lesion denoted by *double tick lines* (on the *sides* of the images) with the *arrow pointing* to the transaxial slices. The front (*FT*) and back (*BK*) of the patient is annotated on the SPECT

Hybrid SPECT/CT is particularly useful in the work-up of back pain. It allows precise anatomical localization of active bone metabolism in facet arthropathy (Fig. 40.3) and/or spondylolysis on the CT portion, which is obtained with a significantly lower radiation dose as compared to the diagnostic CT. Before the advent of hybrid imaging, differentiating between those two pathologies on SPECT alone presented a significant challenge with precise anatomical position of a focal abnormality. It was necessary to correlate with CT obtained at a separate visit. SPECT and SPECT/CT are more sensitive than planar bone scans for scintigraphic lesion detection because of better contrast resolution. Both facet arthropathy and spondylolysis can present either asymptomatically, such as in chronic and stable states when these are discovered incidentally, or symptomatically. While normal or minimal radiotracer uptake is usually seen in the former clinical circumstance, the latter is typically associated with increased accumulation of $Na^{18}F$ (Fig. 40.2) and ^{99m}Tc-PPs (Fig. 40.3).

In spite of its nonspecific nature, the bone scan is very useful because of its high sensitivity. The bone turnover and osteoblastic activity increase well before there is either a bone loss (lytic lesion) or formation of pathologically increased density (blastic lesion). Therefore, metastatic disease can be seen on a bone scan well in advance of its appearance on the plain radiographs and sometime before any CT abnormality becomes obvious. The other advantage of the bone scan is its ability to image the whole body with a single radiotracer injection, which gives a relatively low radiation exposure. In comparison, CT is more specific for skeletal conditions but typically exposes patients to a greater radiation burden, which increases with coverage of every additional body area (not applicable to a bone scan that has radiation exposure determined by injected radiotracer and independent of the number of obtained images).

References

Wikipedia Contributors. Bone scintigraphy. 16 October 2013 08:40 UTC; http://en.wikipedia.org/w/index.php?title=Bone_scintigraphy&oldid=577401413. Accessed 10 Dec 2013, 01:22 UTC, 2013.

Wong KK, Piert M. Dynamic bone imaging with 99mTc-labeled diphosphonates and 18F-NaF: mechanisms and applications. J Nucl Med. 2013;54(4):590–9.

Part VI
Interventional Radiology Section

41 Diagnostic Arteriography

Objectives:
1. Describe in detail the technique for arterial groin and arm punctures.
2. Discuss how catheter design helps in the performance of arteriography.
3. Discuss the complications of arteriography and their relative frequency.

Arteriography involves the placement of a catheter into the arterial system with injection of contrast while obtaining X-ray images. Various catheters and wires are used in combination to cannulate the desired arteries (Fig. 41.1).

Femoral and Brachial Artery Access

Access to the femoral or brachial artery is performed at the level of the femoral head or in line with the humerus above the elbow, respectively. Access is achieved at either of these points for two reasons. First, the artery in these locations is easy to palpate and therefore easier to locate and puncture. Second, the artery is adjacent to a bony structure; when the catheter is removed, hemostasis can be achieved by compressing the artery against the bone directly behind it (Fig. 41.2).

Once access to the artery is obtained, a floppy-tipped guide wire is advanced under fluoroscopy. The stiffer portion of the guide wire follows for an adequate distance. The needle is then exchanged over the wire for either a catheter or a vascular sheath (this is called **Seldinger technique** – you will hear this term over and over again during your medical careers). A vascular sheath is a device which has a hemostatic valve on the portion that remains outside the patient. The sheath stays in the artery and through the sheath, catheter exchanges can be accomplished with

H. Singh et al. (eds.), *Radiology Fundamentals: Introduction to Imaging & Technology*, DOI 10.1007/978-3-319-10362-4_41

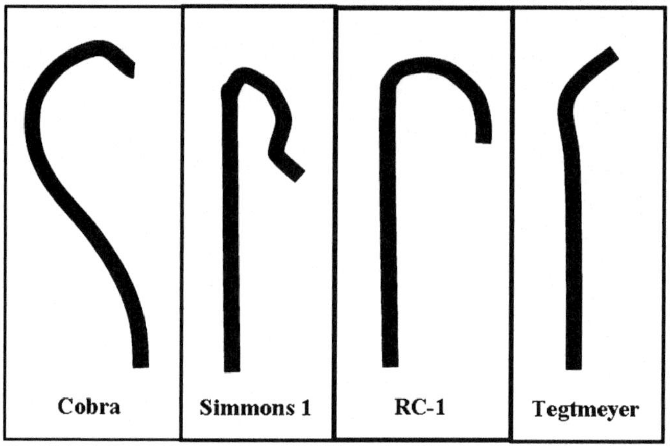

FIGURE 41.1 - CATHETERS AND WIRES
Various catheters and wires are used in combination to cannulate the desired arteries

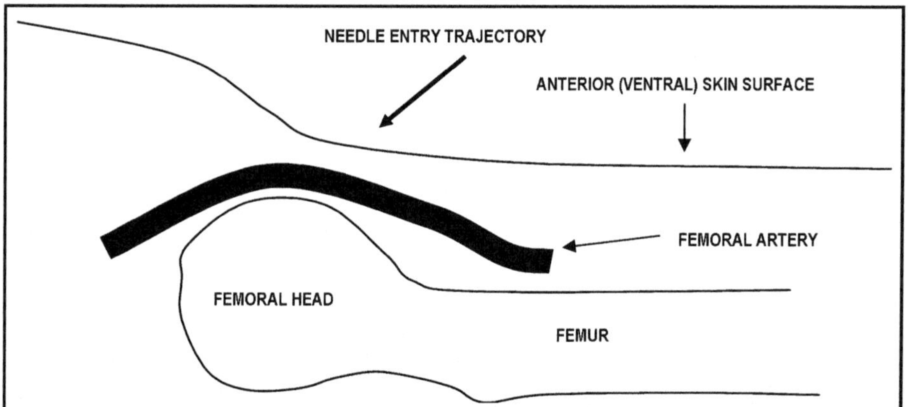

FIGURE 41.2 - COMMON FEMORAL ARTERY ACCESS
In the lateral view, the femoral artery lies just on top of the femoral head. At this point, it is easy to palpate and easy to compress after the catheter is removed

minimal blood loss. A disadvantage of using a sheath is its larger outer diameter and the larger hole it makes in the artery compared to a catheter alone.

If "flush" arteriographic studies are to be performed, particularly of large vessels, a catheter with multiple side holes is used to evenly distribute the contrast in the blood pool. A typical example of this would be aortography using a "pigtail" or "tennis racket" catheter. If selective arteriography is needed, then an appropriately shaped catheter, usually with a single end hole, is used with a guide wire to select the desired arteries and then inject contrast (Fig. 41.1).

Once the catheter is in appropriate position, contrast is injected either by hand or with a power injector using a known rate and pressure. Images are obtained with digital subtraction angiography (DSA) imaging. Diagnostic images are reviewed. Either the study is concluded at that time or, if appropriate, an intervention is undertaken.

At the completion of the procedure, the catheter or sheath is removed and hemostasis is obtained at the puncture site by compressing the artery against the underlying bony structure. Compression is usually held for 15–20 min. Once hemostasis is obtained, the patient must lie flat for 6 h (or maintain the elbow extended after an arm puncture) and the groin or antecubital fossa must be checked frequently to make sure no bleeding has occurred. Using an arterial closure device can significantly shorten the 6-h time period.

Arteriography Complications

Complications of arteriography include:

1. *Groin or arm hematoma*
   In the groin, a hematoma which requires some additional treatment is not uncommon, occurring up to 5 % of the time. In the arm, it can be much more dangerous because of possible compression of the vessels and nerves in the neurovascular bundle requiring urgent attention.
2. *Infection*
   Infection is almost unheard of in arteriography. Because of the small access points and the sterile draping and technique, it occurs in less than 1 % of all cases.
3. *Contrast reaction*
   Injection of contrast media in anyone may result in a contrast reaction. The most common reaction clinically is the onset of itching and hives. Treatment is nearly always successful using known drug algorithms. If a patient has a known contrast allergy, he or she must be pretreated with oral or intravenous steroids (e.g., oral prednisone 50 mg) at 13, 7, and 1 h before the procedure. The patient should also be given Benadryl 50 mg IV or PO one hour prior to the procedure. The most important steroid dose is the dose given 13 h before the procedure. The mechanism of protection is thought to be the stabilization of mast cell membranes thereby preventing the degranulation and release of histamine.
4. *Contrast-induced nephrotoxicity (CIN)*
   Current literature suggests the main risk factors for CIN include preexisting renal insufficiency, diabetes mellitus, and, in some cases, severe congestive heart failure. When ordering an arteriogram (or any study with contrast), the increased risk for CIN should be considered.

5. *Vessel dissection or pseudoaneurysm formation*
   Any time a blood vessel is entered traumatically (as with a puncture for arteriography), there is a definite but small risk of vessel injury, pseudoaneurysm, or arteriovenous fistula formation.

42 Pulmonary Arteriography and IVC Filter Placement

Objectives:
1. List the indications for pulmonary arteriography.
2. Describe the technique for pulmonary arteriography including the contraindications.
3. Describe the technique for inferior vena cava filter placement including what is appropriate for an inferior cava larger than 28 mm.

Although still considered the gold standard for the diagnosis of pulmonary embolism, pulmonary arteriography has largely been supplanted by pulmonary CT scan angiography (CTAP). Nevertheless, pulmonary arteriography may still be indicated in patients with a high clinical suspicion for pulmonary embolism and:

1. A low probability or indeterminate V/Q scan or CTAP
2. An indeterminate V/Q or CTAP and contraindication to anticoagulation
3. Prior to catheter-based pulmonary embolectomy

Conventional pulmonary arteriography is accomplished from the right common femoral vein or right internal jugular vein. Access is obtained in a fashion similar to that described in the arteriography section. Once access has been obtained, a pulmonary artery catheter is advanced to the level of the right atrium. The catheter is gently advanced across the tricuspid valve and, while pushing forward, is rotated (Fig. 42.1). As it crosses through the right ventricle to the pulmonary outflow tract, it is gently pushed farther, usually into the left pulmonary artery. The catheter position in each pulmonary artery is confirmed with a minimal amount of contrast, and *pulmonary artery pressures are recorded.* The contrast injection is tailored, based on the pulmonary artery pressures. If the pressures are normal or only mildly elevated, a standard pulmonary arteriogram is performed. If the pressures are elevated,

H. Singh et al. (eds.), *Radiology Fundamentals: Introduction to Imaging & Technology*, DOI 10.1007/978-3-319-10362-4_42

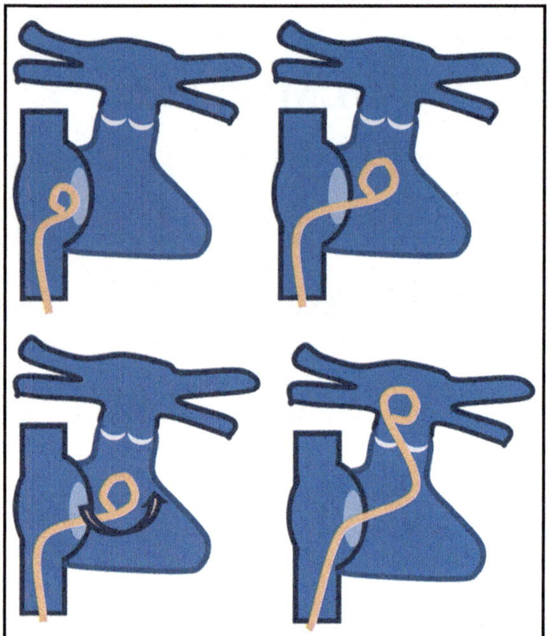

FIGURE 42.1 - TECHNIQUE FOR PULMONARY ARTERY CATHETERIZATION
Diagram depicts technique required to passing the pulmonary artery catheter across the right heart valves and into the main pulmonary artery

the contrast injection volume is decreased or a subselective angiogram is performed. Once images have been obtained on the left, the catheter is then manipulated to the right side.

Images are obtained in the AP and opposite oblique (i.e., for a left pulmonary arteriogram, an AP and right anterior oblique study are performed). If there remains a question, selective magnification views of the area of concern can be performed. Angiographic findings of acute pulmonary embolism include "wormlike" filling defects (clots that are casts of the lower leg veins) that are often draped over vessel bifurcation points, tram-tracking of contrast around clots that are nearly occlusive in the vessel, and complete vessel occlusions characterized by cutoffs with a meniscus.

IVC Filter Placement

Although often thought of as separate entities, deep vein thrombosis (DVT) and pulmonary embolism (PE) are the beginning and ultimate final end result of a single disease process known as venous thromboembolic disease (VTED).

The primary treatment of choice of VTED is anticoagulation therapy. Anticoagulation therapy prevents new clot formation and allows the body's *own mechanisms* to dissolve the blood clot. (NB – anticoagulation therapy does not dissolve clot itself.) It is a generally safe, effective, and affordable means of preventing a DVT from progressing to a PE.

Inferior vena cava (IVC) filters are metallic devices placed in the inferior vena cava that present a mechanical barrier that prevents an embolus from traveling from the lower extremities or pelvis to the pulmonary arteries. Although IVC filters are effective in preventing PE, they remain as second-line therapy for several reasons:

1. IVC filters do nothing to help resolve existing clot and, in some cases, may worsen underlying DVT.
2. IVC Filters are associated with complications that become more likely the longer that the device stays in place. These include:
   (a) Filter fracture
   (b) Perforation of filter elements through the cava and into adjacent structures
   (c) Filter migration/embolization
   (d) Caval thrombosis
3. Some studies suggest that over time, IVC filters lose their protective value (Decousus et al. 1998). After 2 years, when compared with patients who receive anticoagulation, patients with IVC filters have the same rate of recurrent PE with twice the rate of recurrent DVT.

Indications for the placement of an IVC filter in patients with VTED include:

1. Contraindication to anticoagulation
2. PE despite adequate anticoagulation (failed anticoagulation therapy)
3. Significant risk of complication from anticoagulation therapy (e.g., fall risk, planned elective surgery)
4. Trauma with injury patterns known to place the patient at high risk for VTED, such as long bone fracture and spinal cord injuries

Many different filter designs are available in the North American and European markets, but in general, they all fall into one of two categories: permanent and retrievable (Fig. 42.2). A permanent filter, as the name implies, is intended to stay in place permanently. A retrievable filter (also sometimes referred to as an "optional" filter) can be used as a permanent device but has design features that allow it to be removed using percutaneous techniques. These devices are sometimes referred to as "optional" filters because they are permanent devices with the option to be removed.

The rationale for having such a device is simple. Because IVC filters are good at preventing PE in the short term but lose their effectiveness while increasing their complication rate over time, it makes sense to have a device that can be placed to protect a patient during a period of high risk that can then be removed once the risk returns to normal.

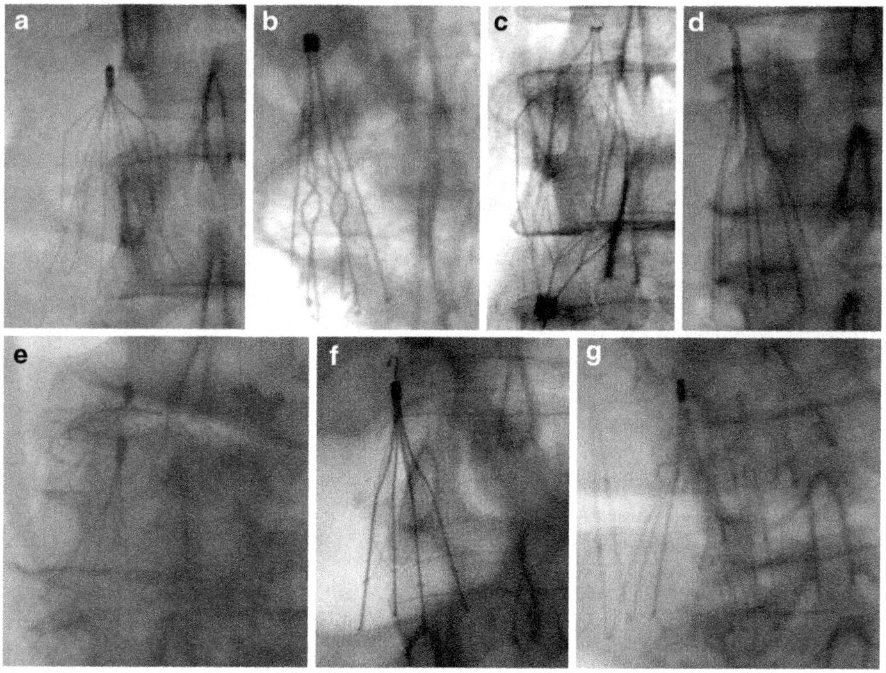

FIGURE 42.2 - EXAMPLES OF SEVERAL IVC FILTERS AVAILABLE TODAY
Clockwise starting from the *upper left*: (**a**) G2 (removable), (**b**) Greenfield (permanent), (**c**) Optease (removable), (**d**) Option (removable), (**e**) Simon Nitinol (permanent), (**f**) Tulip (removable), (**g**) Vena Tech LP (permanent)

IVC filters are placed via common femoral vein or internal jugular vein access. A marker catheter (a catheter with radiopaque markers at an exact distance, usually 20 mm) is placed in the right common iliac vein and a power-injection inferior vena cava study is performed, paying close attention to the iliac vein confluence and the inflow from the renal veins. Most IVC filters are designed to be stable in vena cavas 28 mm or less in diameter. The marks on the catheter serve as a reference distance and allow for accurate measurement of the caval diameter accounting for magnification. The appropriate filter is chosen (based on caval size and configuration) and delivered into position inside of a long deployment sheath. Rather than being pushed out the end of the sheath, the filter is deployed by withdrawing the outer sheath, allowing the filter to expand in place, usually just below the renal veins. A follow-up study is performed to confirm the filter's position (Fig. 42.3).

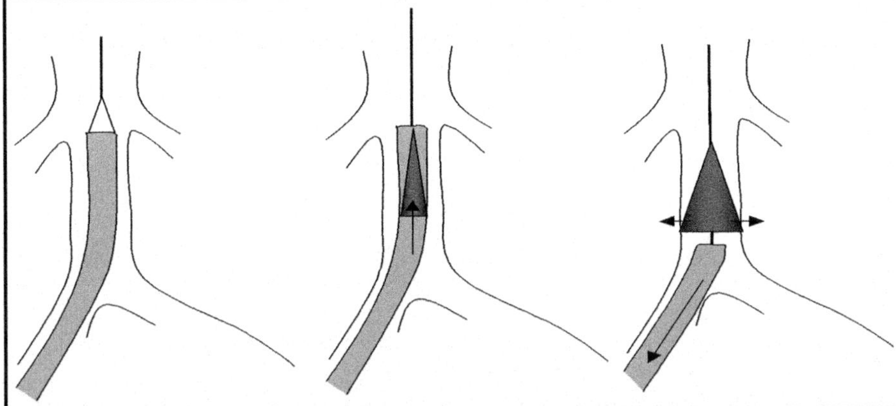

FIGURE 42.3 - DEPLOYMENT OF A VENA CAVA FILTER
On the *left*, a deployment sheath with the introducing cannula is advanced over a wire. The cannula is then removed, and inside the sheath, the filter is advanced to the tip of the sheath. The sheath is then pulled back (big point) and the filter self-deploys. It is very important to know exactly where the renal veins, accessory renal veins, and the iliac vein confluence are, so that optimal deployment is possible

Reference

Decousus H, Leizorovicz A, Parent F, et al. A clinical trial of vena caval filters in the prevention of pulmonary embolism in patients with proximal deep vein thrombosis. N Engl J Med. 1998; 338(7):409–15.

43 Percutaneous Nephrostomy Placement

Objectives:
1. Identify the relevant anatomy of the kidney and how it relates to deciding on access to the kidney.
2. Describe why air is important to the performance of a nephrostomy tube placement.
3. Describe a Cope loop.

Percutaneous drainage of the kidney is performed for several reasons, the most common of which is obstruction from nephrolithiasis, kidney stone disease. Obstructive uropathy secondary to a ureteral stone can be a medical emergency, particularly if there is evidence of urosepsis from ureteral obstruction. In those cases, percutaneous drainage may be a lifesaving measure.

Frequently, renal ultrasound or abdominal CT scan has already been performed to evaluate the cause of the patient's flank pain, fever, etc. These studies are then reviewed carefully to help localize the kidney and any possible intervening structures such as the colon, spleen, or liver prior to drainage.

The three most common methods for initial puncture of the kidney include using anatomic landmarks, using ultrasound guidance, and using a small dose of intravenous contrast to generate a faint nephrogram. With the patient in the prone position, the initial access is achieved with a 22 g Chiba needle.

Once the needle is in the renal pelvis, urine is withdrawn and sent for culture. A small amount of contrast is used to confirm access to the renal pelvis. The renal pelvis can be opacified with contrast (although this may require a large amount of contrast and may distend the collecting system unnecessarily) or air. The air will fill the nondependent posterior calyces that can then be targeted under fluoroscopy for definitive access. Once the appropriate calyx is chosen, the angle of entry should be

H. Singh et al. (eds.), *Radiology Fundamentals: Introduction to Imaging & Technology*, DOI 10.1007/978-3-319-10362-4_43

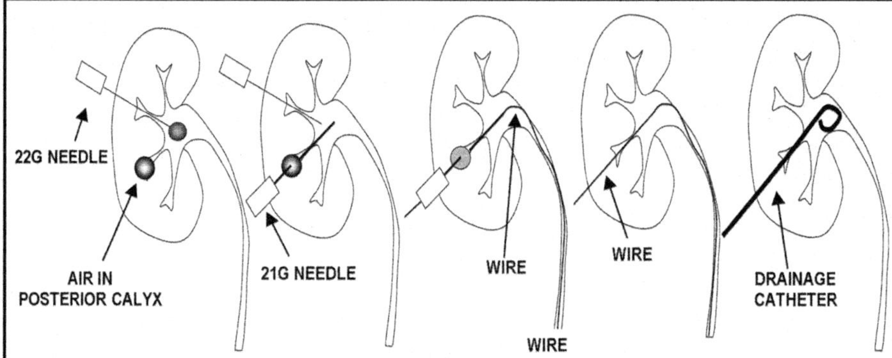

FIGURE 43.1 - PERCUTANEOUS NEPHROSTOMY TUBE PLACEMENT
In the first image, a small-caliber needle (22 g) is advanced into the renal collecting system. The system is opacified with contrast and air is instilled to demonstrate a posterior calyx. This is then accessed with a larger needle (21 g) which accepts an 0.018″ wire. The needle is then removed, the tract dilated over the wire, and a drainage catheter advanced into place (Remember, this is the Seldinger technique). The tip is drawn back by an internal string system, which helps keep the catheter locked in the collecting system, termed "Cope looped" (see below)

determined. The kidney should be accessed along Brödel's avascular line, a plane between the posterior and anterior segmental arteries.

Once the calyx has been accessed, a wire is advanced into the renal collecting system through the access needle. The needle is removed, and over the wire, the tract is dilated to an appropriate caliber. Once the tract is dilated, a stiffer wire is advanced into place, and over the wire, a drainage catheter is advanced into the collecting system, Cope looped, and locked in place. The catheter is placed to external drainage and the output is recorded carefully (Fig. 43.1).

Once the kidney is decompressed, various catheters are available for long-term drainage, including nephroureteral stents and internal double-J stents. The possible combinations are quite extensive (Figs. 43.2 and 43.3).

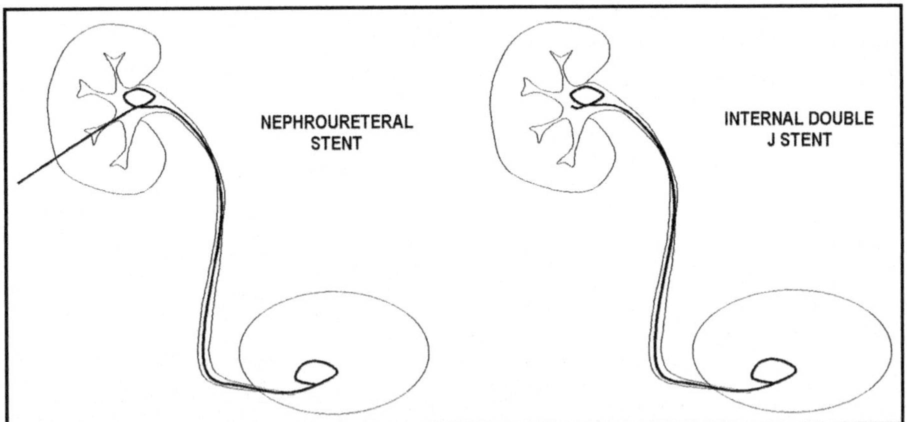

FIGURE 43.2 - TWO TYPES OF UROLOGICAL STENTS
On the *left*, the percutaneous nephrostomy tube has been converted to a nephroureteral stent, from the kidney down to the bladder. On the *right*, there has been percutaneous placement of an internal double-J stent

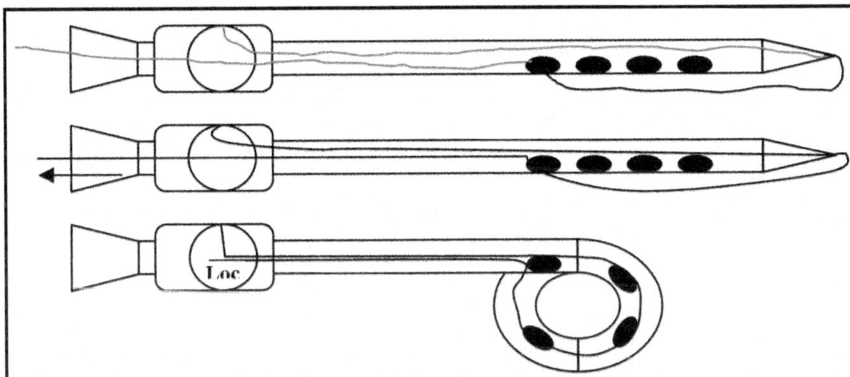

FIGURE 43.3 - COPE LOOP
In the first catheter at the *top*, there is a string extending loosely from the hub, through the end of the catheter and back into a sidehole. Once the catheter is in place, tension is placed on the string which then draws the tip of the catheter back on itself, forming the distal Cope loop. The string is then locked at the hub and the excess string is trimmed

44 TIPS

Objectives:
1. List the indications for TIPS.
2. List the contraindications for TIPS.
3. Describe the steps needed to create a TIPS.
4. Discuss how TIPS placement alters long-term survival.

The transjugular intrahepatic portosystemic shunt (TIPS) is a percutaneous procedure designed to decompress the portal system in patients with portal hypertension.

TIPS Indications

1. Variceal hemorrhage which is refractory to medical management
2. Prophylaxis for recurrent variceal bleeding
3. Ascites or large pleural effusion which is refractory to medical management
4. Budd-Chiari syndrome

TIPS Contraindications

1. Severe hepatic insufficiency
2. Poorly controlled encephalopathy
3. Portal vein occlusion
4. Polycystic liver disease
5. Hypervascular hepatic tumor

H. Singh et al. (eds.), *Radiology Fundamentals: Introduction to Imaging & Technology*, DOI 10.1007/978-3-319-10362-4_44

TIPS-Relative Contraindications

1. Active bleeding
2. Active infection

Once placement of the TIPS has been deemed appropriate, several questions must be answered. Is the portal vein patent by ultrasound or CT scan? If the varices are actively bleeding, TIPS is relatively contraindicated because of the high mortality associated with placement of a TIPS in an actively bleeding patient. Sometimes, however, it is the patient's only option.

TIPS Placement

For placement of the TIPS, the right internal jugular vein is used for access. Once access has been obtained, a large, long sheath (10 French) is placed with its tip in the right atrium. Using an angled catheter, access is obtained to the right hepatic vein (or sometimes the middle hepatic vein). Simultaneous pressures are obtained between the hepatic vein and the right atrium. Next the catheter is "wedged" as peripherally as possible in the hepatic vein. A wedged hepatic vein pressure to right atrial pressure gradient (similar to inflating the balloon of a Swan-Ganz catheter to obtain left atrial pressures) is determined. A hepatic venogram is then obtained. The angled catheter is exchanged for one of several transhepatic needle access systems.

A large, hollow, directional needle is used to gain access through the liver, and via the needle, a wire is advanced into the portal vein. True simultaneous pressures are obtained across the liver in the hepatic vein and the portal vein. The tract is predilated with an 8 mm balloon. A stent of appropriate length is deployed across the liver and dilated (Fig. 44.1). Simultaneous gradients are then obtained. If the gradient is too low, there can be a significant "steal" phenomenon from liver perfusion. If the gradient is too high, improvement in the varices or ascites/effusion may be inadequate. Pressure gradients greater than 12 mmHg are associated with an increased rate of variceal bleeding. If the pressure gradient remains elevated after TIPS placement, the stent may need to be dilated to a larger diameter to reduce the gradient to an acceptable level. If hepatic encephalopathy is not controlled after TIPS placement, the TIPS may actually need to be occluded.

An ultrasound is obtained prior to the patient's discharge and at subsequent regular intervals for follow-up after discharge to ensure patency of the TIPS (Fig. 44.2).

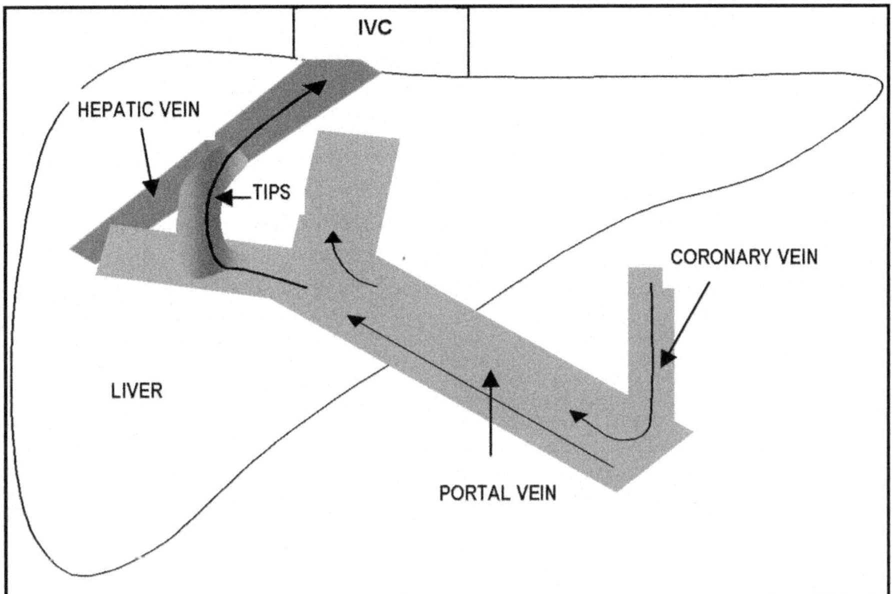

FIGURE 44.1 - DIAGRAM OF A TIPS
Through a percutaneous access from the internal jugular vein, the right hepatic vein is "connected" to the right portal vein branch via a transparenchymal tract. This tract is supported open utilizing a stent, frequently a Viatorr device. This allows the portal venous flow to decompress into the hepatic venous system and the associated varices to bypass the diseased liver

DIAGNOSTIC CRITERIA	1	2	3
ENCEPHALOPATHY	NONE	MODERATE	SEVERE
ASCITES	NONE	MODERATE	SEVERE
BILIRUBIN	<2	2-3	>3
ALBUMIN	>3.5	2.8-3.4	<2.8
PT	<14	15-17	>18

FIGURE 44.2 - CHILD'S SCORE
This classification scheme is used to assess the prognosis of chronic liver disease. To calculate a score, add the points from each category together. A is 5–6 points, B is 7–9 points, while C is greater than 10 points

Long-Term Survival

TIPS placement is successful in 96 % of cases. It is important to understand that TIPS placement does not alter the underlying liver disease. It only alters the manifestations of portal hypertension. Current transplant-free survival after a TIPS is 75.1 % at 6 months, 63.1 % at 12 months, 49 % at 24 months, and 38.1 % at 36 months (Salerno et al. 2007). It is important to calculate the MELD (Model for End Stage Liver Disease) score as this dramatically influences survival. As would be expected the higher the MELD score, the lower the overall survival (Ferral et al. 2004)

References

Ferral H, Gamboa P, et al. Survival after elective transjugular intrahepatic portosystemic shunt creation: prediction with model for end-stage liver disease score. Radiology. 2004;231:231–236.

Salerno F, Camma C, et al. Transjugular intrahepatic portosystemic shunt for refractory ascites: a meta-analysis of individual patient data. Gastroenterology. 2007;133:825–34.

45 Central Venous Access

Objectives:
1. List the types of devices available and their indications for placement.
2. List the different methods of central venous access.

Maintenance of venous access is the cornerstone of many medical therapies. Durable venous access into the central venous systems is essential for most cancer regimens, extended antibiotic therapies, parenteral nutrition, and inotropic therapies. Durable central venous access for patients who require hemodialysis serves as a bridge until a dialysis fistula or graft is established or as a means of last resort when a graft or fistula is no longer possible. Increasingly, the placement of a long-term central venous access device is performed using ultrasound and fluoroscopic image guidance and is most commonly performed by interventional radiology (Fig. 45.1).

There is a great deal of confusion concerning the different types of venous access devices. This situation is complicated by the common practice of referring to catheters by trade names, which are often ambiguous as to form and function. In general, catheters are classified by two attributes: non-tunneled versus tunneled and infusion versus exchange. An exception to this is subcutaneous devices (ports) which are almost always used for infusion therapy and can remain in place for extended periods of time (Fig. 45.2).

Non-tunneled catheters are generally intended for short-term use (days to weeks). These catheters have no subcutaneous tunnel, and their entry site goes directly through the skin and into the access vein. As the name implies, tunneled catheters have a subcutaneous tunnel between the skin entry site and the vein entry site. Often, these devices include one or more fabric cuffs that are positioned along the tunnel and serve to provide a barrier to infection and eventually assist in anchoring

H. Singh et al. (eds.), *Radiology Fundamentals: Introduction to Imaging & Technology*, DOI 10.1007/978-3-319-10362-4_45

CATHETER TYPE	DURATION	ROUTE OF ACCESS	EXPECTED DURATION
CENTRAL VENOUS CATHER (CENTRAL LINE)	SHORT TERM	IJ, Subclavian, Femoral	3-7 DAYS
PERIPHERALLY INSERTED CENTRAL CATHETER	SHORT TERM	Upper Extremity Veins, Usually Basilic Vein	6 WEEKS
DIALYSIS CATHETER (NON TUNNELLED)	SHORT TERM	Usually IJ, rarely Subclavian V. Inpatients - Femoral	4—6 WEEKS
HICKMAN (TUNNELLED)	LONG TERM	Usually IJ or Subclavian	4 -6 MONTHS
P.A.S PORT ® (ARM PORT)	LONG TERM	Usually Basilic V.	6 -12 MONTHS
DIALYSIS CATHETER (TUNNELLED)	LONG TERM	Usually IJ, rarely Subclavian V.	6 MONTHS
CHEST PORTS	LONG TERM	IJ or Subclavian V.	12 - 18 MONTHS

FIGURE 45.1 - CENTRAL VENOUS ACCESS
Indications and route of access for various central venous catheters

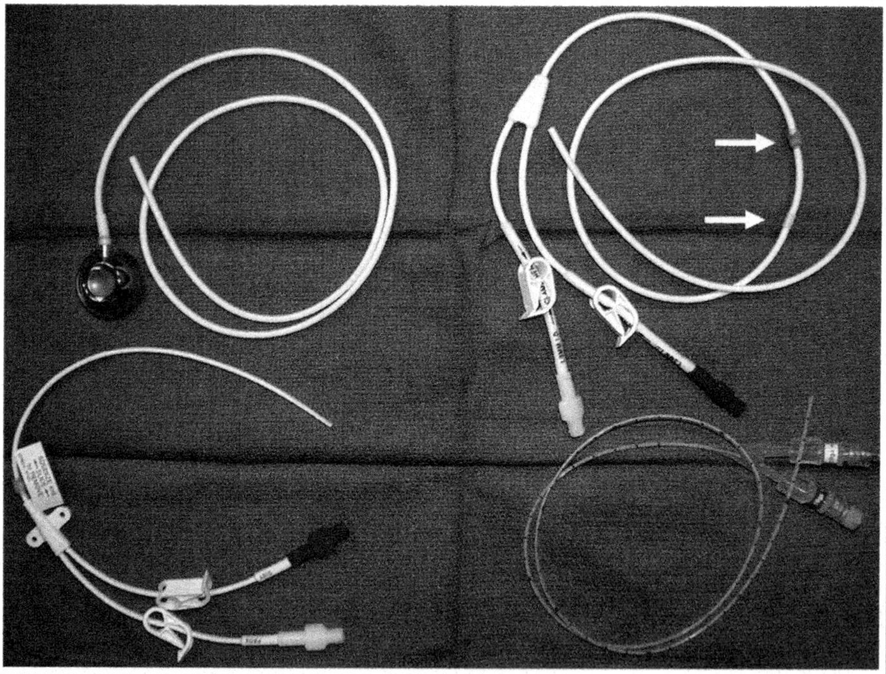

FIGURE 45.2 - EXAMPLES OF INFUSION CATHETERS
From *left* to *right* and *top* to *bottom*, they include a subcutaneous port, a tunneled infusion catheter, a non-tunneled infusion catheter (Hohn), and a percutaneously inserted central catheter (*PICC*). Note the fabric cuffs on the midshaft of the tunneled catheter (*arrows*)

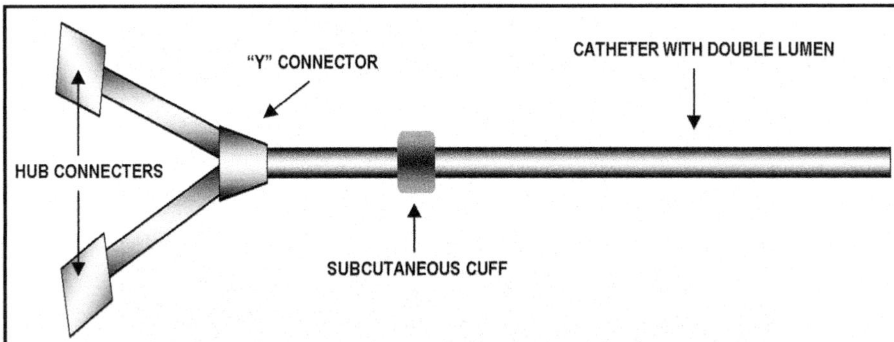

FIGURE 45.3 - TUNNELED CATHETER GENERAL DESIGN
In this dual lumen catheter, the main catheter has an extruded dual lumen. These are divided at the Y connector. The hub connectors are used for access, each equipped with a Luer lock device. The key portion is the subcutaneous cuff which seals the subcutaneous access tunnel when the surrounding tissues grow into the cuff, preventing movement of the catheter and preventing the advancement of skin flora up the tract into the central venous system

the catheter in place (Fig. 45.3). The tunnel and cuff system allow the device to stay in place for weeks to months.

Subcutaneous ports (or mediports) consist of an infusion catheter attached to a reservoir hub. The entire device is placed under the skin, and when accessed or used, a special needle is placed through the skin into the reservoir. Once accessed, the port functions like any other infusion catheter. When not accessed, the port requires little care. These attributes make it ideal for patients whose therapies are characterized by episodes requiring continuous venous access separated by periods where venous access is not required, e.g., chemotherapy.

Catheters intended for infusion therapy are generally small in diameter (5 10 Fr), may have one to three lumens, and have simple end-hole designs. Catheters intended for exchange therapy, such as hemodialysis or plasmapheresis catheter, are much larger in diameter (11–16 Fr), have at least two lumens (one to withdraw and one to return), and have specially designed tips that prevent the blood that is returned from the catheter from being re-aspirated through the other lumen (Fig. 45.4). During exchange therapy, blood flows sometimes up to 600 ml per minute are required through these devices.

The subclavian vein is often used for short-term venous access because of the relative distance of the vein to the mouth reduces the likelihood of infection. Anatomically, the subclavian vein passes through a narrow space at the junction of the first rib and clavicle. This space is further compressed with movement at the shoulder. This compression combined with the presence of the catheter is associated with a high incidence of venous stenosis and even catheter fracture, also known as catheter pinch-off syndrome. Since subclavian vein stenosis may have long-term implications for future venous and hemodialysis access, the preferred site for long-term central venous access is the internal jugular vein.

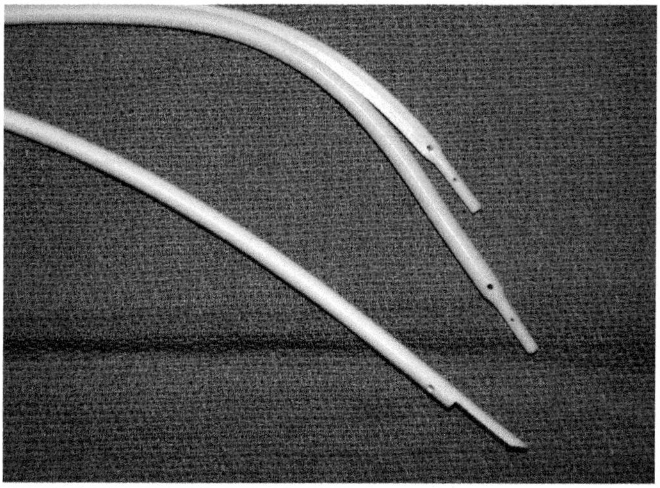

FIGURE 45.4 - EXCHANGE CATHETERS
Two examples of specially designed tips on exchange catheters that prevent recirculation of blood that has already been processed during dialysis or plasmapheresis

The procedure for placement of central venous access is quite straightforward. A preliminary ultrasound of the vein to be accessed is performed to confirm its patency. The neck and the ipsilateral chest are then prepped appropriately. Access is obtained to the vein using vascular ultrasound guidance almost exclusively. Once venous access is established, an appropriate tunnel area is chosen. The tunnel is formed under the skin using a tunneling device, and the catheter is advanced through the tunnel. Finally, the catheter is advanced into the vein. The ideal catheter tip position is at the cavoatrial junction, which is typically 3–4 cm below the carina on chest radiograph.

In unusual circumstances, when a patient may no longer have patent veins in the chest, central venous catheters can still be placed in other locations. Using similar techniques as described above, catheters can be placed in the common femoral veins or even directly into the inferior vena cava through the back. Trans-organ venous access can also be performed percutaneously through the kidneys or liver. Catheters placed in these sites carry high rates of complications and are therefore used as options of last resort for venous access.

46 Interventional Oncology

Objectives:
1. Understand the similarities and differences of and transarterial hepatic chemoembolization and transarterial hepatic radioembolization and when these procedures are indicated.
2. Understand the different ablative therapy options.

Interventional radiology (IR) has always been an incredibly broad field involved with the management of numerous disease states as outlined in the "Introduction to Interventional Radiology" chapter. In the past, IR performed much of the peripheral angiography. Over the last decade vascular surgery has begun to focus on endovascular therapies as an alternative to open surgery. During this same time the IR subspecialty of interventional oncology has blossomed into existence. Interventional oncology (IO) is rapidly growing and expanding. Currently the most common procedures include transarterial hepatic chemoembolization, transarterial hepatic radioembolization, and several types of ablative therapies.

Transarterial Hepatic Chemoembolization

Transarterial hepatic chemoembolization (TACE) is often used to treat unresectable hepatocellular carcinomas (HCC) and other hypervascular tumors. Normal liver parenchyma receives much of its blood supply from the portal vein with a smaller component derived from the hepatic artery. HCCs and other hypervascular tumors desire the highly oxygenated blood in the hepatic arteries and therefore are almost exclusively supplied by the hepatic artery. Because of this property, TACE can

H. Singh et al. (eds.), *Radiology Fundamentals: Introduction to Imaging & Technology*, DOI 10.1007/978-3-319-10362-4_46

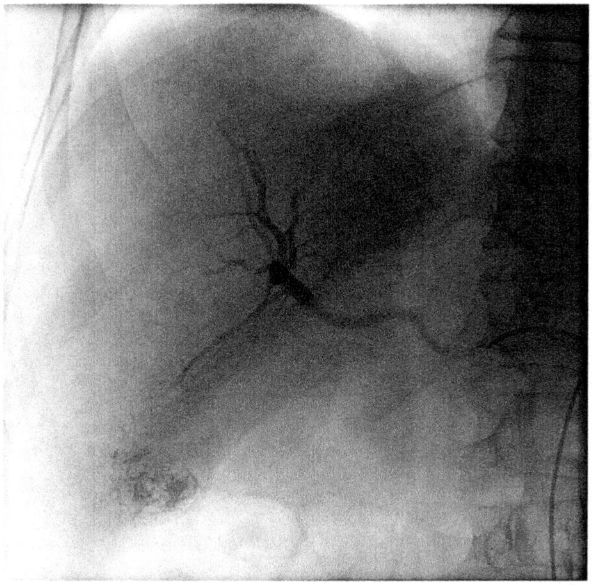

FIGURE 46.1 - TRANSARTERIAL HEPATIC CHEMOEMBOLIZATION
Fluoroscopic image during hepatic chemoembolization demonstrates a post therapy angiogram with a microcatheter positioned in the proper hepatic artery. Note the accumulation of the chemotherapy cocktail within the right lower lobe hypervascular tumor

deliver the chemoembolization mixture directly to the hypervascular tumors. The chemoembolization cocktail is a mixture of one or more chemotherapy drugs, an embolic agent to the slow blood flow through the tumor, and sometimes a special oil called Lipiodol. Vascular access is gained in one of the femoral arteries. Then various wires and catheters are guided into a branch of a hepatic artery that supplies the tumor(s). Finally, the chemoembolization mixture is injected once the catheters are properly positioned (Fig. 46.1).

The indications for TACE include:

1. Patients with unresectable tumors
2. To maintain a patient on the transplant list by controlling the tumor(s) size
3. To downsize a tumor(s) so that a patient can be placed on a transplant list

TACE is contraindicated if the patient has uncompensated, end-stage liver disease or if the bilirubin is elevated greater than 4.

With proper patient selection the major risks are minimized. However, most patients experience some degree of postchemoembolization syndrome. This consists of a triad of abdominal pain, nausea, and fever and is secondary to the effect of embolization and not indicative of a true complication.

Transarterial Hepatic Radioembolization

Transarterial hepatic radioembolization (TARE) is a procedure similar to TACE. It is FDA approved to treat unresectable hepatocellular carcinoma or to treat HCCs as a bridge to transplant. It is also FDA approved for the treatment of hepatic metastases from colorectal carcinoma. The procedure is technically very similar to TACE. However, instead of a chemoembolization mixture, either glass or resin microspheres impregnated with a pure beta-emitting isotope called Yttrium-90 (Y-90) (half-life of 64 h, mean/max tissue penetration of 2.5 mm/10 mm) are injected into the tumor(s). Poor hepatic function with elevated bilirubin is again a contraindication.

The postchemoembolization syndrome seen frequently with TACE is uncommon with radioembolization. However, radioembolization is not free of complications. Nontarget embolization is a phrase which refers to the delivery of chemoembolization mixture or radioembolization particles to unintended areas. This occurs due to reflux of the agent into other vessels, such as those that supply the stomach or bowel. Nontarget embolization is a potential complication with either TACE or radioembolization, but it is associated with much greater morbidity with radioembolization due to the long half-life of Y-90. For this reason, radioembolization requires extensive pretreatment planning and meticulous attention to detail during treatment, factors that are beyond the scope of this discussion.

Ablative Therapy

Ablative technology is another rapidly growing and expanding modality for the treatment of locoregional lesions in malignant and benign diseases of the kidneys, liver, lung, breast, prostate, and bones. Historically, ablation therapy was limited to chemical ablation where either alcohol or acetic acid was injected into tumors in order to cause tissue necrosis. Currently, the most commonly used ablative therapies use extremes of temperature to cause tissue necrosis. The three most commonly used ablative therapies are radiofrequency ablation (RFA), microwave ablation, and cryoablation.

Radiofrequency ablation generates high temperatures by passing high-frequency electrical current through an electrode. Microwave ablation utilizes high-frequency electromagnetic waves to cause rapid vibration of molecules. The friction generated

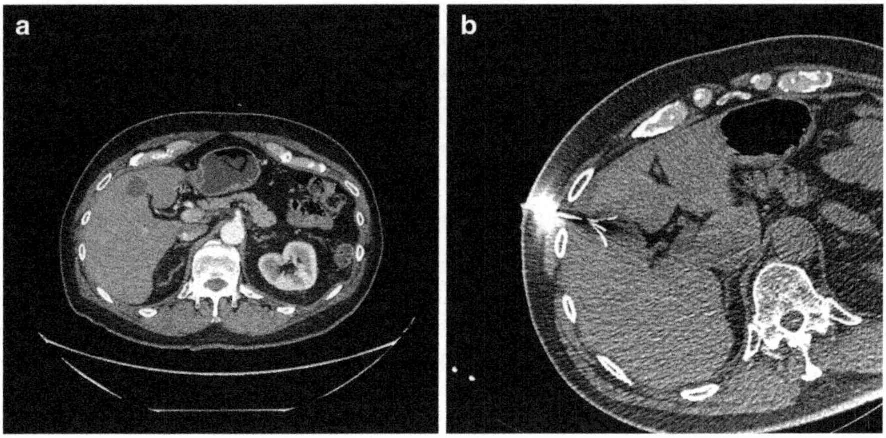

FIGURE 46.2 - RADIOFREQUENCY ABLATION
Image (**a**) demonstrates a round hypodensity in the liver. Image (**b**) shows a radiofrequency (*RF*) probe deployed into the lesion during ablation

by the vibration causes extreme heat (temperatures greater than 50 °C). The heat generated by RFA and microwave ablation disrupts cellular activity and produces coagulative necrosis. Alternatively, cryoablation freezes tissues to less than -20 °C. Cellular injury and death results from direct injury from ice formation, shifting of cellular solutes and solvents resulting in dehydration and cell rupture, as well as microvascular thrombosis resulting in ischemia.

Each of these three techniques requires image-guided (CT, US, MRI, or fluoroscopy) placement of one or several probes, through which either electrical current, electromagnetic waves, or a cryogen is delivered to the probes in order to generate the desired temperature extreme for cellular destruction (Fig. 46.2).

Part VII
Musculoskeletal Section

47 Fractures 1

Objectives:

1. List five major categories of description when evaluating a fracture.
2. Identify internal and external rotation views of the shoulder.
3. Define normal and abnormal anatomy on the "Y" view of the shoulder.
4. Discuss the significance of a joint effusion in the elbow in the presence of acute trauma.
5. State the mechanism of injury in a Colles' fracture.
6. Discuss the concept of the "Scottie dog" in evaluating the lumbar spine.
7. Describe the "bony ring" principle and relate its importance to acute trauma involving the pelvis.

Fractures are ubiquitous in medical practice. Radiographs have been used to evaluate fractures from the earliest days of diagnostic radiology and remain a cornerstone of clinical care in the diagnosis and treatment of skeletal trauma.

The Simple Fracture

Figure 47.1 demonstrates an acute fracture of the fourth proximal phalanx in the left foot. Note the presence of a linear lucency, sharp edges without marginal sclerosis, and soft tissue swelling.

H. Singh et al. (eds.), *Radiology Fundamentals: Introduction to Imaging & Technology*, DOI 10.1007/978-3-319-10362-4_47

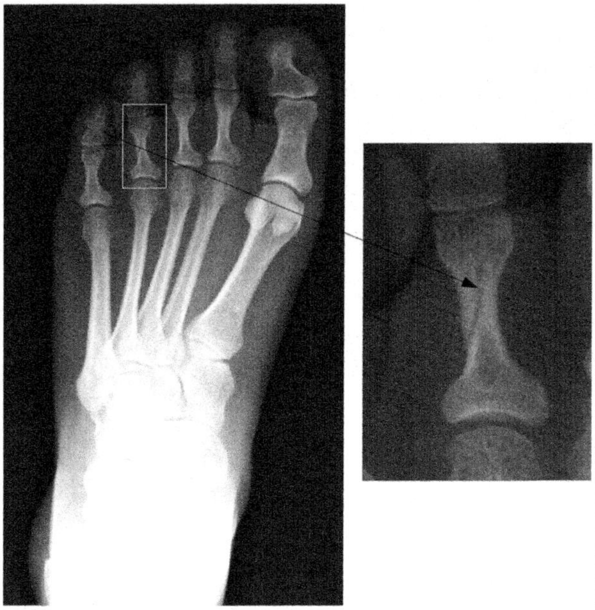

FIGURE 47.1 - SIMPLE FRACTURE
Oblique, nondisplaced fracture of the fourth proximal phalanx of the left foot

Fracture Nomenclature

It is important to verbally describe a fracture since you will often need to communicate the radiographic findings to other healthcare professionals. Features that must be mentioned include the following:

1. *Location:* The name and part of the bone involved. In long bones, the fracture can involve the epiphysis, metaphysis, diaphysis, and even the physis (growth plate). Other designations such as head, neck, body, waist, etc. (depending on the bone) may be employed (Fig. 47.2).
2. *Types of fracture:* Transverse, oblique, spiral, and butterfly are all appropriate descriptors. Comminuted is used when there are multiple fracture fragments. It is also important to note any intra-articular extension of the fracture (extension into the joint) (Fig. 47.3).
3. *Displacement (nonalignment of periosteal surfaces of the bone):* Displacement is described using the location of the distal fragment with respect to the proximal fragment. Hence, if the distal fragment is medially displaced, the fracture is medially displaced. Open or compound fractures are fractures which penetrate the skin (Fig. 47.4).

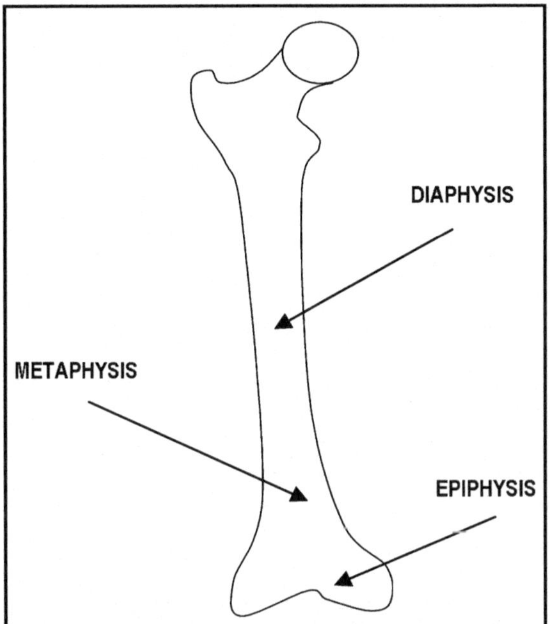

FIGURE 47.2 - BASIC LONG BONE ANATOMY
It is important to have familiarity with the long bone anatomy

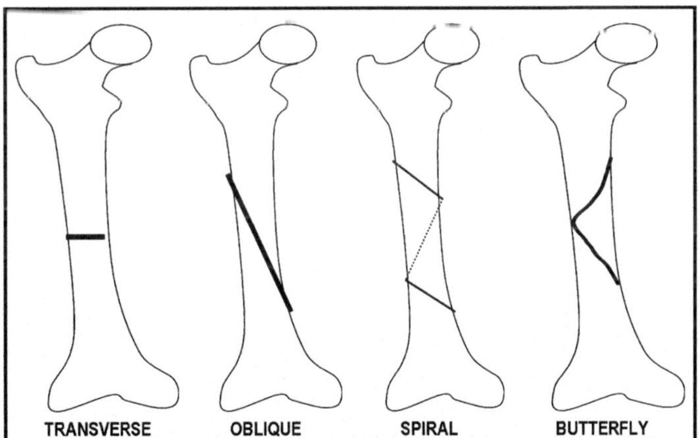

FIGURE 47.3 - FRACTURE NOMENCLATURE
In describing fractures, the referring physician should be able to visualize the fracture without the x-rays. Knowing the nomenclature greatly facilitates this communication

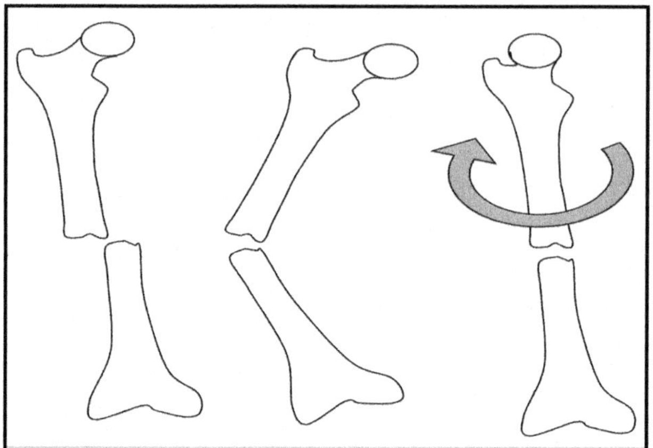

FIGURE 47.4 - FRACTURE FRAGMENT ORIENTATION
In the image on the *left*, there is one shaft width medial displacement of the distal fracture fragment. In the *middle* image, there is lateral angulation of the fracture apex. In the image on the *right*, there is rotation of the fracture fragments

4. *Angulation of the "apex" of the fracture:* The direction that the angle of the fracture points is used to describe the fracture position. A common phrase used would be "the apex of the fracture is directed laterally" (Fig. 47.4).
5. *Rotation of the distal fragment:* If the distal fragment is rotated relative to the proximal fragment, this should be included in the description (Fig. 47.4).

Note that at least two views are required to completely visualize and describe the position of a fracture. An example of a complete description of a fracture would be: "There is a comminuted fracture of the diaphysis of the left femur with medial displacement of the distal fragment, apex lateral angulation, and internal rotation of the distal fragment."

Shoulder Views

Figure 47.5 shows a normal two-view study of the shoulder as might be obtained in the emergency room.

Note the difference between the internal and external rotation views. On internal rotation views, the appearance of the humeral head is similar to the smooth round top of an ice cream cone (**I**ce cream = **I**nternal). On external rotation views, the greater tuberosity is seen clearly in profile. These two views will usually suffice to exclude a fracture. However, dislocation may be more difficult to exclude without views from another projection.

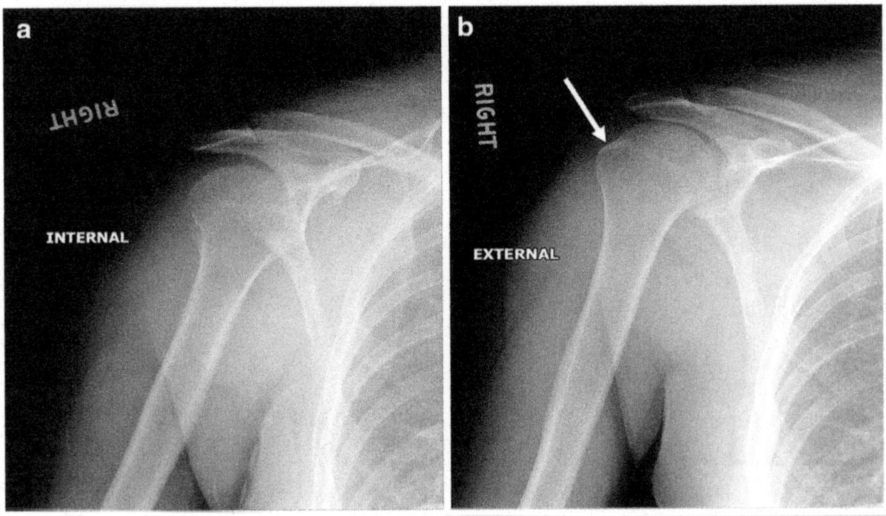

FIGURE 47.5 - INTERNAL AND EXTERNAL ROTATION VIEWS OF THE RIGHT SHOULDER
Arrow shows the greater tuberosity of the humeral head

Figure 47.6 shows an axillary and scapular "Y" view of the shoulder. The axillary view is projected so that you are looking upward through the axilla toward the ceiling in a standing patient. You should be able to visualize the clavicle and acromion process anteriorly, the acromioclavicular joint, and the glenohumeral articulation. Because of the projection of the axillary view, anterior or posterior dislocations are usually well demonstrated. The problem with this view is that it is often very uncomfortable for a patient with an acutely injured shoulder.

A different way of imaging the shoulder in a plane perpendicular to the anterior posterior projection is called a scapular Y view. In this case, the patient is obliqued slightly, and a "lateral view" of the shoulder is obtained. The stem of the Y is the scapular body, while the two upper arms of the Y are the acromion and coracoid processes. At the center of the Y is a circle corresponding to the glenoid fossa. The humeral head should project over the confluence of the three arms of the Y. If the humeral head is posterior to the intersection of the arms of the Y, a posterior dislocation may be diagnosed. Again, remember that posterior dislocation may look normal in the AP view. Note that the scapular Y view is not as good as the axillary lateral view for assessing dislocations or subluxation.

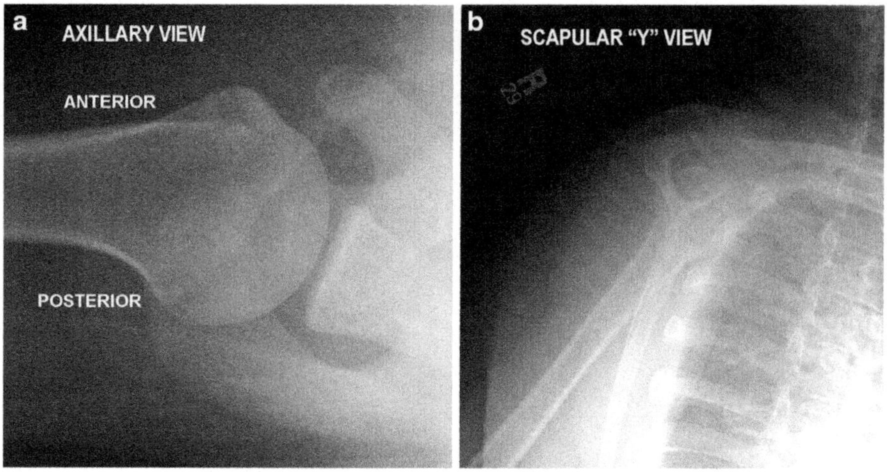

FIGURE 47.6 - (a) AXILLARY AND (b) SCAPULAR Y VIEWS OF THE RIGHT SHOULDER

Shoulder Dislocation

Figure 47.7 shows a typical anterior (most common) dislocation of the humerus. In anterior dislocation, the humeral head moves inferiorly under the coracoid and slightly medially. This can usually be identified on the routine anterior views (a). The axillary view (b) demonstrates the humeral head anterior to the glenoid.

Figure 47.8 demonstrates a typical posterior dislocation of the humerus. The dislocation is hard to appreciate on the AP view (a), but in posterior dislocations the humerus is always internally rotated (patient cannot externally rotate). Image (b) shows the axillary view with the humeral head posterior to the glenoid. The Grashey view (c) reveals overlap of the humeral head at the glenohumeral joint.

Fat Pad Sign

Figure 47.9 shows a normal and abnormal lateral view of the elbow. In the image on the right, note the presence of the triangular-shaped lucency just anterior to the distal humerus representing the anterior fat pad of the elbow. Fat pads serve as markers for elbow joint effusions. Fluid or blood within the joint will displace them. Elbow joint effusions in the setting of acute trauma almost always indicate a fracture. In the image on the right, no obvious fracture is seen. However, there is evidence of an elbow joint effusion since the anterior fat pad is displaced (compare to normal). In addition, a posterior fat pad along the posterior aspect of the distal humerus is seen. This always indicates the presence of a joint effusion and usually indicates a

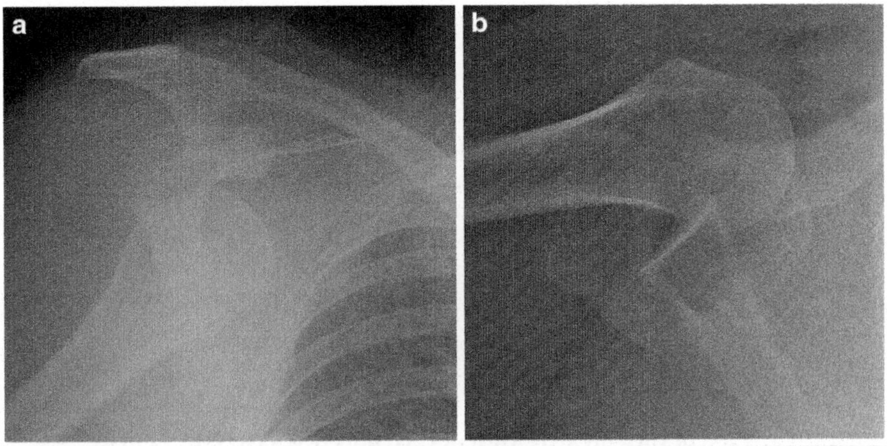

FIGURE 47.7 - ANTERIOR DISLOCATION OF THE SHOULDER

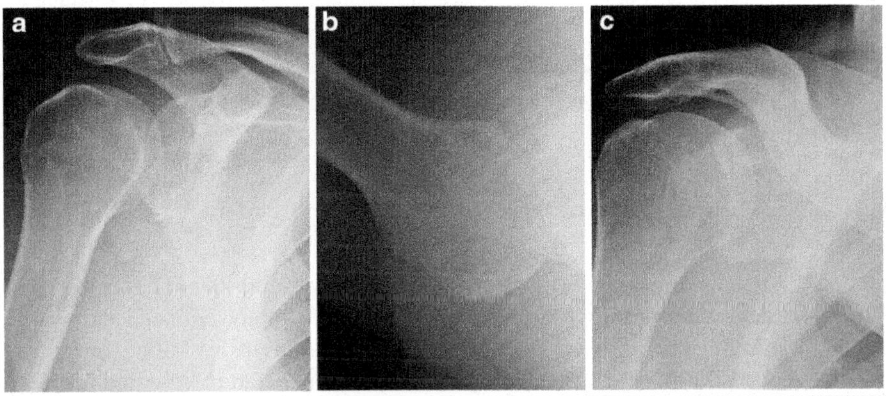

FIGURE 47.8 - POSTERIOR DISLOCATIONS OF THE SHOULDER

fracture, in the proper clinical situation. It is important to understand that while an anterior fat pad sign is more sensitive for joint pathology, a posterior fat pad sign is more specific for occult fracture.

The elbow is not the only joint in which fat pads can be useful. For instance, ankle injuries may reveal a fat pad anterior to the joint between the talus and tibia which may suggest fracture.

These fractures may be occult radiographically. Occasionally, a small fracture of the radial head can be demonstrated with further or follow-up views. Again, whenever an elbow joint effusion is seen in the setting of acute trauma (and in the absence of other preexisting reasons for an elbow joint effusion such as rheumatoid arthritis, hemophilia, etc.), the patient should be treated for a fracture.

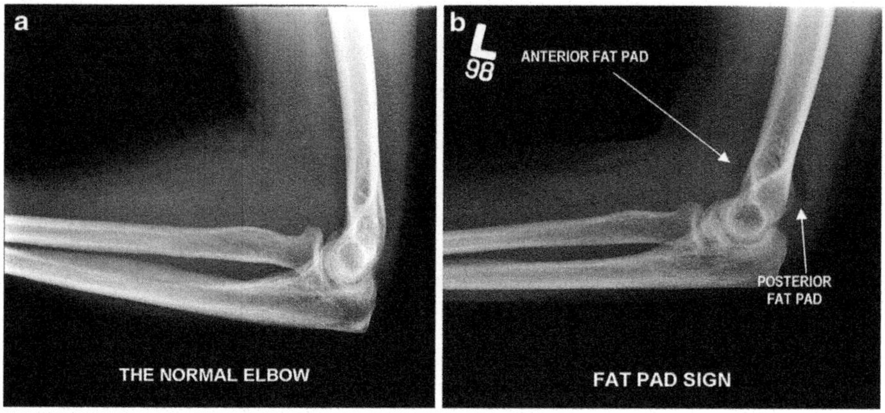

FIGURE 47.9 - NORMAL (a) AND ABNORMAL (b) VIEWS OF THE ELBOW AND FAT PAD SIGN
The image on the left is a normal lateral elbow. The triangular lucencies anterior and posterior to the humerus on the right image represent displaced fat (fat pad sign) when there is fluid in the elbow joint. Fluid in the joint can be seen in inflammatory conditions. In the setting of trauma, displaced fat pads have a high association with fracture even if the fracture is not immediately visualized

Colles' Fracture

Figure 47.10 demonstrates one of the most common wrist injuries. The Colles' fracture is defined as a transverse fracture of the distal metaphysis of the radius with dorsal angulation of the distal fragment commonly caused by falling on an outstretched hand. Based on the previously described nomenclature, it would be appropriate to describe this fracture as apex volar (palmar) angulation. However, in the case of a fracture near an articular surface, the direction of the articular surface is used to describe angulation. Often a Colles' fracture will have an associated fracture of the ulnar styloid process.

The Scottie Dog

Another term you should be familiar with is the Scottie dog. This refers to the outline of a dog that can be seen on an oblique view of the lumbar spine. As depicted in the figures below, the eye of the dog corresponds to the pedicle, the snout the transverse process, the neck the pars interarticularis, the ear the superior articular facet, and the front leg the inferior articular facet.

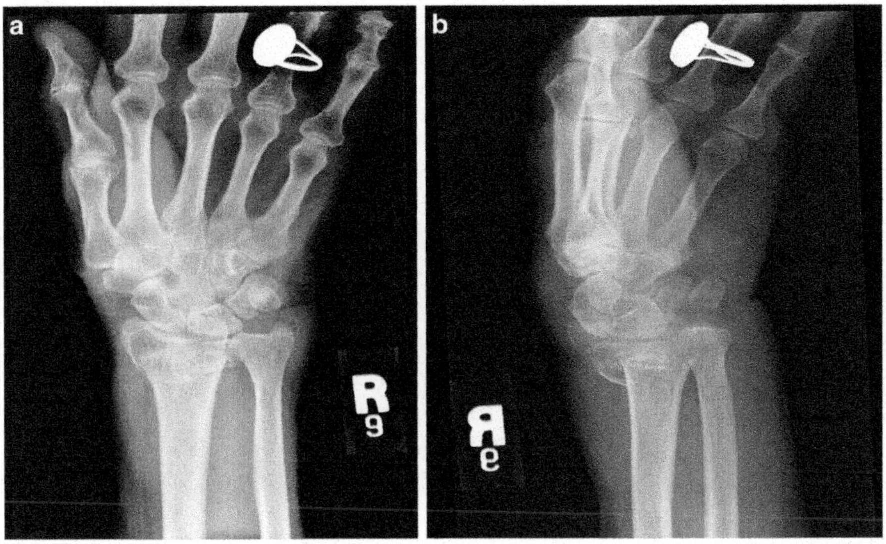

FIGURE 47.10 - COLLES' FRACTURE
AP (**a**) and lateral views (**b**) of the right wrist demonstrate a comminuted, impacted, and intra-articular fracture of the right distal radius, with approximately 20° of dorsal angulation of the distal fragment. Note that there is also deformity and marked soft tissue swelling at the site of injury

It is important to evaluate these structures, especially the pars interarticularis. A fracture or congenital defect in this region will manifest itself as a lucent (dark) line in the neck of the dog (it looks like a dog collar). This is termed spondylolysis. Spondylolysis can lead to spondylolisthesis which is a slippage of the superior vertebra on the inferior one, most often in the anterior direction. There is a grading system based upon what percentage of the vertebra has slipped forward, but for now, just understand the concept.

Roughly 5 % of the population has L5 spondylolisthesis, and of those, roughly 5 % are symptomatic. In general, spondylolysis with spondylolisthesis is more likely to be symptomatic (Fig. 47.11).

Pelvic Fractures

Evaluation of the pelvis is often a part of the radiographic evaluation of acute trauma patients. One helpful principle in looking for fractures of the pelvis is the "bony ring" concept. This concept states that a bony ring will always break in two places. A fracture or separation in a bony ring is usually associated with at least one other fracture in that ring. Figure 47.12 illustrates this principle. Remember that pelvic fractures also occur in the elderly with much less force of trauma secondary to osteoporosis.

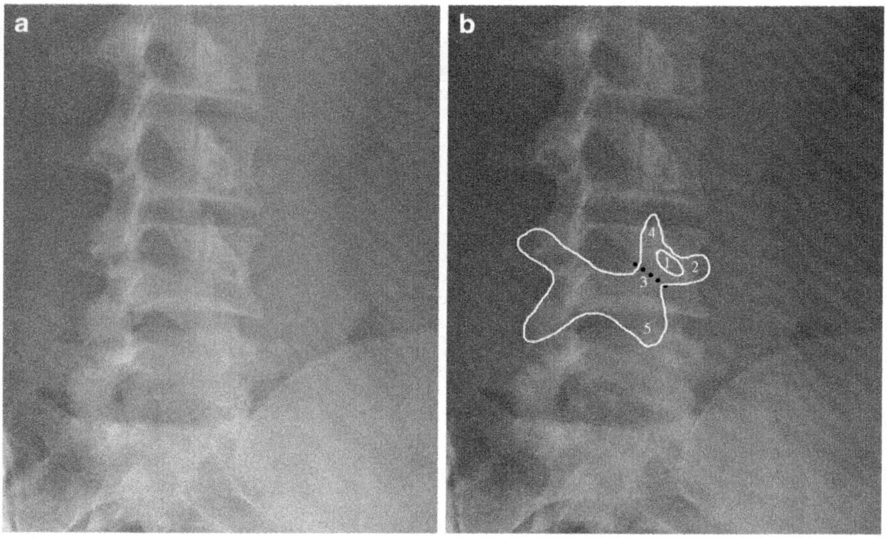

FIGURE 47.11 - THE SCOTTIE DOG CONCEPT
This figure outlines the Scottie dog on an oblique lumbar radiograph: *1* pedicle, *2* transverse process, *3* pars interarticularis, *4* superior articular facet, and *5* inferior articular facet. The *dashed line* through the neck that looks like a collar represents what a pars fracture would look like

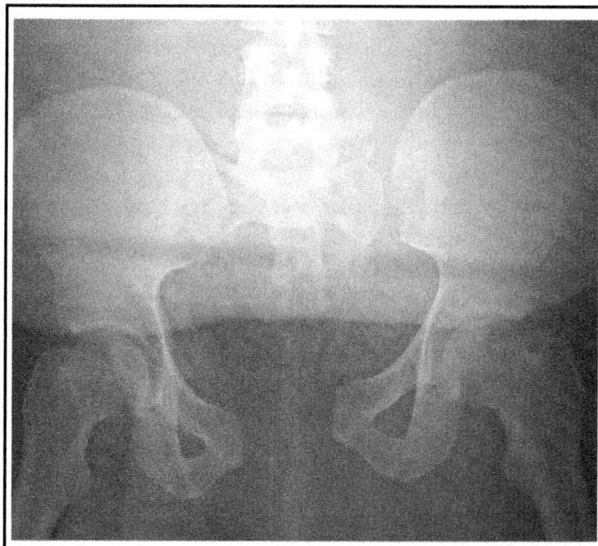

FIGURE 47.12 - PELVIC FRACTURE
There is marked widening of the left sacroiliac joint and the pubic symphysis. Also note that there is extensive soft tissue density in the pelvis consistent with hematoma

48 FRACTURES 2

Objectives:

1. Describe the classification of femoral neck fractures.
2. Describe the radiographic features of a suprapatellar knee joint effusion.
3. Discuss the imaging of tibial plateau fractures and the significance of a fat fluid level within the knee joint space.
4. List the two main mechanisms of injury in ankle fractures.
5. Define Bohler's angle and its pathologic significance in regard to fractures of the calcaneus.
6. Define the phrase pathologic fracture.

Femoral Neck Fractures

The femoral neck is a very common site for acute skeletal trauma. Femoral neck fractures range from quite obvious both clinically and radiographically to very subtle abnormalities radiographically. Fractures are classified according to the site of the fracture within the proximal femur. The most common locations for femoral neck fractures are in the intertrochanteric area extending between the greater and lesser trochanters and in the subcapital region, that area of the femoral neck just distal to the femoral head. Mid-cervical or basi-cervical femoral neck fractures are less common. Internal rotation of the hip will improve evaluation of the femoral neck (Fig. 48.1).

Fractures of the hip may be more extensive than is evident on plain radiograph alone, and further imaging, commonly with computed tomography, is often performed. Of course, as with all fractures, two plain film views are required to assess the fracture. A commonly used view with hips is called the cross table lateral view. An example of this view is shown in Fig. 48.2.

H. Singh et al. (eds.), *Radiology Fundamentals: Introduction to Imaging & Technology*, DOI 10.1007/978-3-319-10362-4_48

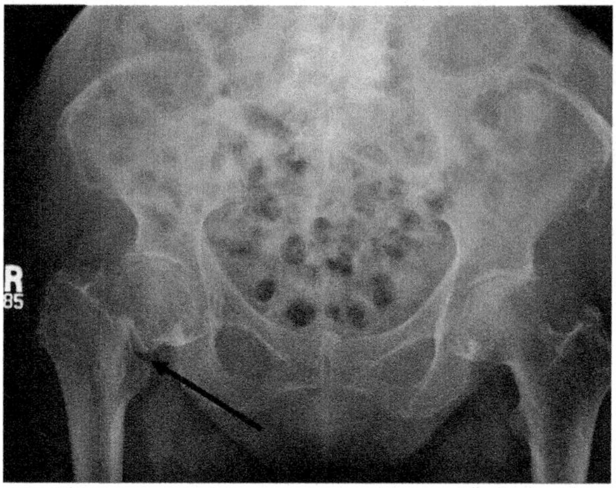

FIGURE 48.1 - FEMORAL NECK FRACTURE
Displaced subcapital fracture in an osteopenic elderly female. Femoral necks are best evaluated with the hips internally rotated

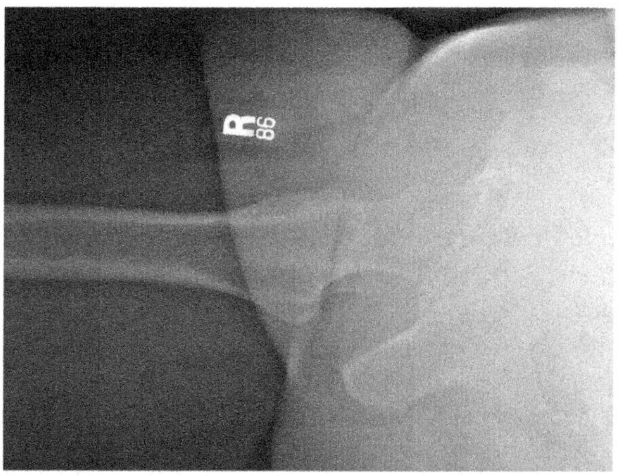

FIGURE 48.2 - CROSS-TABLE LATERAL VIEW OF THE HIP

Knee Joint Effusion

Many abnormalities of the knee are associated with a knee joint effusion. The relationship of effusion to fracture is not as strong as that discussed in a previous section in relation to the elbow. However, the presence of a knee joint effusion

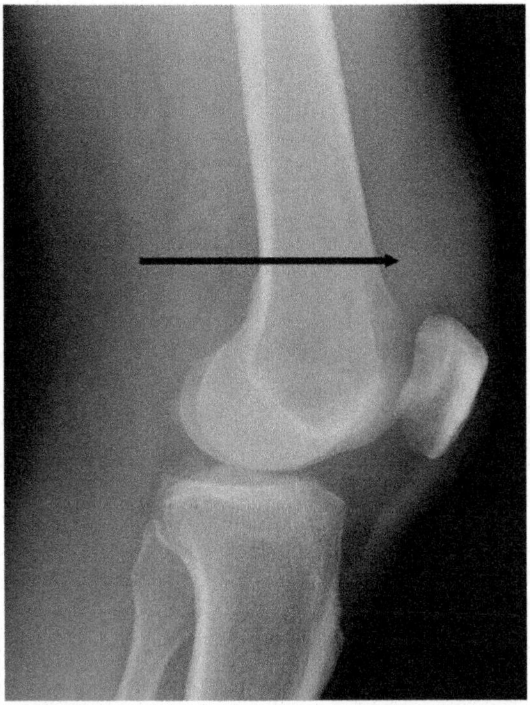

FIGURE 48.3 - KNEE JOINT EFFUSION
Large left knee joint effusion with associated soft tissue swelling (*arrow*)

may be the only manifestation of a cartilaginous or ligamentous injury in the absence of fracture. On the lateral view, the suprapatellar fat pad is a dark triangle with its apex directed superiorly and its base situated along the superior aspect of the patella itself. The pre-femoral fat pad is a broad, anteriorly convex area of decreased density along the anterior aspect of the distal femur. The suprapatellar pouch of the knee joint is between these fat pads. When there is a knee joint effusion, these two fat pads are separated by more than 5 mm. It is important that on the lateral view, the knee be appropriately flexed at approximately 30° and that a true lateral view (non-rotated) be obtained when evaluating for a joint effusion (Fig. 48.3).

In some patients who have undergone significant trauma involving the knee, a cross-table lateral view may be performed with the knee straight. When this occurs, a transverse interface may be oriented horizontally and represents a fat fluid level. Remember that fat is less dense (darker) radiographically than fluid. Also, fat is of lesser physical density than fluid and tends to rise to the top of the joint compartment, while the fluid sinks to the bottom. The fat represents marrow contents which

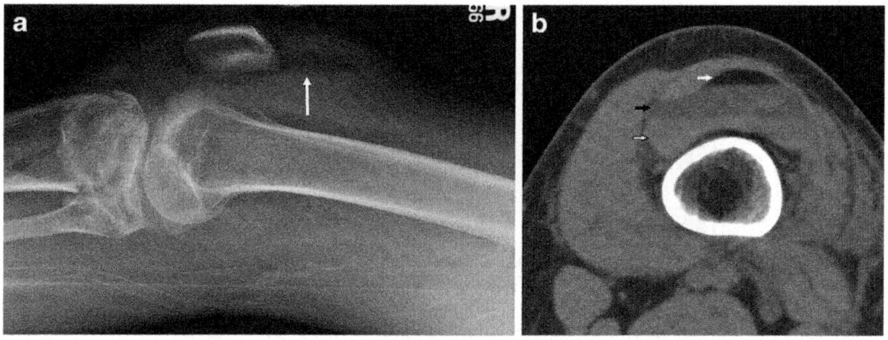

FIGURE 48.4 - LIPOHEMARTHROSIS
Image (**a**) shows a cross-table lateral view demonstrating a fat fluid level (*white arrow*). Image (**b**) shows the corresponding axial CT slice revealing lipohemarthrosis with fat (*top white arrow*), serum (*black arrow*), and hematocrit fluid levels (*bottom white arrow*)

have leaked into the joint space as the result of a fracture, usually of the proximal tibia, which involves the articular surface. In patients with a fat fluid level, an intra-articular fracture will invariably be present (Fig. 48.4).

Tibial Plateau Fractures

A common intra-articular fracture involving the proximal tibia is a so-called tibial plateau fracture. The lateral and medial tibial plateaus may be injured by impact from the femoral condyles. This results in a depression of the plateau with subsequent fracture of the underlying bone. The radiographic features of a tibial plateau fracture may be quite subtle with only a small cortical irregularity or plateau depression noted on plain radiographs. Further imaging with computerized tomography is commonly performed to delineate the true extent of the fracture which may be much more extensive than appreciated on the radiograph alone (Fig. 48.5).

Ankle Fractures

Figure 48.6 shows a trimalleolar fracture. There is an oblique fracture of the lateral malleolus (distal fibula), a transverse fracture of the medial malleolus, and, seen best on the lateral film, a fracture of the posterior malleolus. In some cases, there may only be a tear of the deltoid ligament (medial aspect of ankle). In these cases, only nonspecific soft tissue swelling may be seen on the radiograph.

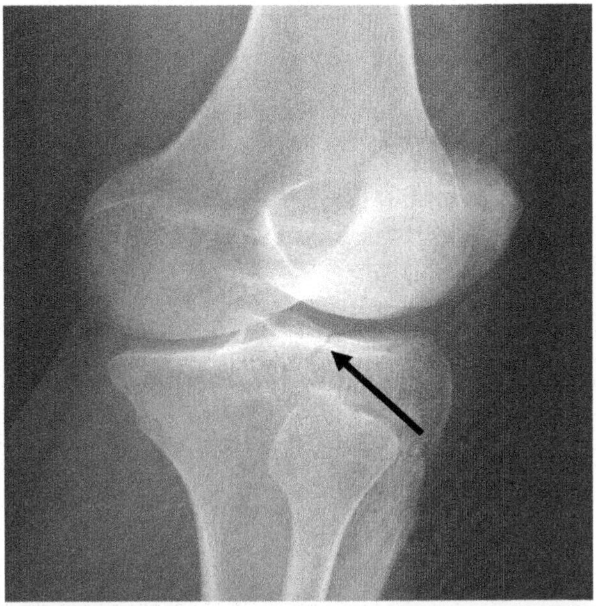

FIGURE 48.5 - TIBIAL PLATEAU FRACTURE
Non-displaced intra-articular fracture of the lateral tibial plateau

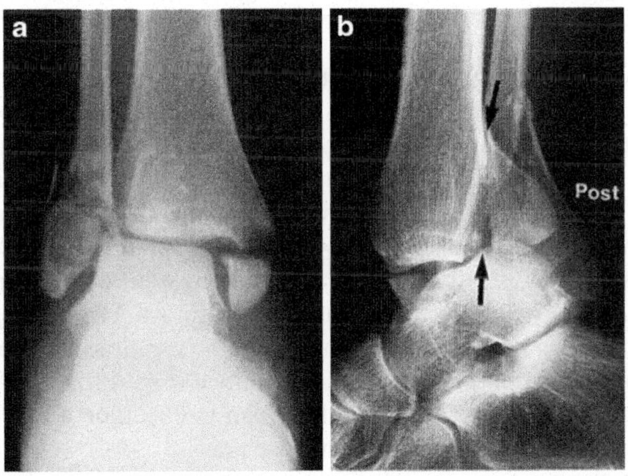

FIGURE 48.6 - AP AND LATERAL VIEWS OF A TRIMALLEOLAR ANKLE FRACTURE
Note that all three malleoli are fractured

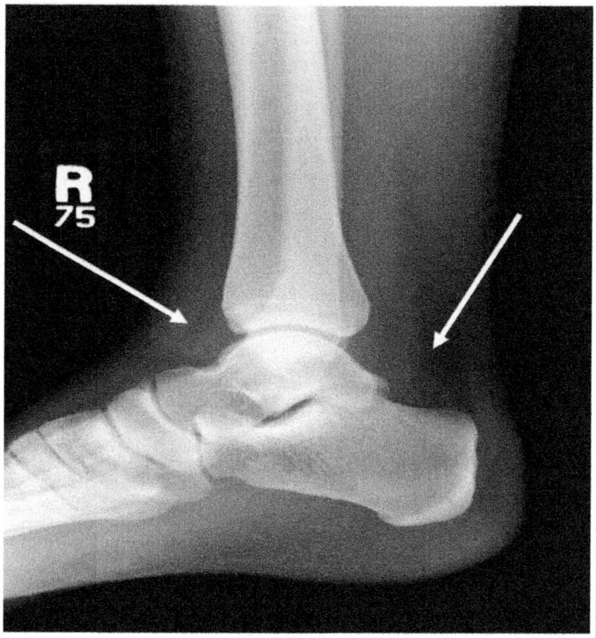

FIGURE 48.7 - ANKLE SPRAIN
This patient presented following an ankle sprain with significant swelling. The *arrows* denote the significant soft tissue swelling over the anterior and posterior-lateral aspects of the ankle joint

During the injury process, different types of rotation stress can result in fractures of the mid or even high fibula. High fractures of the fibula are especially common in eversion (or pronation)-type injuries, are called Maisonneuve fractures, and can easily be missed if only ankle radiographs are taken. For this reason, understanding the mechanism of injury is important in deciding which radiographs should be performed.

Ankle injuries may be divided into inversion and eversion types. One can further subdivide these fractures into inversion (adduction) with or without rotation and eversion (abduction) with or without rotation. The most common type of "twisted ankle" is the inversion injury with rotation. From the location and appearance of the injuries, the mechanism of injury can be ascertained (Fig. 48.7).

There are four areas that are always important to check on a foot or ankle view because fractures can easily be missed in these areas.

They are:

1. Base of the fifth metatarsal
2. Lateral talus
3. Superior part of the talus/talar neck
4. Anterior calcaneus

Another term important to be familiar with is Lisfranc injury or fracture. The Lisfranc ligament connects the medial cuneiform to the bases of the first and second metatarsals. Lisfranc injuries tend to be quite difficult to evaluate with plain films. As with most radiographs, it is important to provide a good clinical history which can greatly help the radiologist when attempting to determine if an injury or fracture has occurred.

Since ankle injuries are so common and often imaged, the Ottawa ankle rules were developed (Wofle et al. 2001) These are recommendations to determine when radiographs are necessary to evaluate an ankle injury based on physical exam findings. These recommendations have a sensitivity of nearly 100 %. These rules do not apply to pregnant females, children under the age of 18, or patients that cannot follow the test commands (intoxication, dementia, cognitive deficit, etc.)

Ankle radiographs are indicated if there is any pain in the malleolar zone and any one of the following:

1. Bone tenderness along the distal 6 cm of the posterior edge of the tibia or tip of the medial malleolus
2. Bone tenderness along the distal 6 cm of the posterior edge of the fibula or tip of the lateral malleolus
3. An inability to bear weight for four steps

The Ottawa foot rules are followed for assessing whether a foot X-ray series is indicated. Foot radiographs are indicated if there is any pain in the midfoot zone and any one of the following:

1. Bone tenderness at the base of the fifth metatarsal
2. Bone tenderness at the navicular bone
3. An inability to bear weight for four steps

A common foot injury occurs when a patient jumps from a high location, landing on his/her feet. Often the bone that bears the brunt of the initial impact is the calcaneus. The calcaneus may be evaluated on the lateral view by calculating Bohler's angle, normal between 20° and 40°. See Fig. 48.8 where the angle is reduced when a fracture is present. The fracture line(s) itself may not be evident on the radiograph.

Note that calcaneal injuries are often bilateral and can be associated with other axial loading injuries such as tibial plateau or thoracolumbar spine fractures.

Pathologic Fracture

Figure 48.9 shows a patient with a lytic lesion in the bone as a result of metastatic lung cancer. Because this has thinned the cortex of the bone and weakened it structurally, a fracture has occurred. This is termed a pathologic fracture. A pathologic fracture is the result of normal stresses in an abnormal bone. The pathologic process can be benign or malignant.

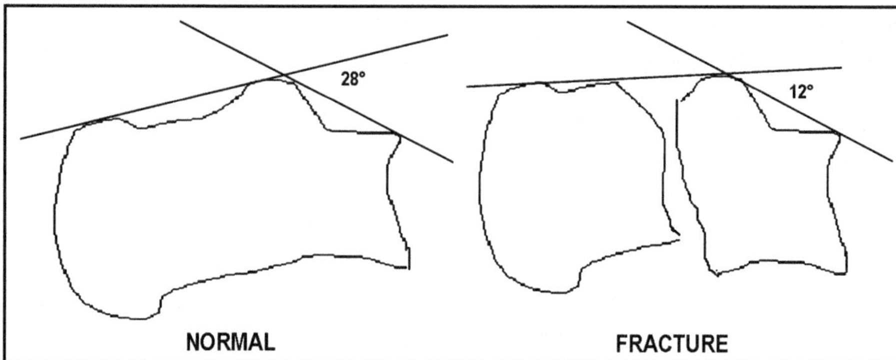

FIGURE 48.8 - BOHLER'S ANGLE
On the *left*, the diagram demonstrates the normal angle of 28° formed by the intersection of the anterior and the posterior aspect of the calcaneus. With axial loading injuries (i.e., landing feet first), the calcaneus is fractured. The angle then is reduced and is noted to be less than 28°

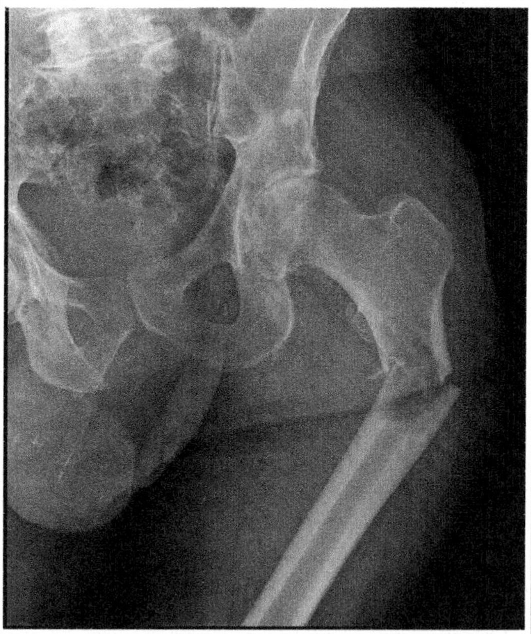

FIGURE 48.9 - PATHOLOGIC FRACTURE
Lytic lesion in the proximal left femoral metaphysis with a mildly comminuted pathologic fracture. Pathology at the time of fixation revealed metastatic squamous cell carcinoma of lung primary

A useful mnemonic for remembering which tumors spread to bone is PB KTL (Lead Kettle – remember lead's symbol is Pb).

P = **P**rostate
B = **B**reast
K = **K**idney
T = **T**hyroid
L = **L**ung

Osteoporosis

Osteoporosis refers to decreased bone density which is most often associated with aging. Screening for osteoporosis is accomplished with a modality called dual-energy X-ray absorptiometry (DEXA). All women over age 65 are counseled to get a baseline DEXA exam. It is also recommended that men with a history of vertebral fracture or long-term corticosteroid use get a DEXA scan. A DEXA scan uses approximately 1/10th the radiation dose of a chest X-ray. Figure 48.10 shows an example of an osteoporotic vertebral column. Note how lucent the vertebrae appear. Figure 48.11 shows an example of a DEXA scan printout.

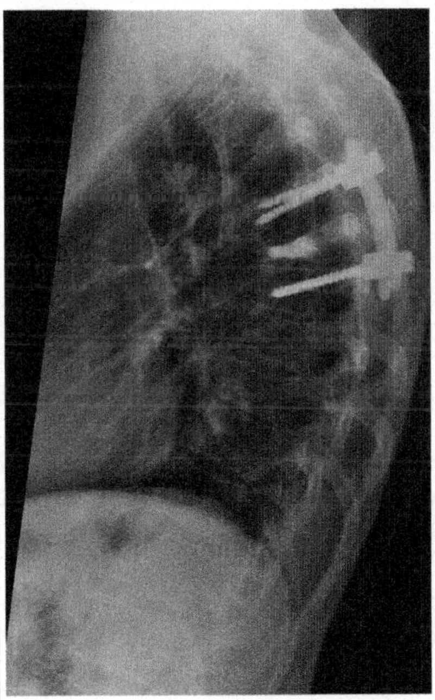

FIGURE 48.10 - OSTEOPOROSIS
Note the lucency of the vertebral column

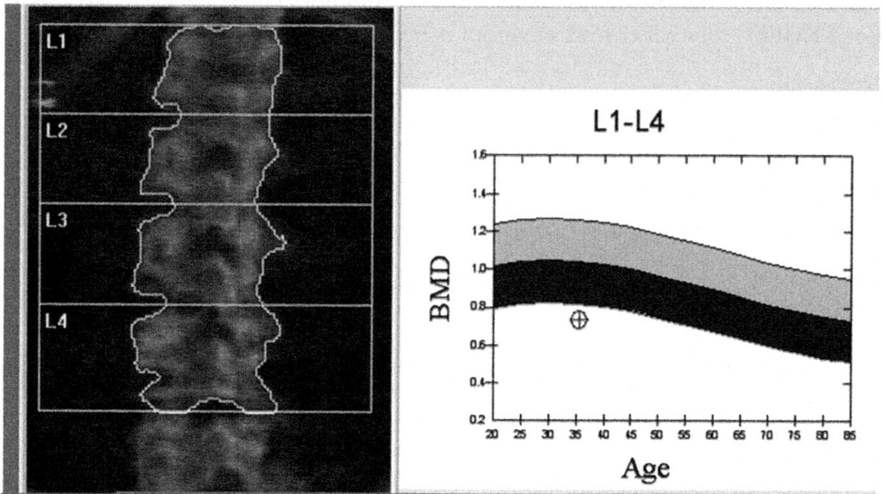

Region	T-Score	PR (Peak Reference)	Z-Score	AM (Age Matched)
L1	-3.0	65	-2.9	65
L2	-2.8	70	-2.7	71
L3	-2.8	71	-2.8	72
L4	-2.8	72	-2.7	73
Total	**-2.8**	**70**	**-2.8**	**71**

FIGURE 48.11 - DXA SCAN
Both T- and Z-scores are reported. Note that the risk of fracture is high in this patient

The patient's bone mineral density (BMD) is compared to two norms. These are calculated as T-scores and Z-scores and reported as standard deviations. T-scores compare the patient's BMD to a healthy 35-year-old's BMD. Meanwhile, Z-scores compare a patient's BMD to an age-matched control. While a Z-score is often measured, the T-score is the number used to define osteopenia and osteoporosis. On the scale, anything above zero is normal. Negative 1 to negative 2.5 is considered osteopenia, which means low bone density. Anything more negative than negative 2.5 is defined as osteoporosis. A general rule of thumb is that for every standard deviation below normal, the risk of fracture doubles (T-score of negative 1 has double the risk, T-score of negative 2 has four times the risk).

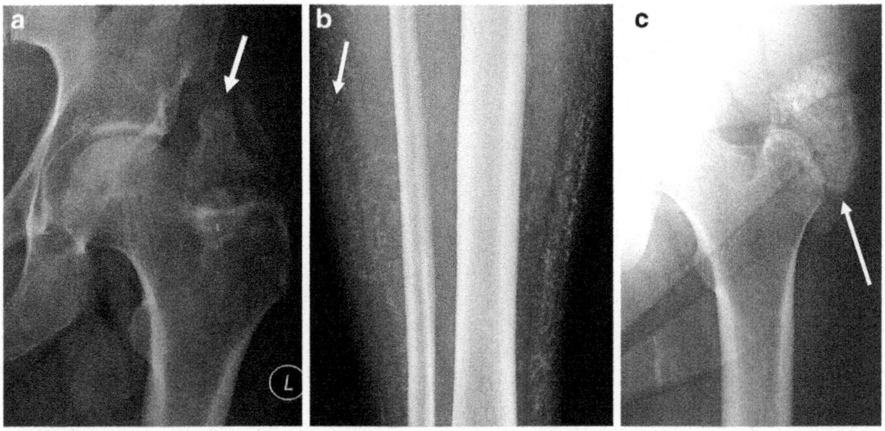

FIGURE 48.12 - SEVERAL TYPES OF CALCIFICATION
(**a**) Heterotopic ossification (*arrows*) (**b**) Dystrophic calcifications are noted in the skin of a patient with peripheral vascular disease (**c**) Metastatic calcification (tumoral calcinosis) is present above the greater trochanter in a patient with chronic renal failure on dialysis (*arrow*)

There are three abnormal types of calcifications that you should be familiar with:

1. **Heterotopic ossification** is an abnormal deposition of true bone within soft tissues. It is formed by dormant osteoprogenitor cells in the soft tissue that are caused to differentiate into osteoblasts by a variety of bone morphogenetic proteins (BMPs).
2. **Dystrophic calcification** refers to an accumulation of calcium salts in dying tissues (any area of necrosis, AVN, damaged heart valves). This calcification can become heterotopic. Serum calcium is normal.
3. **Metastatic calcification** refers to the deposition of calcium in tissues secondary to hypercalcemia. This may be due to increased parathyroid hormone, destruction of bone by tumors, chronic renal failure, and increased vitamin D (Fig. 48.12).

Reference

Wofle M, Uhl T, Mccluskey L. Management of ankle sprains. Am Fam Physician. 2001;63(1): 93–105.

49 Bone Tumor Characteristics

Objectives:

1. Name the two most important variables when creating a differential for bone tumors.
2. Name three lesional characteristics that further refine a differential of bone tumors.
3. Understand the difference between aggressive/nonaggressive and benign/malignant.

This chapter is not an exhaustive description detailing the characteristics of various types of bone tumors. It does however provide a paradigm to evaluate and classify types of bone tumors which allows for the creation of a useful differential diagnosis when a new bone tumor is encountered in clinical practice.

First, it is imperative to understand the concept that aggressive and nonaggressive are not synonymous with malignant and benign. Though an aggressive appearing lesion is more likely malignant than a nonaggressive one, certain lesions can be aggressive and not malignant and vice versa. For example, osteomyelitis often appears aggressive but is not malignant, whereas a giant cell tumor may look nonaggressive but can be malignant.

The two most important aspects when evaluating a bone tumor lesion and creating a differential diagnosis are to note the age of the patient and the location of the lesion.

Skeletal maturity is the most important variable used to classify bone tumors. That is, certain tumors have a predilection for certain age ranges (less than 20 years old, between 20 and 40 and older than 40 years old). For instance, primary bone malignancies are uncommon in patients older than 40 years old. In this age group, a bony malignancy is much more likely to be a metastatic lesion or multiple myeloma.

H. Singh et al. (eds.), *Radiology Fundamentals: Introduction to Imaging & Technology*, DOI 10.1007/978-3-319-10362-4_49

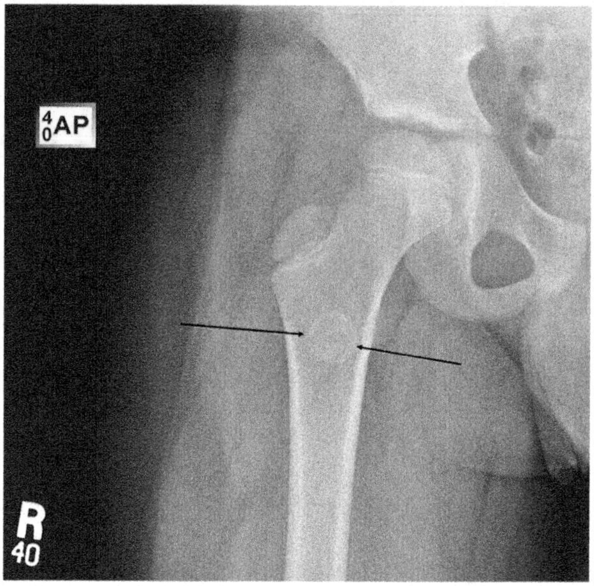

FIGURE 49.1 - NONAGGRESSIVE MARGINS
Thin white (sclerotic) rim margins indicate a nonaggressive lesion

The second most important way to classify a bone tumor is based upon the tumor's location. Most tumors have a predilection for specific locations within bone, i.e., diaphysis, metaphysis (site of rapid bone growth), and epiphysis. Axial skeleton versus appendicular skeleton or long versus flat bones are other important factors regarding location. As an example, a Ewing sarcoma follows the course of red marrow. Therefore, in children, it is often found in the diaphysis of long bones, and in young adults, it has a predilection for flat bones such as the pelvis reflecting the normal evolution of red marrow distribution.

Certain features of the lesion itself are quite important. Most notable is the margins of the lesion. The sharper the margins, especially if there is a sclerotic (white) rim, the less aggressive the lesion (Fig. 49.1). The more indistinct and ill defined the margin, the more aggressive the lesion. The most aggressive lesions have a characteristic appearance called "moth eaten" or "permeative" (Fig. 49.2). These terms refer to small, patchy, ill-defined areas of destruction.

Furthermore, the presence of periosteal reaction and its appearance is an important characteristic in evaluating a bone lesion. A solid or unilamellar periosteal reaction signifies that a tumor is slow growing, allowing the bone to "wall off" the lesion (Fig. 49.3). A multilamellated appearance, also known as "onionskin appearance," suggests an intermediate aggressiveness. Periosteal reaction that is spiculated in

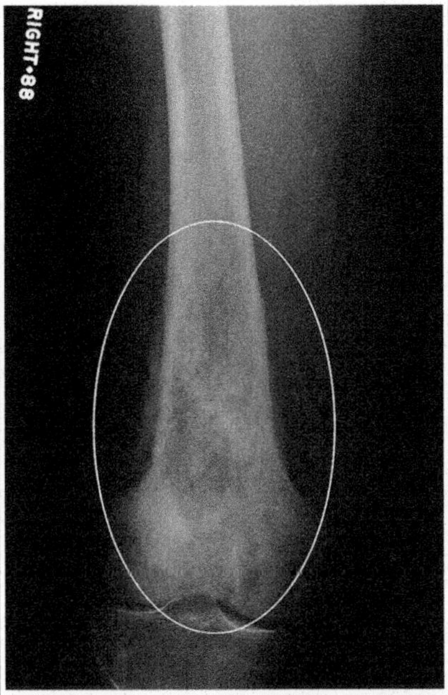

FIGURE 49.2 - AGGRESSIVE MARGINS
Example of permeative or "moth-eaten" appearance of an aggressive lesion

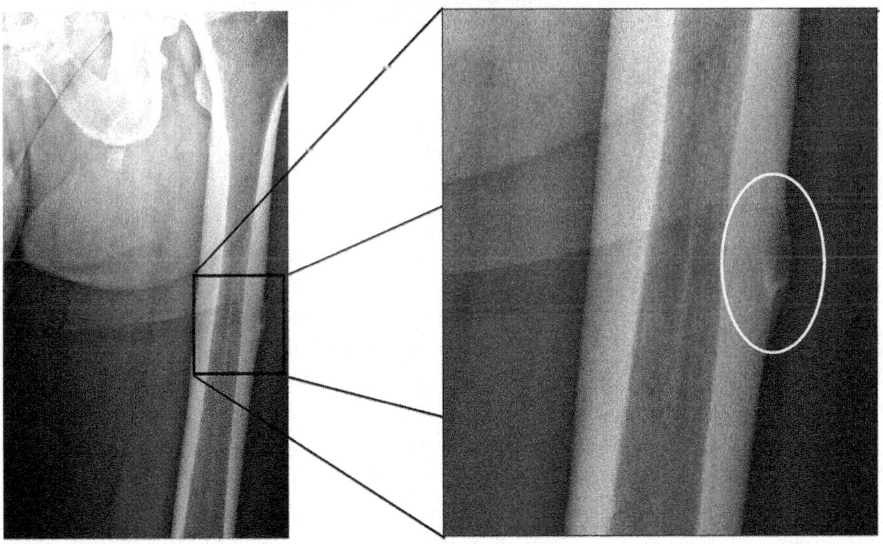

FIGURE 49.3 - NONAGGRESSIVE PERIOSTEAL REACTION
Unilamellated or solid periosteal reaction usually found with nonaggressive lesions

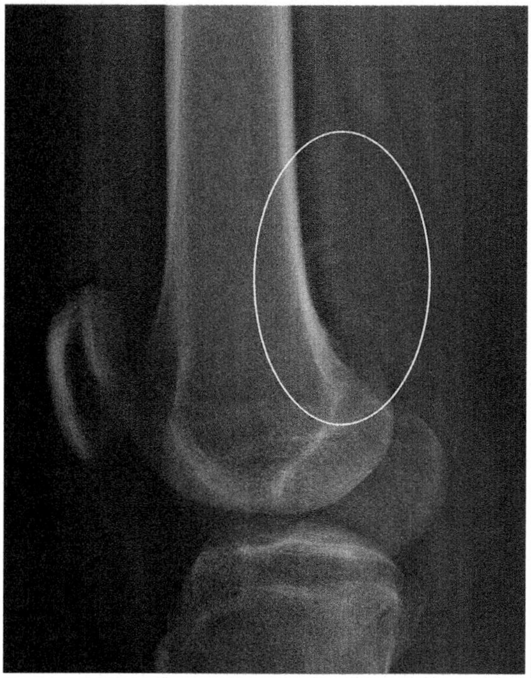

FIGURE 49.4 - AGGRESSIVE PERIOSTEAL REACTION
Radiographic appearance of the classic "hair-on-end" periosteal reaction characteristic of aggressive lesions

appearance, "hair on end," is the most aggressive type (Fig. 49.4). A Codman triangle refers to an elevation of the periosteum away from the cortex. This term is classically associated with an osteosarcoma but is not limited to this as any number of malignant or benign processes can cause this feature.

Evaluating the matrix mineralization of a bone tumor can help classify the lesion and further refine the differential diagnosis. A tumor producing new bone will have a fluffy or cloudlike amorphous matrix appearance (Fig. 49.5). Whereas a chondral (cartilaginous) tumor will have matrix mineralization that appears as punctate arc and ring calcifications (Fig. 49.6). CT is often better than plain film at delineating the type of matrix mineralization.

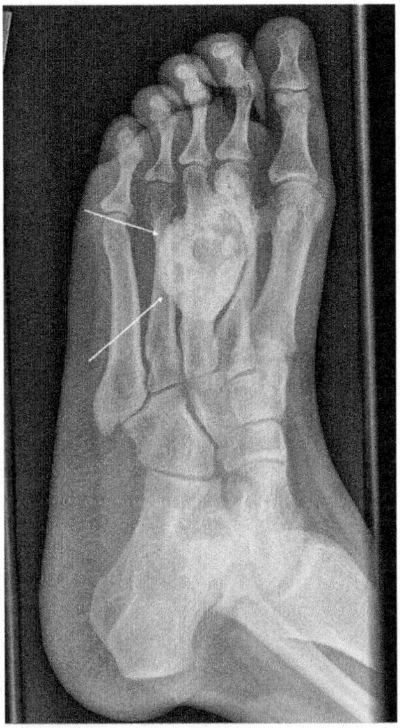

FIGURE 49.5 - OSTEOID MATRIX
Lesion arising from the second metatarsal which has an osteoid matrix characterized by the fluffy, cloud-like appearance

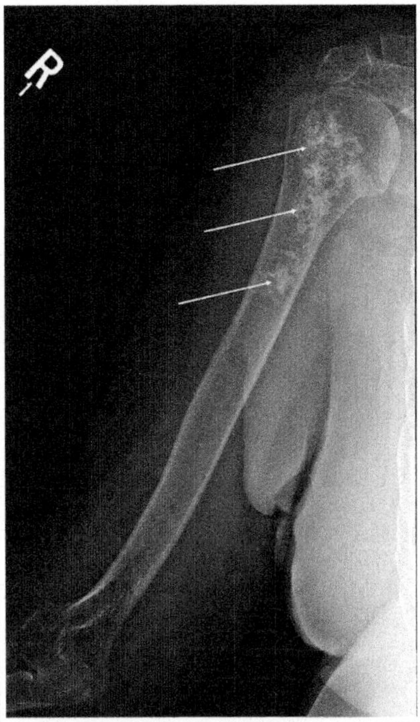

FIGURE 49.6 - CHONDROID MATRIX
Lesion arising in the proximal humerus with chondroid matrix characterized by arc and ring calcifications

Reference

Miller TT. Bone tumors and tumor like conditions: analysis with conventional radiography. Radiology. 2008;246(3):662–74.

50 Arthritides

Objectives:

1. List four features which allow distinctions between rheumatoid arthritis/ rheumatic variants and osteoarthritis.
2. List three findings seen in the skeleton in gout and explain how they differ from those seen in rheumatoid arthritis.

Osteoarthritis

The typical radiographic characteristics of osteoarthritis include:

1. *Asymmetric joint space narrowing* – This indicates loss of articular cartilage. For example, the hip migrates superiorly because of the loss of cartilage superiorly along the weight-bearing surface.
2. *Subchondral sclerosis (also called eburnation)* – This is caused by trabecular compression and fracture with callus formation.
3. *Osteophyte formation.*

Figure 50.1 is an example of asymmetric joint space narrowing which reflects thinning of the cartilage in the medial aspect of the joint, the area of maximal weight bearing. The body reacts to this change in its weight-bearing surface by increasing the thickness at the margins of the weight-bearing area resulting in subchondral sclerosis and reinforcement of the ligamentous support of the knee through the formation of spurs or osteophytes.

This new bone formation is what characterizes degenerative or osteoarthritis and allows the radiographic changes to be separated from rheumatoid arthritis and the rheumatoid variants.

H. Singh et al. (eds.), *Radiology Fundamentals: Introduction to Imaging & Technology*, DOI 10.1007/978-3-319-10362-4_50

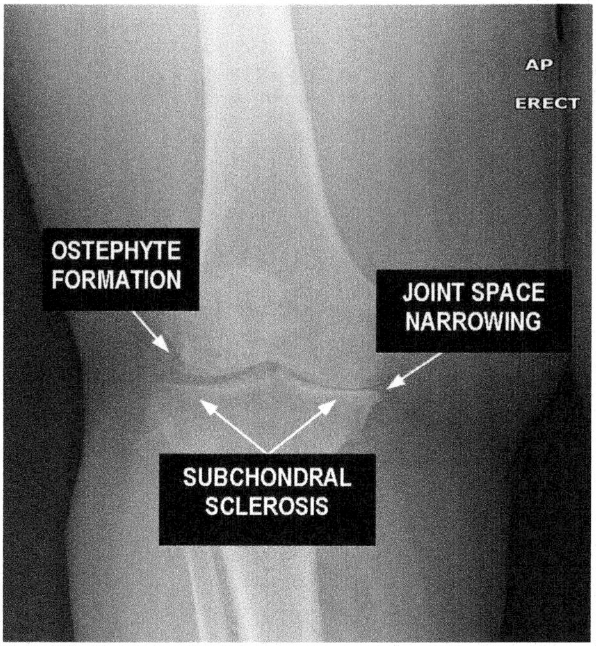

FIGURE 50.1 - OSTEOARTHRITIC KNEE
Right knee displaying osteophyte formation, joint space narrowing, and subchondral sclerosis, consistent with severe osteoarthritis

Rheumatoid Arthritis

Figure 50.2 demonstrates a case of rheumatoid arthritis (RA). In rheumatoid arthritis, there is symmetric joint space narrowing and loss of bone density. These findings help distinguish rheumatoid arthritis from osteoarthritis.

In addition, look for marginal erosions along the edges of articular surfaces in RA. Erosions first occur along the edges of the articular surface because these areas lack articular cartilage. Articular cartilage offers protection from the inflammation. Therefore, the edges of the articular surface not covered by cartilage are the first areas susceptible to the inflammatory pannus. The locations of these erosions help distinguish rheumatoid arthritis from other arthritides.

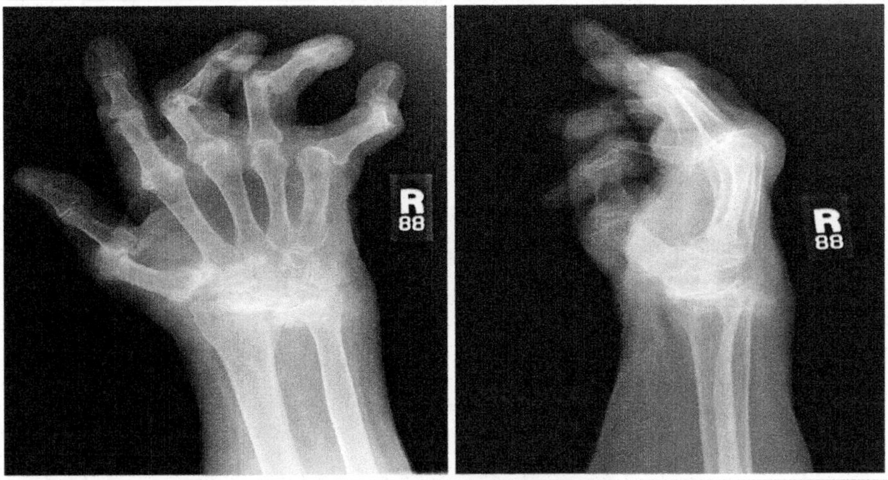

FIGURE 50.2 - SEVERE RHEUMATOID ARTHRITIS
Boutonniere deformity of the fifth digit is noted, with hyperflexion at the PIP joint and hyperextension at the DIP joint. There are severe ulnar subluxations and marginal erosions. Diffuse joint space narrowing is noted at the carpal joints and the metacarpal-phalangeal joints

Distinctions Between Osteoarthritis and Rheumatoid Arthritis

Note again that in osteoarthritis (OA), there is asymmetric joint space narrowing, subchondral sclerosis, and osteophyte formation. Also note that the main areas of involvement are in the distal interphalangeal joints with relative sparing of the metacarpophalangeal joints and intercarpal joints. Osteophytes formed about the DIP joints are referred to as Heberden's nodes, while those at the PIP joints are referred to as Bouchard's nodes. Osteoarthritis begins peripherally and, as it becomes more severe, progresses to involve the PIP joints. The only exception from the distal to proximal migration of osteoarthritis would be the first (thumb) carpometacarpal joint. This is a common site of osteoarthritis proximally.

On the other hand, in rheumatoid arthritis (RA), there is symmetric joint space narrowing and periarticular erosions (which can be quite subtle in the early stages). RA usually involves the intercarpal joints and metacarpophalangeal joints at an early stage (Fig. 50.3). There is ulnar deviation and erosions in the late stages of RA. You should be able to distinguish osteoarthritis from the rheumatoid-type arthritides in most cases. However, in very advanced disease, degenerative arthritis may be superimposed on preexisting rheumatoid-type arthritis. Other arthritides, which may look like osteoarthritis, include the arthritis produced by pseudogout (calcium pyrophosphate deposition disease) and hemochromatosis. Other than

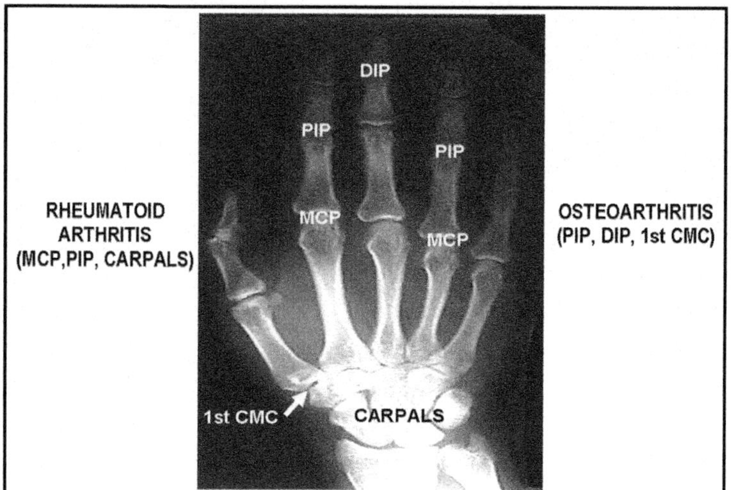

FIGURE 50.3 - DISTRIBUTION OF OSTEOARTHRITIS VERSUS RHEUMATOID ARTHRITIS
Osteoarthritis, characterized by joint space narrowing, subchondral sclerosis (also called eburnation), and osteophyte formation, tends to affect the proximal and distal interphalangeal joints as well as the first carpometacarpal joint. Rheumatoid arthritis, characterized by periarticular osteoporosis, marginal erosions, boutonniere deformity, swan neck deformity, subluxations, and dislocations, tends to affect the metacarpophalangeal joints and proximal interphalangeal joints

rheumatoid arthritis, arthritides which produce erosions include psoriatic arthritis and enteropathic arthritis (associated with Crohn's disease and ulcerative colitis).

Gout

Figure 50.4 demonstrates a patient with gout. You should note the following:

1. *Soft tissue tophi:* Lumpy bumpy pattern of soft tissue swelling that may mineralize in a small percentage of cases.
2. *Juxta-articular erosions:* Erosions occur in the regions of soft tissue tophi. Unlike the marginal erosions of rheumatoid arthritis, gouty erosions are located further from the joint and have characteristic sharply defined overhanging edges.

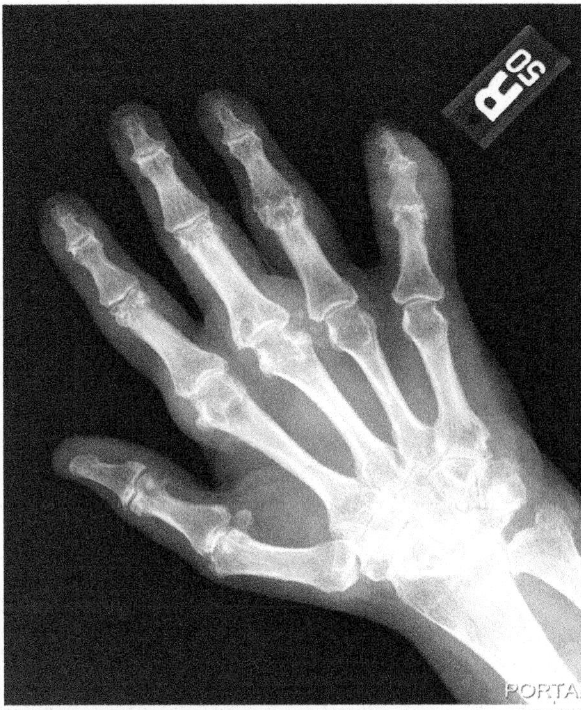

FIGURE 50.4 - GOUT
Nodular soft tissue swelling most impressive in the distal little finger, but also involving the ring, middle, and index fingers. Also note juxta-articular erosions in multiple joints, most conspicuous in the 3rd MCP and 5th PIP. These findings are consistent with tophaceous gout

3. *Joint destruction:* This usually occurs late in the disease and contiguous to the tophus. The joint spaces are characteristically normal in joints that are not destroyed.

In summary, gout is a disease of the soft tissues near the joints, not of the intra-articular portions of the joint itself.

Part VIII
Neuroradiology Section

51 CNS Anatomy

Objectives:

1. Identify the important normal anatomic landmarks on brain CT and MRI.
2. Describe how you would differentiate an enhanced (intravenous contrast) from an unenhanced CT scan of the head.
3. Understand the basic principle of image formation in MRI.

Figures 51.1 and 51.2 demonstrate a normal CT and MRI of the brain. Be sure to become familiar with the labeled structures. An in-depth discussion of the CNS anatomy is beyond the scope of this introductory text.

Note that on CT scans which are performed after administration of intravenous contrast, the circle of Willis as well as other various cortical vascular structures are prominently displayed. You should be able to identify the anterior cerebral artery, the middle cerebral artery, the posterior cerebral artery, and the region of the anterior and posterior communicating arteries.

MRI technology uses powerful magnets with magnetic fields several times more powerful than the earth's gravitational field. Hydrogen atoms are normally spinning in a random fashion. When a magnetic field is applied to the atoms, the magnetic poles of the hydrogen atoms are aligned. The magnetic field is then turned off, and the alignment of the hydrogen atoms degrades. With the degradation, a radiofrequency signal is given off which is then recorded and analyzed by the computer. From this information, an image is formed.

H. Singh et al. (eds.), *Radiology Fundamentals: Introduction to Imaging & Technology*, DOI 10.1007/978-3-319-10362-4_51

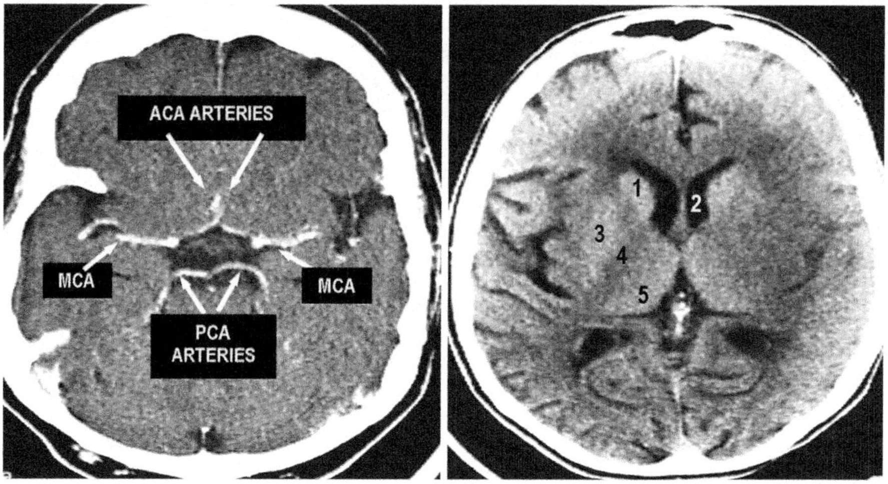

FIGURE 51.1 - BASIC CT NEUROANATOMY
The image on the *left* shows the intracerebral circulation (circle of Willis), which is clearly evident post-contrast. On the *right*, a non-contrast image, the following structures have been labeled: (*1*) caudate, (*2*) lateral ventricle frontal horn, (*3*) putamen and globus pallidus, (*4*) internal capsule (extends anteriorly), and (*5*) thalamus

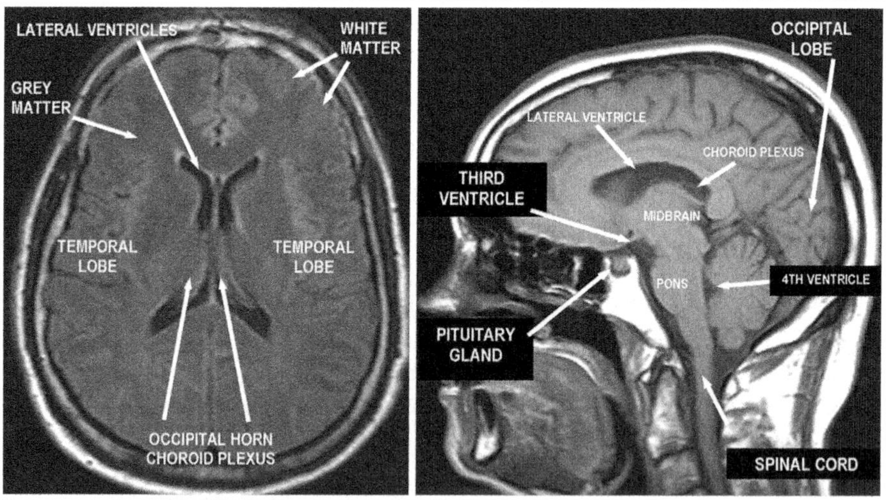

FIGURE 51.2 - BASIC MRI NEUROANATOMY

52 The Cervical Spine

Objectives:
1. Be able to list the various imaging modalities in evaluation of the cervical spine.
2. Describe a systematic approach to evaluating the cervical spine.

Plain radiographs of the cervical spine are the initial imaging modality, where the frontal, lateral, and AP views may be supplemented by additional views (like the "openmouthed" and extension/flexion views). Screening in spine trauma may begin with plain radiographs as traumatic injuries must be ruled out prior to moving the patient for other views and further treatment. Bony evaluation is now more commonly performed with CT which has much higher resolution and can provide multiplanar reformations. MRI is the modality of choice when spinal cord injury or ligamentous or soft tissue injury is suspected. A systematic and thorough review as outlined in the following steps is mandatory.

Systematic Approach to Evaluating the Cervical Spine with CT or Plain Film (Figs. 52.1 and 52.2)

Step 1: Count the visualized cervical vertebral bodies. It is mandatory that all seven cervical vertebrae (both the body and posterior elements) as well as the relationship of the inferior aspect of C7 with T1 are visualized.

Step 2: Check the alignment of the anterior aspects of the vertebral bodies: the anterior vertebral line. There should be a smooth curve that is convex anteriorly as one progresses from superior to inferior in the cervical spine. Loss of this curvature may indicate muscle spasm or soft tissue injury if the curvature is straightened or reversed. If the curvature changes abruptly, a fracture is likely.

H. Singh et al. (eds.), *Radiology Fundamentals: Introduction to Imaging & Technology*, DOI 10.1007/978-3-319-10362-4_52

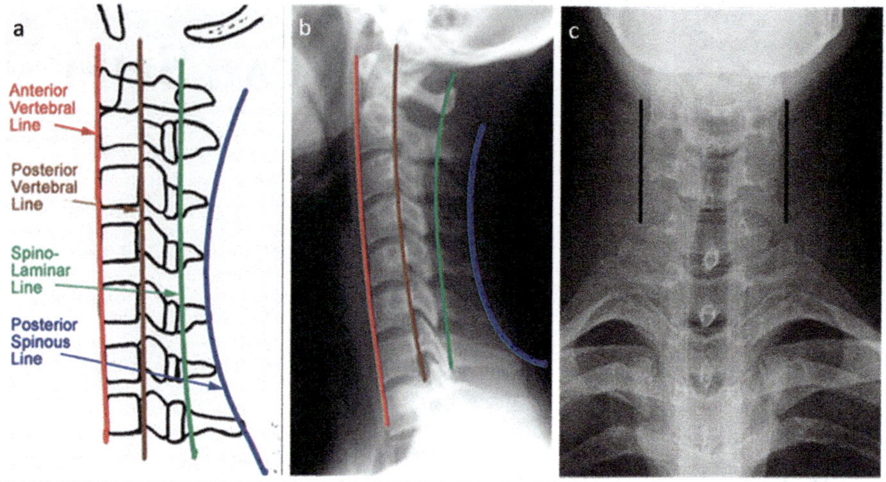

FIGURE 52.1 - CERVICAL SPINE LATERAL AND AP VIEWS
The anatomical landmarks are labeled on the diagram (**a**) and subsequently shown on the lateral radiograph (**b**). Note the undulating, rhythmic appearance of the lateral aspects of the cervical spine, bilaterally (**c**)

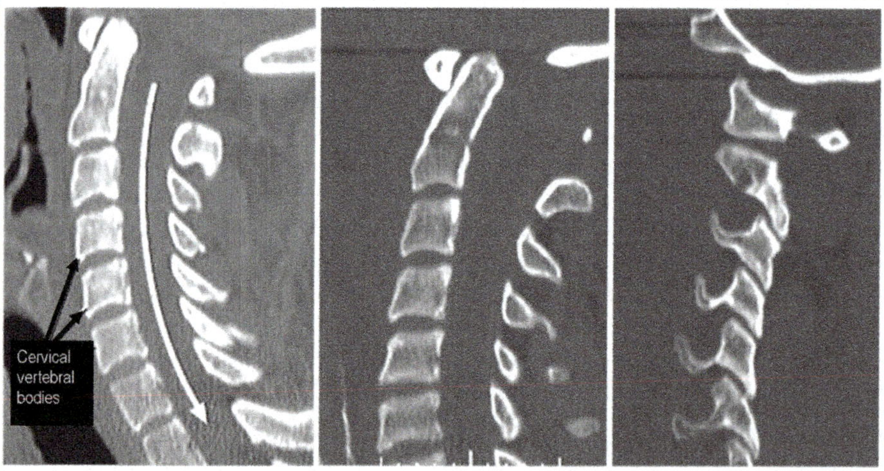

FIGURE 52.2 - CERVICAL SPINE CT SAGITTAL VIEWS
Normal alignment of the vertebrae with maintained body heights and normal facet articulations

Step 3: Check the alignment of the posterior aspects of the vertebral bodies (posterior vertebral line, which represents the anterior aspect of the bony spinal canal). For obvious reasons, this curvature should parallel the curvature of the anterior aspect of the vertebral bodies. Abnormalities of this curvature have the same significance as those of the anterior vertebral body curvature.

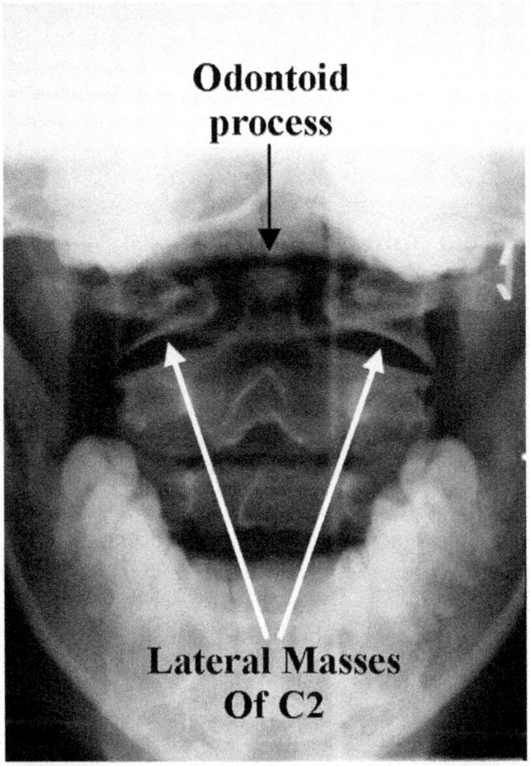

FIGURE 52.3 - OPENMOUTHED ODONTOID VIEW
The AP openmouthed odontoid view provides an unobstructed view of both the odontoid process of C2 and the lateral masses of C1

Step 4: Check the alignment of the spino-laminar line. This is a smooth line drawn along the anterior aspect of the spinous processes (which represents the posterior aspect of the bony spinal canal). Again, any disruption of this smooth curvature should be viewed with suspicion.

Step 5: Check the distance between the posterior aspect of the anterior arch of C1 and the anterior aspect of the odontoid process. This is the atlantoaxial space (sometimes called the predental space). Any increase in this distance may represent disruption of the transverse ligament that secures the posterior aspect of the dens to the atlas. The upper limit of normal for adults is 2.5 mm. Check the prevertebral soft tissues. As a general rule, think 6 and 2: at C2 they should be maximally 6 mm wide, and at C6 they should be maximally 22 mm wide. An openmouthed odontoid view is helpful to look for fractures of the odontoid process of C1 and the status of the lateral masses of C2 (Fig. 52.3).

The approach in evaluating a cervical spine CT is similar to that of a radiograph. However, with multiplanar reformats and better resolution, CT is much more sensitive than plain radiography. With the advent of multidetector CT, bony evaluation of the cervical spine is now done with CT, but the principles outlined above can be applied to any imaging modality.

MRI in the Cervical Spine Evaluation

MRI is very useful for evaluating spinal injuries. It is especially helpful for diagnosing or ruling out spinal cord injuries and acute compression of the spinal cord when clinical examination shows muscle weakness or paralysis. MRI is able to detect subtle changes in the vertebral column that may be an early stage of fracture, infection, or tumor. The imaging modality may be better than CT scanning for evaluating tumors, abscesses, and other masses near the spinal cord (Fig. 52.4).

Evaluation of cervical spine MRI begins with the assessment of alignment, vertebral body heights, and presence abnormal marrow signal. Disc and ligaments are much better seen on MRI as compared to CT. Next, evaluation should include assessment of the cord for compression, canal stenosis, or abnormal signal within the cord. Finally, the pre-/para-vertebral soft tissues and muscles are evaluated for hematoma or pathologic masses.

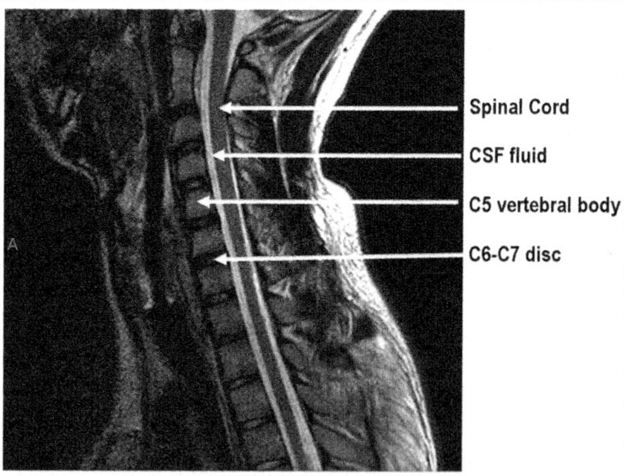

FIGURE 52.4 - SAGITTAL CERVICAL SPINE MRI
T2-weighted MRI of the cervical spine shows normal alignment of the vertebrae with normal bone marrow and spinal cord signal

53 Head Trauma

Objectives:
1. Understand the role of skull radiographs in head trauma.
2. Describe the appearance of an epidural hematoma on a head CT scan.
3. Describe the appearance of a subdural hematoma on a head CT scan.
4. Describe the appearance of a subarachnoid hemorrhage on a head CT and MRI.
5. Be able to list the findings on CT/MRI in a patient with cerebral contusion.
6. Describe the appearance of diffuse axonal injury on CT/MRI.

Skull Radiograph

With the advent of CT scans, the role of routine skull radiographs in neurologic trauma has become limited. In moderate and severe head trauma, a CT scan is the study of choice. Skull radiographs are only indicated in minor head trauma patients where a CT scan is otherwise not clinically indicated during the initial evaluation.

Skull radiograph may be helpful and can complement other imaging modalities in the following conditions:

1. Depressed fracture is suspected clinically or by the nature of the injury.
2. Penetrating injury by metal or glass is suspected.
3. Radiodense foreign body is suspected.

The basic skull projections used in evaluation of head trauma are the lateral and the fronto-occipital (AP) views (Fig. 53.1).

H. Singh et al. (eds.), *Radiology Fundamentals: Introduction to Imaging & Technology*, DOI 10.1007/978-3-319-10362-4_53

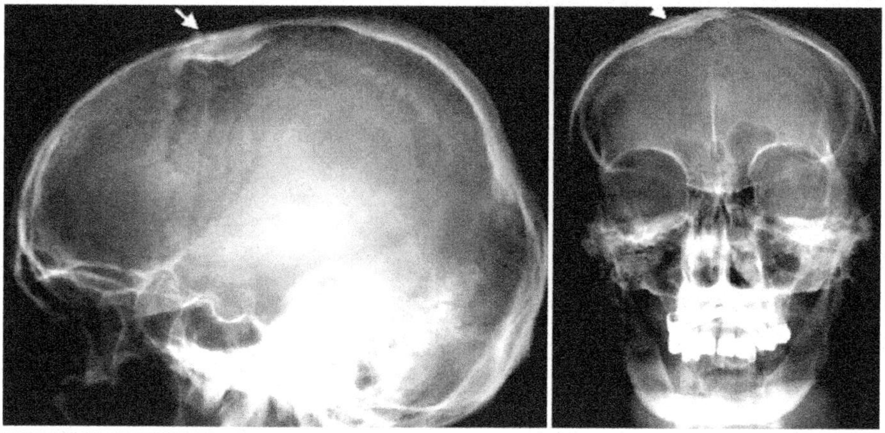

FIGURE 53.1 - SKULL RADIOGRAPH
Lateral and AP views show a depressed fracture of the right parietal bone with displacement of the bone fragment into the skull

Epidural Hematoma

Figure 53.2 shows a CT of a patient with a known skull fracture and acute hemorrhage. Blood appears as white material on head CT. The biconvex appearance of the epidural blood is caused by the tight attachment of the dura to the skull. Midline shift is present secondary to the mass effect of the hematoma.

Subdural Hematoma

Figure 53.3 demonstrates a subdural hematoma which is hemorrhage under the dura. Note that the blood is free to follow the contour of the brain so that it has a flat or concave inner surface.

In the normal evolution of a subdural hematoma, the collection becomes hypodense (more gray) with respect to brain tissue. As more time passes, it becomes isodense (equally dense) with respect to the brain tissue. Diagnosis during this period of isodensity can be difficult. Chronic subdural hematomas that are hypodense with respect to the brain substance are referred to as subdural hygromas.

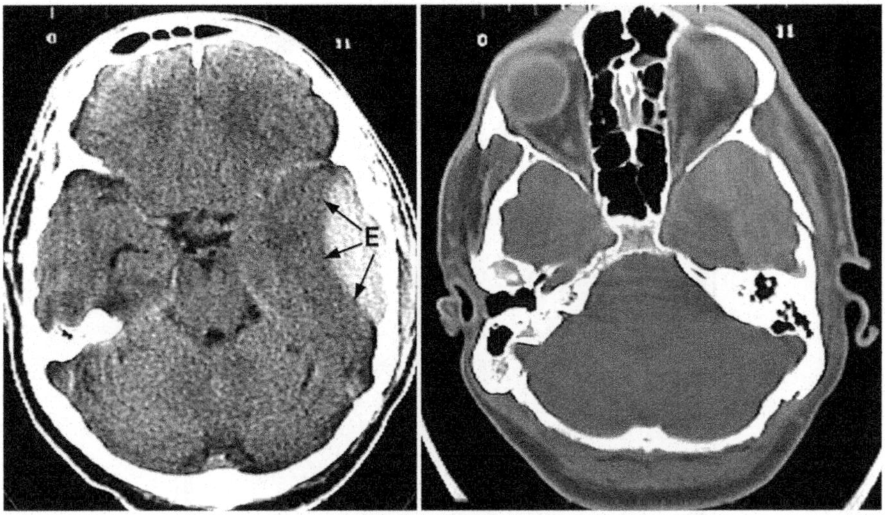

FIGURE 53.2 - EPIDURAL HEMATOMA WITH SKULL FRACTURE
In this trauma victim, there is an epidural hematoma (*E*). It has the typical elliptical shape. There is mass effect, centered on the bleed (*arrows*). The image on the *right* is further evidence of head trauma and the likely cause of the epidural hematoma. Did you notice the left temporal bone fracture?

Subarachnoid Hemorrhage

Trauma is the most common cause of subarachnoid hemorrhage (SAH) overall. A large percentage of traumatic brain injuries include of this type of bleeding. On CT scans, SAH appears as a high-attenuating (white), amorphous substance that fills the normally dark, CSF-filled subarachnoid spaces around the brain (Fig. 53.4). These findings are most evident in the largest subarachnoid spaces, such as the suprasellar cistern and sylvian fissures. It can also be seen tracking along the sulci, outlining the gray matter. MRI is more sensitive in diagnosing subarachnoid bleed, especially in hyperacute and chronic phases where CT may be completely negative because blood in those states is equal density to brain on CT.

Parenchymal Contusion

Figure 53.5 shows an area of generally decreased attenuation (gray) with an area of lobular increased densities. There is subtle mass effect with contralateral midline shift (to the patient's right). This displacement and low density are caused by edema

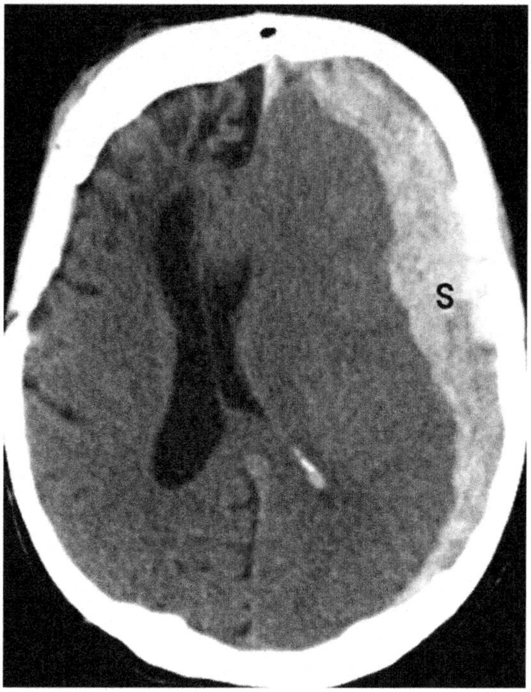

FIGURE 53.3 - SUBDURAL HEMATOMA
In this trauma victim, there is a large left holohemispheric subdural hematoma (*S*). It has a distinctly flat/concave inner surface which allows one to distinguish it from an epidural hematoma

with the lobular areas representing hemorrhage. This is the radiographic appearance of a cerebral contusion or, literally, "a bruise of the brain." In all of the above diagnoses, there may be associated findings such as a skull fracture and associated soft tissue swelling external to the skull. These abnormalities may give you a clue as to where to look within the brain for abnormalities, as these findings can sometimes be quite subtle.

Diffuse Axonal Injury

Diffuse axonal injury (DAI) is a frequent result of traumatic deceleration injuries and a frequent cause of a persistent vegetative state. Typically, the process is diffuse and bilateral, involving the lobar white matter at the gray-white matter interface

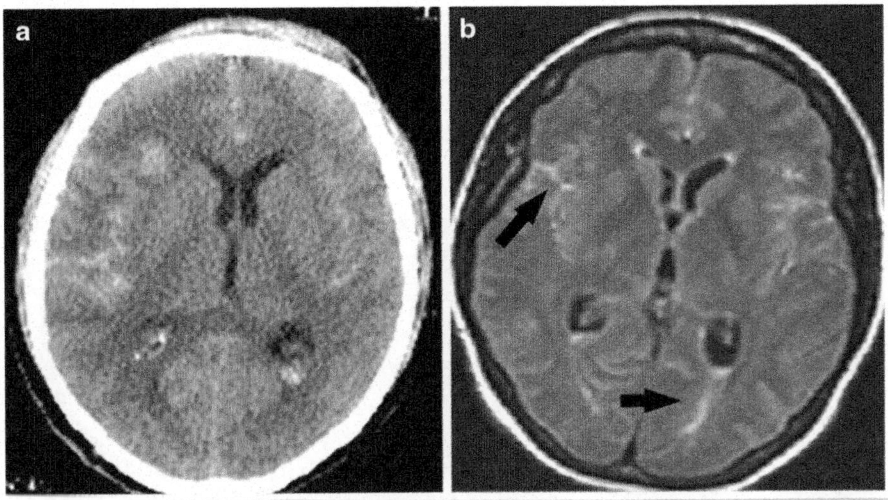

FIGURE 53.4 - CT AND MRI OF SUBARACHNOID HEMORRHAGE
(**a**) CT shows hyperdensity within the CSF sulci spaces, most prominently along the sylvian fissures (*arrow*), consistent with subarachnoid hemorrhage. (**b**) MRI on the same patient shows corresponding areas of T2 hyperintensity within the sylvian fissures along with intraventricular hemorrhage

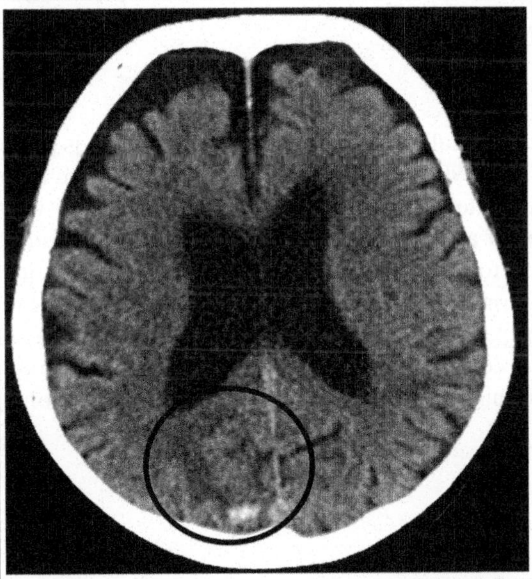

FIGURE 53.5 - PARENCHYMAL CONTUSION
There is blood in the parenchyma with some surrounding edema consistent with a contusion. Note the subtle mass effect at this level

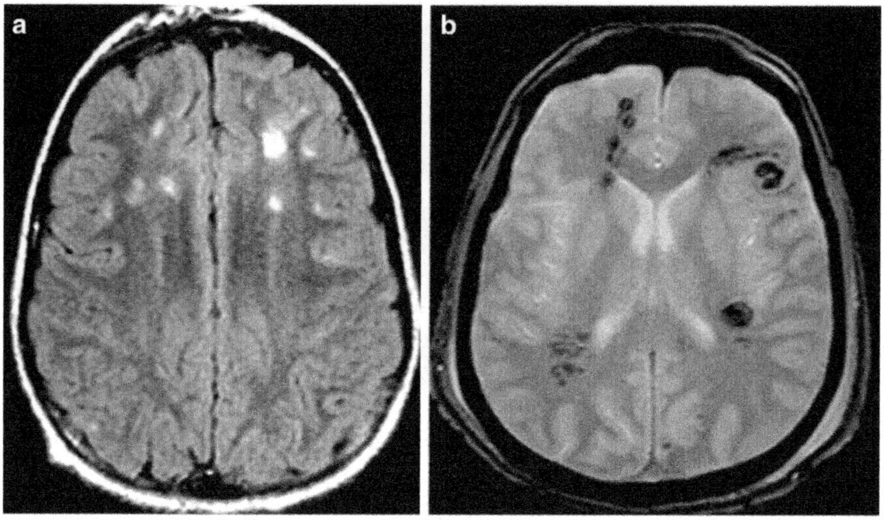

FIGURE 53.6 - HEAD TRAUMA IMAGING
MRI in a young patient with trauma and negative head CT shows multiple areas of T2 hyperintensity at the gray-white matter junction (**a**). The petechial hemorrhages are seen as low signal areas on gradient images (**b**). (Gradient echo is a MRI sequence which is very sensitive to blood products)

(Fig. 53.6). The corpus callosum frequently is involved, as is the dorsolateral rostral brainstem. On CT, 60–90 % of patients with DAI may have a normal CT scan on presentation. Small petechial hemorrhages located at the grey-white matter junction and corpus callosum are characteristic but only occur in about 20 %. MRI is the modality of choice for diagnosing DAI. Most common MRI findings are multiple focal areas of abnormally bright signal on T2-weighted images in the white matter of the temporal or parietal corticomedullary junction or in the splenium of corpus callosum. Gradient echo sequences are very useful in demonstrating petechial hemorrhages. The paramagnetic properties of blood cause a loss of signal, represented by black areas.

54 STROKE

Objectives:
1. State the definition of stroke.
2. Understand the role of imaging in stroke.
3. Be able to describe major CT and MRI findings in stroke.

Introduction

Stroke is a clinical syndrome. It is used to refer to a group of clinical syndromes that present with acute mental status change including ischemic infarction, hemorrhage, seizure, tumor, encephalopathy, etc.

Imaging in stroke is used to differentiate:

1. Vascular process from other mimics such as hemorrhage, tumor, vascular malformation, and encephalopathy
2. Hemorrhagic from nonhemorrhagic infarction
3. Arterial from venous infarction
4. Large territory infarct from lacunar-type infarctions

In addition, more advanced CT and MRI techniques can be applied (i.e., CT perfusion, CT angiography, MRI angiography) to guide treatment options and potentially predict outcome.

H. Singh et al. (eds.), *Radiology Fundamentals: Introduction to Imaging & Technology*, DOI 10.1007/978-3-319-10362-4_54

Imaging Findings in Stroke

When is the optimal time to image "stroke?" The answer generally is "as soon as possible," although this depends on the treatment options available to the patient at the presenting medical care facility. Treatment options include conservative management, intravenous tissue plasminogen activator (t-PA), intra-arterial t-PA, and mechanical thrombolysis. Treatment depends on the timing of onset of symptoms and the clinical status of the patient. The patient's clinical status is assessed using the National Institutes of Health Stroke Scale (NIHSS), a systematic assessment tool that provides a quantitative measure of stroke-related neurologic deficit, based on a 15-item scale measuring the patient's level of consciousness, language, neglect, visual field loss, extraocular movement, motor strength, ataxia, dysarthria, and sensory loss.

Noncontrast CT is usually first obtained (Fig. 54.1). This is a very fast and widely available study. Quite a bit of information can be gained from the basic CT, such as the following: Is there a discernible abnormality? Does it appear to be ischemia or something else, like a mass? Is there bleeding? How much brain tissue is involved? Is there herniation/mass effect that would constitute a neurosurgical emergency?

Ischemia/infarction is not always immediately evident on CT, especially if the patient is imaged very early after the onset of symptoms or if the area of brain involved is small (lacunar infarct).

The early signs of ischemia on CT are:

1. Hypoattenuation (low density) in the affected tissue
2. Loss of gray-white matter differentiation (insular ribbon sign)

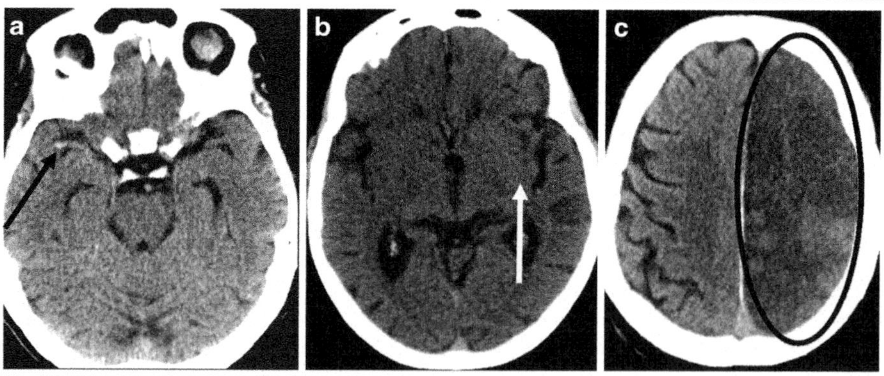

FIGURE 54.1 - CT FINDINGS OF ACUTE ISCHEMIA
The above images represent CT findings of acute ischemia: (**a**) hyperdense MCA, (**b**) loss of grey-white matter differentiation in the insula, and (**c**) sulcal effacement and hyperdensity in the MCA territory

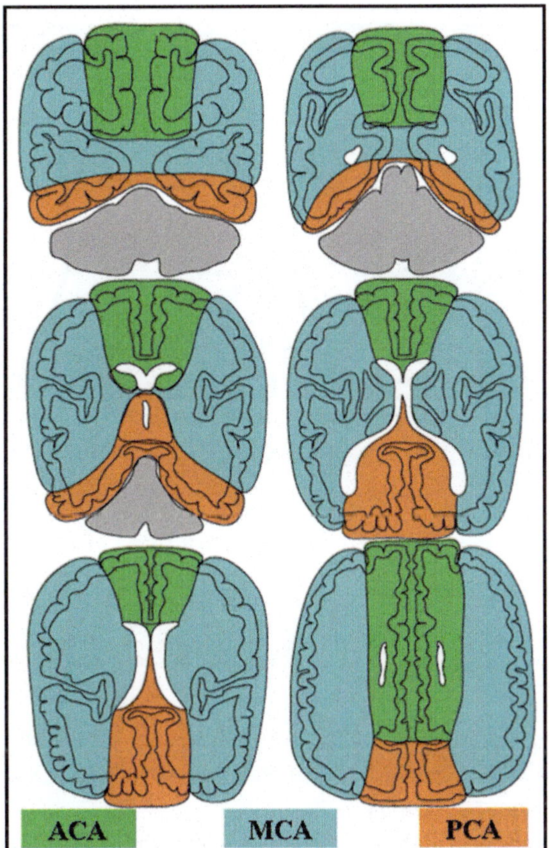

FIGURE 54.2 - VASCULAR AREAS OF CEREBRAL ARTERIES
Based on the distribution of infarcted or ischemic tissue, one can infer the vessel that is affected based on the arterial supply to the brain

3. Sulcal effacement due to brain swelling
4. Hyperdensity in a large vessel (hyperdense MCA sign) or "dot sign" due to acute clot in the diseased vessel.

Seeing the distribution of infarcted or ischemic tissue and knowing the arterial supply (Fig. 54.2) to the different parts of the brain, one can infer the vessel(s) affected. The vascular territories of the cerebral arteries described in the figure include: ACA = anterior cerebral artery, MCA = middle cerebral artery, PCA = posterior cerebral artery.

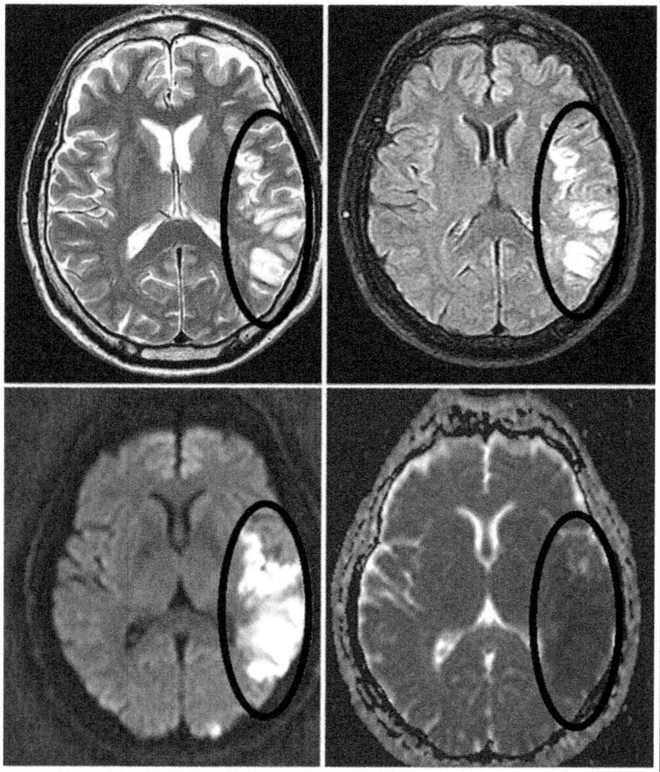

FIGURE 54.3 - ACUTE ISCHEMIA
MRI findings of acute ischemia in the left MCA distribution: (**a**) T2W, (**b**) FLAIR, (**c**) DWI, and (**d**) ADC map

Although in many instances subtle findings can be seen on CT, sometimes the study can appear essentially normal, especially early on. If this is the case, the patient could clinically still have a "stroke" syndrome and will be treated as such.

MRI is more sensitive for detection of early ischemia and is better at detecting small infarctions, especially in patients with cerebrovascular disease who have chronic small infarcts (Fig. 54.3). Diffusion-weighted imaging can detect ischemia within minutes of the acute event and is generally agreed to be the best indicator of the total infarcted volume. Also, MRI is better at finding other processes which may be causing the symptoms; however, disadvantages of MRI include less availability, higher price, and longer scanning time (a major drawback given the previously discussed treatment window). MRI is not safe for some patients who have metallic foreign bodies or certain devices, most notably older model pacemakers, certain models of artificial valves, cochlear implants, and spinal stimulators.

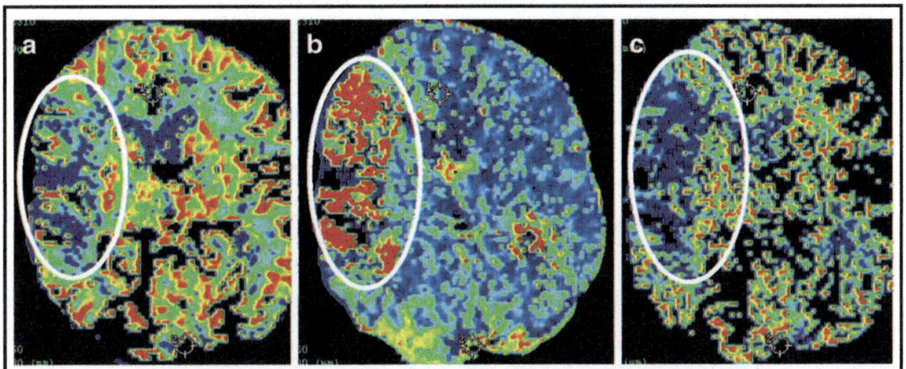

FIGURE 54.4 - CT IMAGES OF AN ACUTE INFARCT
CT perfusion in acute right MCA infarct with all three parameters being abnormal in the affected distribution: (**a**) CBV, (**b**) CBF, and (**c**) MTT

CT perfusion (CTP) is performed by monitoring the first pass of the contrast bolus through the cerebral circulation (Fig. 54.4). Information can be obtained at four representative levels in the brain or be obtained through a volume of brain tissue. Using this information, color maps of cerebral blood volume (CBV), cerebral blood flow (CBF), mean transit time (MTT), and time to peak (TTP) are generated. This information is used to look for areas of perfusion defect and mismatch, which, in addition to the region of the infarction core, indicate other areas of ischemia and potential infarction, the "penumbra." This may influence further treatment decisions. MRI perfusion operates on basically the same principles, except gadolinium-based contrast is used and perfusion maps are compared with diffusion-weighted images to determine if there is tissue that can potentially be saved. Although the information is similar, CTP is much faster and therefore more commonly used in acute settings, although there is some disagreement among the stroke community as to the added value of perfusion imaging.

CT angiography or venography (CTA or CTV) are noninvasive techniques using thin section techniques and contrast to image the intracranial and extracranial (neck) vasculature. This is useful for identifying sites of occlusion, stenosis, dissection, and/or aneurysm (Fig. 54.5).

Although infarction is more frequently caused by arterial occlusion, venous thrombosis can also lead to ischemia and hemorrhage. Venous infarcts do not follow arterial territories and occur in younger patients with hypercoagulable states or other risk factors. CT venography or MR venography can evaluate the patency of major dural sinuses.

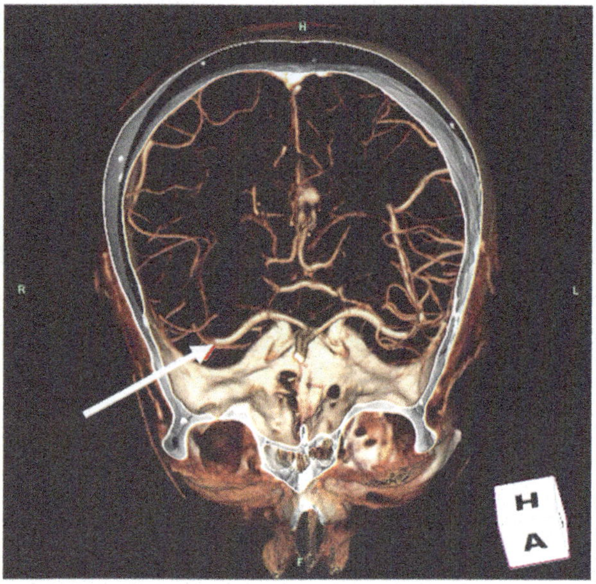

FIGURE 54.5 - OCCLUSION OF MIDDLE CEREBRAL ARTERY
CTA shows acute occlusion of the right MCA (*arrow*)

Summary

Options for imaging stroke include CT, CT perfusion, CT angiography, MRI, MR perfusion, and MRI angiography. Not all of these studies are indicated on every patient. CT is faster, more readily available, and, in some ways, easier to interpret. MRI is more expensive, less available, slower, but more sensitive for acute ischemia and useful for finding other causes of patient's symptoms that may not be evident on CT.

55 Headache and Back Pain

Objectives:
1. Understand the role of imaging in the patient with headache and back pain.
2. Be able to describe the major CT findings of subarachnoid hemorrhage.
3. Be able to state other causes of headache.

Introduction

Many disease processes manifest as headache. While headaches are mostly benign and self-limited, imaging is often obtained to exclude acute or life-threatening processes, such as a hemorrhage or mass.

Back pain is one of the most common complaints in health care. It is important to remember that back pain is not a diagnosis but a symptom of a medical condition. Most causes are benign. Imaging is often obtained when there is no response to rest, exercise, and medication to ensure there is no process that needs further intervention.

Intracranial Hemorrhage

Classically, the presentation of "the worst headache of my life" with sudden onset is concerning for subarachnoid hemorrhage (SAH). The most common cause of *nontraumatic* subarachnoid hemorrhage is a ruptured intracerebral aneurysm. Acute blood products are hyperdense (white) on CT, and therefore CT is useful for detection of SAH. CT angiography (CTA) is highly sensitive for the diagnosis of the underlying aneurysm, although catheter angiography remains the gold standard (Fig. 55.1). CSF sampling by lumbar puncture can be done in cases of CT-negative suspected SAH.

H. Singh et al. (eds.), *Radiology Fundamentals: Introduction to Imaging & Technology*, DOI 10.1007/978-3-319-10362-4_55

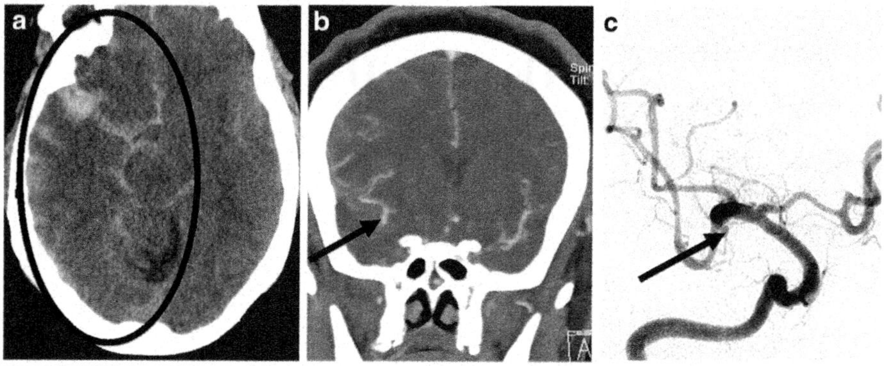

FIGURE 55.1 - SUBARACHNOID HEMORRHAGE
Image (**a**) is a CT which shows predominantly right hemispheric SAH. Image (**b**) is a coronal CTA reformat showing a very small aneurysm of the right M2 segment of the MCA, while the digital subtraction image (*DSA*) shown in image (**c**) shows the same aneurysm

There are other types of intracranial hemorrhage which could cause headache though they are frequently associated with trauma. These include subdural and epidural hematomas and hemorrhagic contusions (see Chap. 53, "Head Trauma").

Other Common Causes of Headache on Imaging

Any disease process which alters the intracranial pressure (ICP) or causes hydrocephalus, midline shift, or cerebral edema can cause a headache. This includes brain tumors (primary or metastatic), non-neoplastic masses which can have mass effect or obstruct the ventricles, or idiopathic processes such as pseudotumor cerebri. Infectious processes, including meningitis and encephalitis, can present with headache but often have no or little findings on imaging; rather, the diagnosis is dependent on CSF and serum assay (Fig. 55.2).

Back Pain

Causes of back pain include mechanical problems, injuries, neoplasms, infections, and many other conditions. Intervertebral disc degeneration and herniation, facet arthritis, and muscle spasm are examples of mechanical problems that result in back pain. Injuries to bones, muscles, tendons, and ligaments from sports, trauma such as car accidents, and improper lifting and twisting can result in back pain.

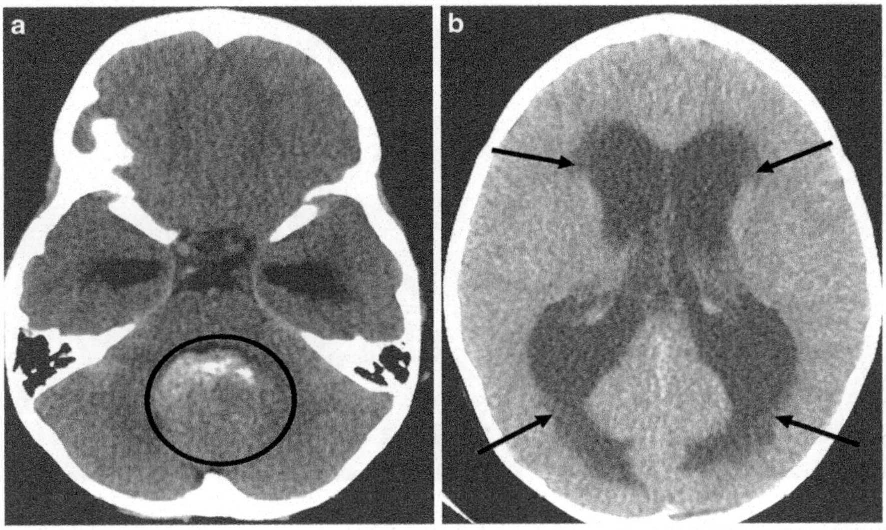

FIGURE 55.2 - HYDROCEPHALUS
CT showing a dense posterior fossa mass (**a**) causing hydrocephalus (**b**)

Compression fractures in osteoporotic patients may manifest as back pain. Permanent and progressive conditions such are inflammatory and osteoarthritis, scoliosis, and fibromyalgia cause or contribute to back pain. Patients with renal calculi, pancreatitis, pregnancy, and endometriosis may have back pain. Leaking aortic aneurysm and aortic dissection may present as back pain. Osteomyelitis/ discitis, primary tumors of the spinal cord or vertebral bodies, and metastatic disease may also cause back pain. And while most causes of back pain are physical, stress, anxiety, depression, and insomnia can present as back pain or exacerbate underlying back pain conditions.

In the absence of underlying conditions such as malignancy or trauma, appropriate treatment may first be exercise, mild medication, physical therapy, and lifestyle modification such as weight loss and management of stress and depression. If these interventions do not help, imaging should be considered. Plain films of the lumbar spine will demonstrate alignment, compression or traumatic fractures and disc space height, and changes of arthritis and serve as a road map. CT scan, particularly if other conditions are suspected, will frequently demonstrate other causes such as kidney stones, aortic aneurysm, pelvic mass, etc. MRI is sensitive for the detection of infections of the bone, discs, and spinal cord; tumors; disc herniation; and nerve root impingement (Fig. 55.3).

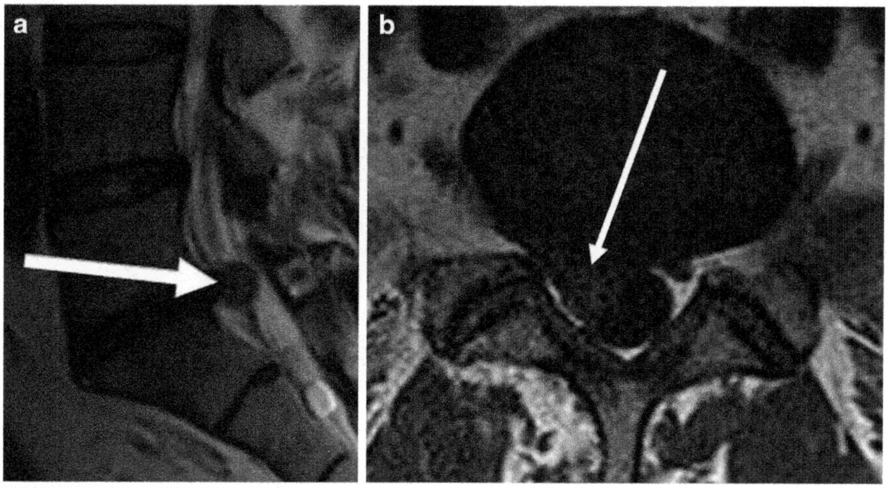

FIGURE 55.3 - LUMBAR DISC HERNIATION
Sagittal (**a**) and axial (**b**) MRI images showing a focal protrusion of the L5–S1 disc (*arrows*) causing moderate mass effect on the thecal sac

Summary

Headache is a very common complaint. Patients with simple headache often have no imaging findings. Moreover, imaging is not needed in the majority of cases of headache. Imaging is used when there is clinical suspicion for a more complicated or acute process, such as hemorrhage, mass, or hydrocephalus. Noncontrast CT is excellent for the initial evaluation of headache to exclude life-threatening processes, with the caveat that some very serious disease processes, especially infectious diseases affecting the central nervous system, can have little or no imaging findings.

Back pain is also very common and imaging is also not always required. Acute situations such as loss of bowel or bladder control or acute muscle weakness should prompt a consideration of imaging with CT and/or MRI. Clinical acumen remains of the utmost importance in the evaluation and treatment of patients presenting with either complaints.

Part IX
Pediatrics Section

56 Pediatric Radiology Pearls

Objectives:

1. Recognize the need for greater radiation safety precautions in children.
2. Be familiar with appreciate common imaging appearances of the pediatric chest and abdomen.
3. Identify the differences between pediatric fractures and adult fractures.
4. Recognize the role of radiologic imaging in non-accidental injuries.

Many of the principles of imaging you have learned in the preceding chapters are directly applicable to the pediatric patient. Remember, though, that children are not small versions of adults! While a full discussion of pediatric radiology cannot be covered in a single chapter, there are a few "special topics" in pediatric imaging which are included in this section.

Radiation Concerns in Diagnostic Imaging: We are judicious about the use of imaging modalities which use ionizing radiation in all patients, but particular awareness is needed when making imaging decisions in children. Simply put, ionizing radiation is energy packets in the form of subatomic particles or electromagnetic waves (including x-rays!) which can penetrate various materials and has the capability to detach electrons from atoms. The ensuing free radicals have the potential to create breaks in DNA which could lead to carcinogenesis. Children are more sensitive because they are growing (rapid cell division). They also have a longer life expectancy and thus a larger window of opportunity to express damage caused by radiation. That said, the individual risk is small, estimated risk 1/1,000 excess (i.e., over baseline lifetime risk) fatal cancer from a single CT scan. For the individual child, risk is low, and the child benefits when imaging decisions are made appropriately. Ask these questions:

1. Will the test change management?
2. What is the best test? (Can I use an imaging modality which does not use radiation –US or MRI?)

H. Singh et al. (eds.), *Radiology Fundamentals: Introduction to Imaging & Technology*, DOI 10.1007/978-3-319-10362-4_56

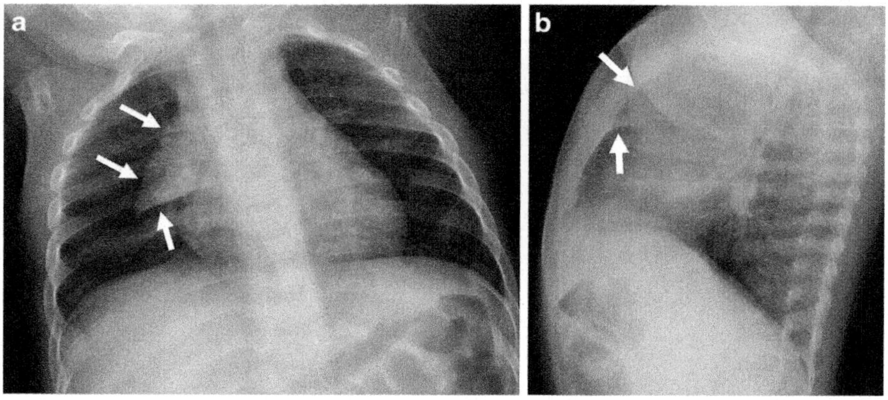

FIGURE 56.1 - (a AND b) CHARACTERISTIC SAIL SIGN ON AP VIEW AND ANTERIOR LOCATION ON LATERAL VIEW (*ARROWS*)

Once the test is deemed appropriate, there are behind-the-scenes factors under the control of the technologist/radiation physicist/radiologist (KVP, mAs, etc.) to use an x-ray dose appropriate for the size of the child. There are many resources available which provide additional information on this topic. www.imagegently.org is an excellent website which provides specific guidance to patients, parents, and physicians.

Thymus: The thymus is a bilobed organ located in the anterior mediastinum and important in immune function. It is large in infants and young children, often "border forming" on a chest x-ray and could potentially be mistaken for a mediastinal mass. To distinguish the thymus from a mass:

1. Look for the characteristic "wave" or "sail" shape (Fig. 56.1a and b).
2. Look through it: You should be able to see lung parenchymal markings through it.
3. Look for absence of mass effect on adjacent structures.

Lung Infections in Children: While it is impossible to determine what specific organism is causing a respiratory infection from the chest x-ray (CXR), there are clues to distinguish between viral and bacterial causes (which can affect patient management, i.e., are antibiotics needed?). The causes of pneumonia vary with age. Infants and preschool children are much more likely to have viral etiologies (about 95 %). The virus infects the airways causing inflammation and peribronchial edema which we see on CXR as hyperinflation and symmetric, coarse interstitial and peribronchial opacities (bronchiolitis and bronchopneumonia) (Fig. 56.2). Secretions occlude airways causing atelectasis. Pleural fluid is rare. In school-age children, while viral infection is still more common, bacterial pneumonia is a bigger player (accounting for 30 % of pneumonias). Bacteria cause their damage in the airspaces

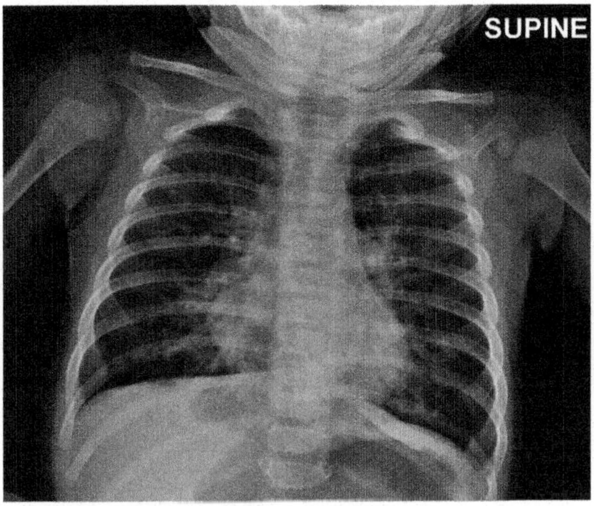

FIGURE 56.2 - PERIBRONCHIAL THICKENING, HYPERINFLATION, AND CENTRAL NON-SEGMENTAL SITES OF ATELECTASIS

with inflammatory exudates leading to alveolar opacities with air bronchograms. In children, consolidations may be round in appearance due to incompletely developed collateral pathways of air drift, the pores of Kohn, and the canals of Lambert (Fig. 56.3a and b). Diagnosis is by CXR (in addition to history/physical exam/laboratory results). CT is reserved for evaluating the complications of pneumonia (empyema, abscess) or look for anatomic abnormality predisposing to recurrent pneumonia.

Child with Stridor: Stridor is noisy breathing that occurs as a result of an obstructed or turbulent airflow through a narrowed airway. Stridor is not in and of itself a diagnosis but rather a symptom that points to a specific airway disorder. The age of the patient and the timing in relation to the respiratory cycle are clues to the etiology of the noisy breathing.

Inspiratory stridor occurs during inspiration and indicates a collapse of the airway above the vocal cords.

Expiratory stridor occurs when a child breaths out and indicates an intrathoracic obstruction.

Biphasic stridor suggests an obstruction in an area between the glottis and subglottis or a fixed obstruction at any level.

The causes of stridor can be congenital or acquired and acute or persistent. Acute stridor is commonly caused by infection (croup) (Fig. 56.4), trauma, or a foreign body. Causes of persistent stridor include congenital laryngeal or tracheal anomalies

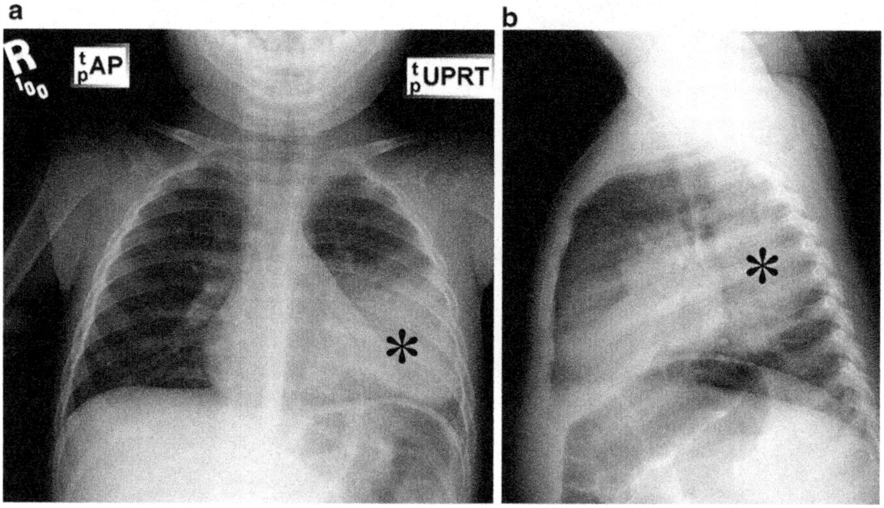

FIGURE 56.3 - (a AND b) LOBAR CONSOLIDATION (*)

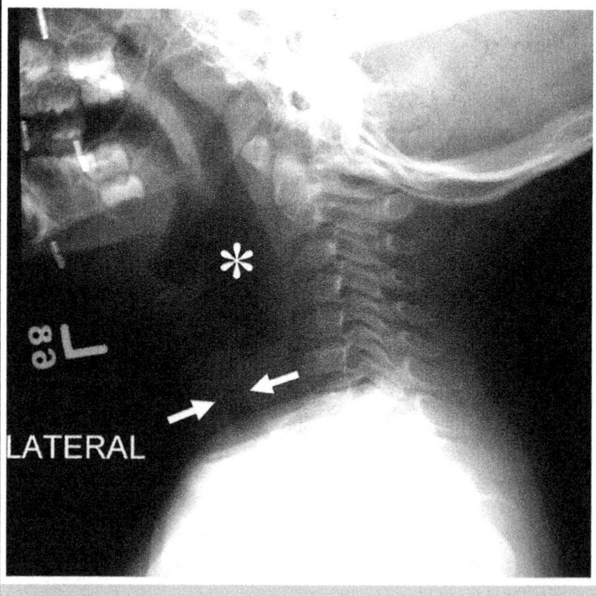

FIGURE 56.4 - AIR-DISTENDED HYPOPHARYNX (*) AND SUBGLOTTIC EDEMA (*ARROWS*)

such as laryngomalacia or tracheomalacia, vocal cord paralysis, or a vascular ring. Subglottic hemangiomas may present with croup-like cough.

The initial investigation begins with a good history and physical examination. Features to be assessed include: onset, duration, and associated symptoms such as fever, feeding, and voice abnormalities. The imaging assessment of stridor begins with AP and lateral views of the neck and chest. Further evaluation is dictated by the most likely diagnosis, based on the age of the child and key historical and exam findings. Look for the following:

1. X-ray of the neck may reveal edema or mass in the subglottic trachea. Further assessment with flexible laryngoscopy and CT/MRI may be performed for surgical planning in the case of subglottic hemangioma.
2. X-ray of the chest should be assessed for tracheal caliber (look for narrowing or abnormal mass effect) and evidence of a right aortic arch. Confirmation with upper GI imaging (UGI)/barium swallow in the case of vascular ring is useful. Again, CT or MRI is helpful for surgical planning.
3. Acute foreign body aspiration into a main stem bronchus may reveal air trapping on the affected side. Bilateral decubitus radiographs show the lack of collapse (air trapping) on the dependent affected side and appropriate collapse of the lung on the contralateral dependent side.

Teaching Points

- Chronic or persistent stridor lasts for more than 3 weeks or recurs on more than three occasions.
- Flexible laryngoscopy can be performed for evaluation of the upper airway. The lower airway and mediastinum are better evaluated with a UGI or cross-sectional imaging (CT and MRI).
- Airway fluoroscopy is helpful in the evaluation of laryngomalacia and tracheomalacia. A UGI can be performed afterward to assess the pattern of airway and esophageal compression particularly when vascular rings and slings are suspected and to assess for reflux.
- CT and MRI are very helpful in demonstrating detailed relationships between soft tissues and vascular anatomy. CT is better in identification of associated tracheal anomalies such as complete tracheal rings. MRI can characterize soft tissue and vascular anomalies without ionizing radiation.
- The choice of cross-sectional imaging modalities depends on the particular question and patient's condition. MDCT (multidetector CT) is preferred over MRI because of the shorter scanning times. High-pitch, rapid volume MDCT can in some cases obviate the need for sedation in young children.

Imaging the Vomiting Child: The causes of vomiting in infants and young children are numerous and diverse. Two diagnoses are worth mentioning: one because of its relative frequency and the other because of the importance of prompt identification and surgical intervention to prevent catastrophic bowel loss and potentially death. It is important to distinguish between bilious and nonbilious vomiting as the

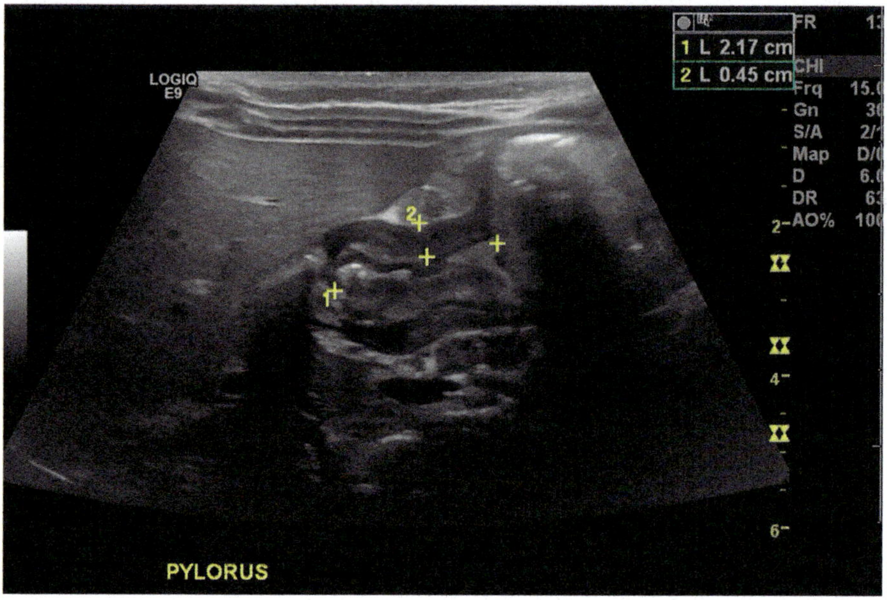

FIGURE 56.5 - HYPERTROPHIED PYLORUS 22 MM LENGTH AND 5 MM THICKNESS

differential diagnosis is dependent upon this factor and patient age. While GERD is the more common cause of nonbilious vomiting in infants, in those 2–8 weeks in age, hypertrophic pyloric stenosis (HPS) (Fig. 56.5) should be considered. Infants typically present with nonbilious projectile vomiting. Using ultrasonography, we can look at the thickness and length of the pyloric channel (for HPS look for muscle thickness of 3–4 mm and channel length of 16 mm+) and make an assessment of whether the pyloric channel is patent. Malrotation with midgut volvulus is an important cause of bilious vomiting. While it can be seen at any age, it commonly occurs in young infants. The diagnosis is made on UGI. High obstruction is identified with distention of the stomach and proximal duodenum. At the site of the twist, typically in the distal second or third portion of the duodenum, a beak will be identified (Fig. 56.6). Depending on the tightness of the twist, a small amount of contrast may pass distally into a "corkscrewed" distal decompressed duodenum.

Intussusception: Intussusception is the most common cause of intestinal obstruction between the ages of 3 months and 4 years. In this condition, part of the intestine invaginates into an adjacent portion of the intestine, similar to a collapsing telescope. If left untreated, it can cause serious ischemia to the intestine. The vascular compromise can lead to a cascade of events from edema to obstruction

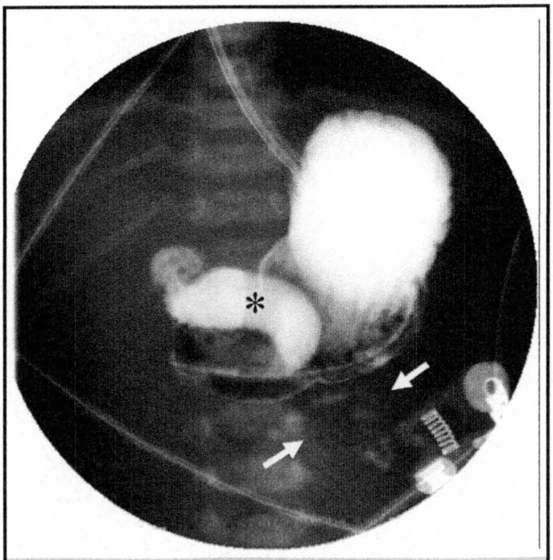

FIGURE 56.6 - DILATED 1ST AND 2ND PORTIONS OF THE DUODENUM (*) WITH CORKSCREW APPEARANCE OF DISTAL DUODENUM AND MIDGUT (*ARROWS*)

and eventually peritonitis. The ischemia can lead to dark bloody stools ("currant jelly" stools).

The presenting symptoms are intermittent abdominal pain in a previously well child. The symptoms may be mistaken for gastroenteritis initially. Intussusception should be considered when a child draws their knees up to their chest, is very irritable, and is inconsolable. The child may recover and become playful between bouts of pain. Once the intussusception is established, the child may become tired and weak from crying.

The initial radiographic study is typically abdominal radiographs. The radiographs may be normal or may show paucity of bowel gas in the right lower quadrant and an area of increased density in the region of intussusception. In some cases, the films may reveal a small bowel obstruction. When clinical suspicion is high, an ultrasound should be performed to confirm the diagnosis. On ultrasonography, an intussusception looks like a mass which is target-like, created by the cross-sectional appearance of one bowel loop within another, often in the right abdomen (Fig. 56.7). Ultrasound may identify a "lead point" and can confirm the presence or lack of blood flow. Once the diagnosis is established, an air enema can be performed to reduce (correct) the intussusception and obviate the need for surgery.

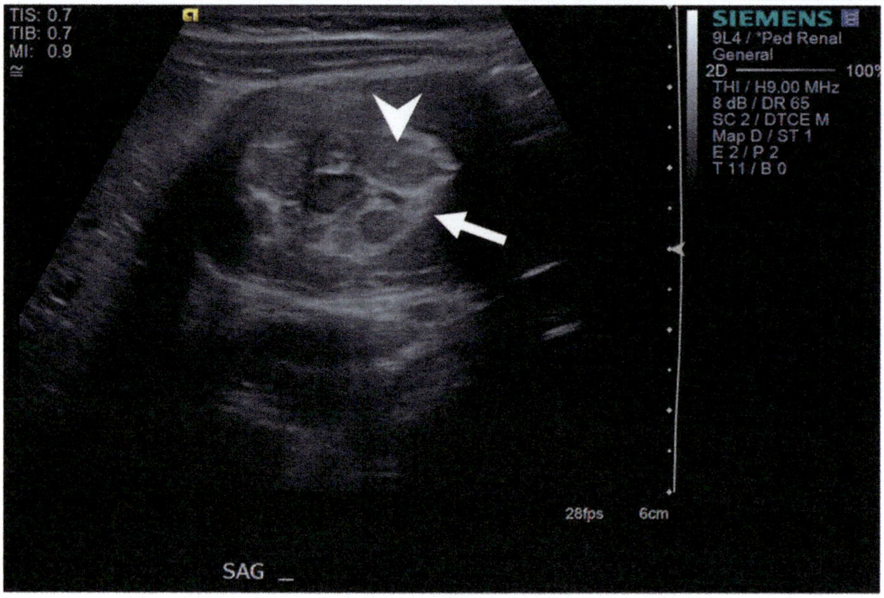

FIGURE 56.7 - TARGET APPEARANCE WITH ECHOGENIC MESENTERY (*ARROW*) WITH SMALL LYMPH NODES (*ARROWHEAD*)

Teaching Points

- Infants and young children with high clinical suspicion for intussusception should have abdominal radiographs followed by screening ultrasound.
- Once the diagnosis of intussusception has been established, pediatric surgery consultation is required before fluoroscopy-guided air reduction enema.
- The intussusception can recur within 24 h, and for that reason, the child remains in observation over night to ensure there is not a recurrence.
- Air enema has a high success rate; however, in 10–15 % of cases, the intussusception cannot be reduced and surgery is necessary.

Child with a UTI: Young children with urinary tract infection, specifically pyelonephritis, present with nonspecific symptoms including high fevers, decreased appetite, irritability, and vomiting. Older children may have back pain, high fever, and nausea and vomiting. The initial imaging study is a renal ultrasound to assess the size and shape of the kidney and the presence of hydronephrosis or congenital renal anomaly (such as duplication or malposition). A voiding cystogram is performed in young infants up to 24 months after the second febrile UTI to look at the anatomy of the urethra (boys) and assess for vesicoureteral reflux (VUR) (boys and girls). In addition, a VCUG is indicated if the renal and bladder ultrasound reveals hydronephrosis,

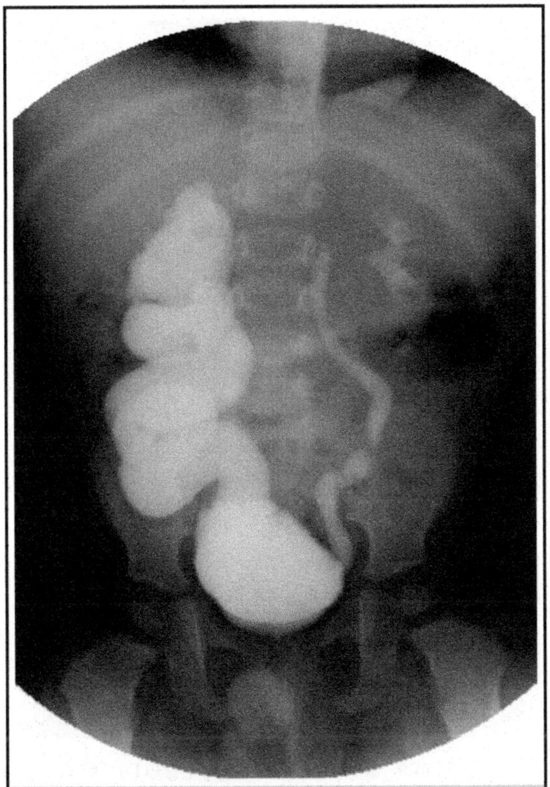

FIGURE 56.8 - GRADE 5 RIGHT VUR AND GRADE 2 LEFT VUR

scarring, or other findings that suggest high-grade VUR or obstructive uropathy. The severity of VUR is based on level and degree of collecting system distention and is graded I–V (Fig. 56.8). The results of the imaging evaluation guide treatment decisions and follow-up. Those patients with persistent high-grade VUR are candidates for surgical intervention.

Teaching Points

- Febrile infants and young children with a UTI should undergo renal and bladder ultrasonography.
- VCUG should not be performed routinely after the first febrile UTI. It is indicated if renal and bladder ultrasonography is abnormal.
- Majority of VCUGs are normal, about a third have grade I to III VUR, and small percentage have grade IV and grade V. Of those with a recurrent UTI, ¼ did not have VUR, little over half had grade I to III VUR, and remaining had grade IV or grade V.

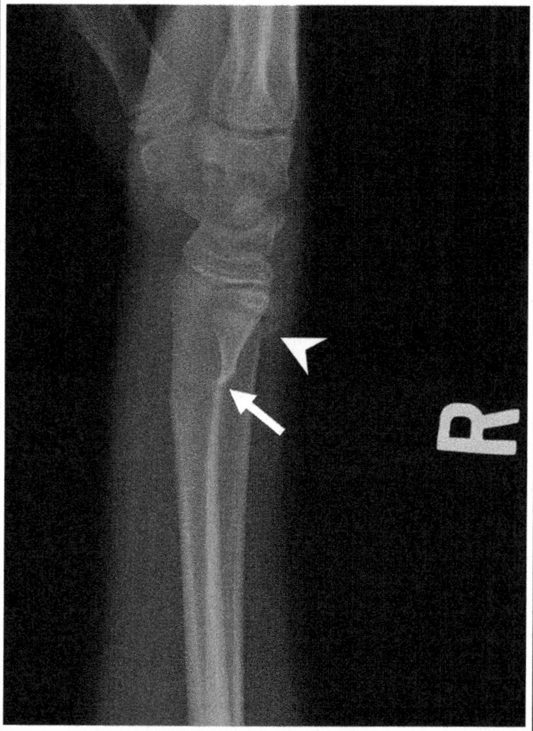

FIGURE 56.9 - BUCKLE FRACTURE DISTAL RADIAL DIAPHYSIS (*ARROW*) AND SALTER II FRACTURE DISTAL ULNA (*ARROWHEAD*)

Pediatric Fractures: Children's bones differ from those of adults. Their composition is different; pediatric bones contain proportionally more woven than lamellar bone. Strong periosteum is loosely attached to underlying cortex by Sharpey's fibers and can act as a splint. Pediatric bones have growth plates (physes). These features lend the bone to characteristic fractures seen in childhood: the torus fracture, the greenstick fracture, and the Salter-Harris fractures. Torus fractures are incomplete fractures in which the cortex has subtle angulation or appears buckled (Fig. 56.9). Greenstick fractures involve disruption of one cortex and bending of the other. Salter-Harris fractures involve the physis and the portions of the bone around them. They are classified I–V (Fig. 56.10) with increasing number portending higher chance of complications (growth arrest). Salter-Harris I fractures involve fracture through the growth plate alone and can be difficult to identify radiographically. Look for soft tissue swelling adjacent to the growth plate and possible displacement of the epiphysis. Salter II fractures involve the metaphysis

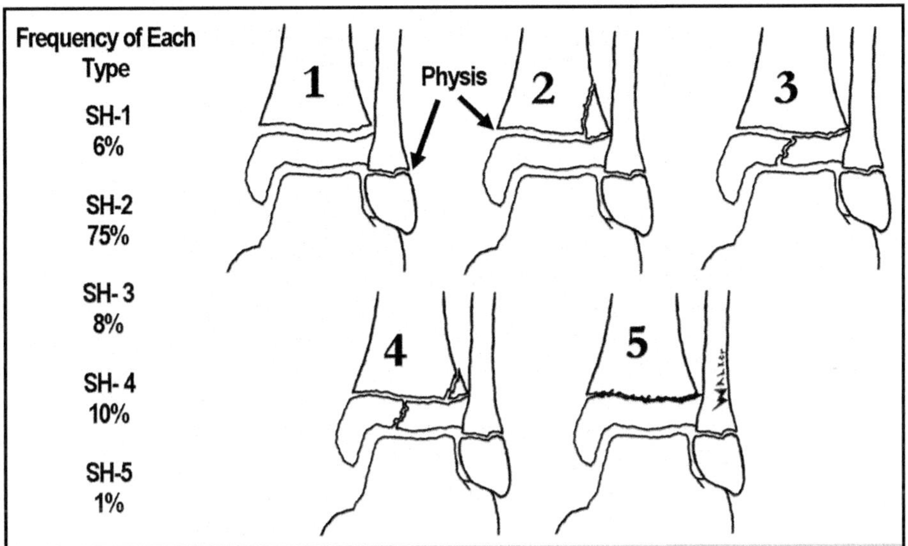

FIGURE 56.10 - SALTER-HARRIS CLASSIFICATION

and extend to the physis. Salter III fractures involve the epiphysis and the physis and Salter IV the metaphysis, physis, and epiphysis. Salter V fractures are crush injuries to the physis and are subject to development of premature physeal closure and growth arrest.

Child Abuse: There are musculoskeletal, visceral, and neurologic manifestations of inflicted injury. Distinguishing accidental from non-accidental injury can be challenging. The types of accidental injury for which a child is at risk are closely related to their development and what milestones they have achieved. Identification of the following should raise concern for inflicted injury: multiple fractures in different stages of healing and fractures in which the history does not fit with the injury. There are also a few high specificity fractures for abuse including metaphyseal corner fractures and multiple rib fractures (Fig. 56.11). Visceral injuries are relatively uncommon out potentially lethal and include pancreatic injury (with pancreatitis and pseudocyst formation) and duodenal hematoma. Neurologic manifestations include subdural hematoma formation, contusion, and cerebral edema.

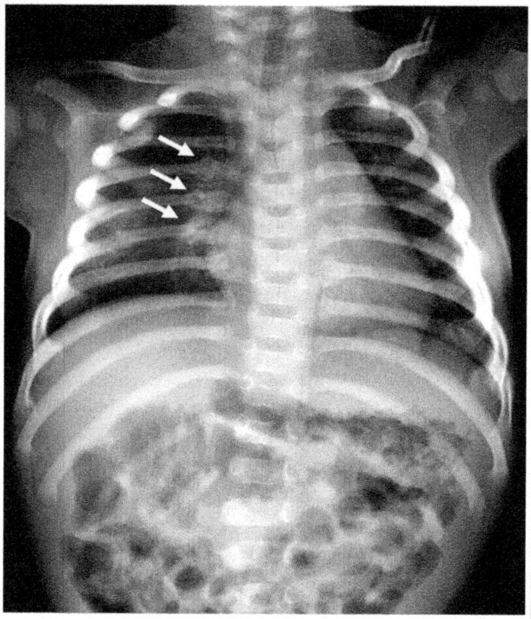

FIGURE 56.11 - MULTIPLE HEALING RIB FRACTURES
Arrows indicate a few examples of the many scattered healing fractures

INDEX

H. Singh et al. (eds.), *Radiology Fundamentals: Introduction to Imaging & Technology*, DOI 10.1007/978-3-319-10362-4

W

Y

Printed by Printforce, the Netherlands